THE MACMILLAN GUIDE TO
HOME NURSING

THE MACMILLAN GUIDE TO
HOME NURSING

DIANA HASTINGS RGN RCNT

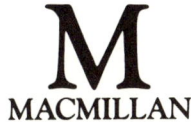

MACMILLAN

AUTHOR'S ACKNOWLEDGMENTS

I should like to thank everybody at Frances Lincoln for giving me the opportunity to write this book and for all their help and advice.

My special thanks to my husband and family for all their help and encouragement; to Jennifer Baker RGN RMN RNT for patiently checking the entire contents of the book and for her positive encouragement and support; also to Noel Gormley RGN MBE, Sister Mary Stemp RGN, Sister Susan Bartlam RGN, Susan Pikesley RGN DipN RCNT and Edward Dolman SRN RNT, all of Dorset County Hospital, Dorset; to Maureen Tuke-Hastings, physiotherapist; to Sandra Crofts for typing the manuscript; to the Library at Dorset County Hospital for all their help in researching this book; to the Spastics Society, Mencap and the Health Education Council for all the very useful information that they sent me; to the Royal College of Nursing; and to Mary Gostelow Enterprises.

I would also like to thank Louise Templeton, dietitian at the Glasgow Homeopathic Hospital, for assistance on the Diet and Nutrition chapter; Barbara Whiteford, senior physiotherapist at St Mary's Hospital, London, for assistance on the Lifting and Moving chapter; and Jim Williams, of the National Head Quarters Training Department of the British Red Cross Society, for assistance on the First Aid chapter.

Finally, my thanks to the Arthritis and Rheumatism Council, British United Provident Association and the American Red Cross for kindly giving me permission to reproduce some of their illustrations.

DIANA HASTINGS RGN RCNT

Text © Diana Hastings 1986

Photographs © Nancy Durrell McKenna 1986

Illustrations © Frances Lincoln Limited 1986

The Macmillan Guide to Home Nursing was edited and designed by Frances Lincoln Limited, Apollo Works, 5 Charlton Kings Road, London NW5 2SB

First published in the United Kingdom 1986 by MACMILLAN LONDON LIMITED 4 Little Essex Street London WCR2 3LF and Basingstoke Associated companies in Auckland, Delhi, Dublin, Gaborone, Hamburg, Harare, Hong Kong, Johannesburg, Kuala Lumpur, Lagos, Manzini, Melbourne, Mexico City, Nairobi, New York, Singapore and Tokyo

British Library Cataloguing in Publication Data

Hastings, Diana
  The Macmillan guide to home nursing.
  1. Home nursing
  I. Title
  649.8   RT61

  ISBN 0-333-42252-X

Printed by Mladinska Knjiga, Yugoslavia

Contents

Introduction

The majority of people who are ill are cared for in their own homes. Only a small minority are looked after in hospital and these days hospital stays are usually fairly short, lasting only while highly technical treatment is given. Nursing homes, supervised hostels or other forms of care outside the home may be prohibitively expensive, unavailable or unsuitable for the family's emotional needs.

Ideally, home nursing care should meet the sick person's physical, mental, social and spiritual needs so that he or she can get well again as quickly as possible, or happily adjust to the limitations of an illness, or in the case of a terminal illness, be allowed to die with dignity and in comfort. Most of this book is concerned with how you, as caregiver, can meet the sick person's needs while lightening the load of your practical responsibilities. However, for yourself and the sick person, your own well-being is essential and in order to maintain your spirits you need to organize practical and emotional support for yourself.

Assessing the situation

From the sick person's point of view, there is no place like home. Most invalids are much happier being nursed by people that they love and trust, in familiar surroundings. However, for the caregiver, looking after a sick person can be a frightening and anxious burden. You may find yourself feeling angry, frustrated, resentful and exhausted, and unable to see a way of improving your circumstances. The first step toward avoiding this is to take a step back and to assess your situation as objectively as possible, reviewing all the choices open to you.

The illnesses described in this book range from short-term, minor ailments to diseases that require long-term, intensive care: it is in the latter case that you need to plan most carefully. Work out your own needs and capabilities, weigh up how caring for a sick person will affect the rest of your family and find out what the sick person's preferences are. Everyone needs to discuss the problem honestly and then come to a conclusion. It helps to talk to a health professional, such as your doctor or a nurse, so that your fears can be allayed and so that you and the other members of the family really understand what caring for the sick person will entail. If you are planning to look after someone who is coming home from hospital, talk to the staff at the hospital and find out exactly what care is needed and for how long. Evaluate what care will be needed, what help is available and where and how to get it. The appendices at the end of the book give advice on the types of help available.

Establish a good working relationship with your doctor: he or she can be an invaluable support and can also direct you to many other sources of help. If you do not find your doctor sympathetic or easy to get along with, it is worth changing to another.

Caring for someone at home does not always have to be the responsibility of one member of the family. If, for example, you are looking after a

For a child, being at home in familiar surroundings with the family is especially important.

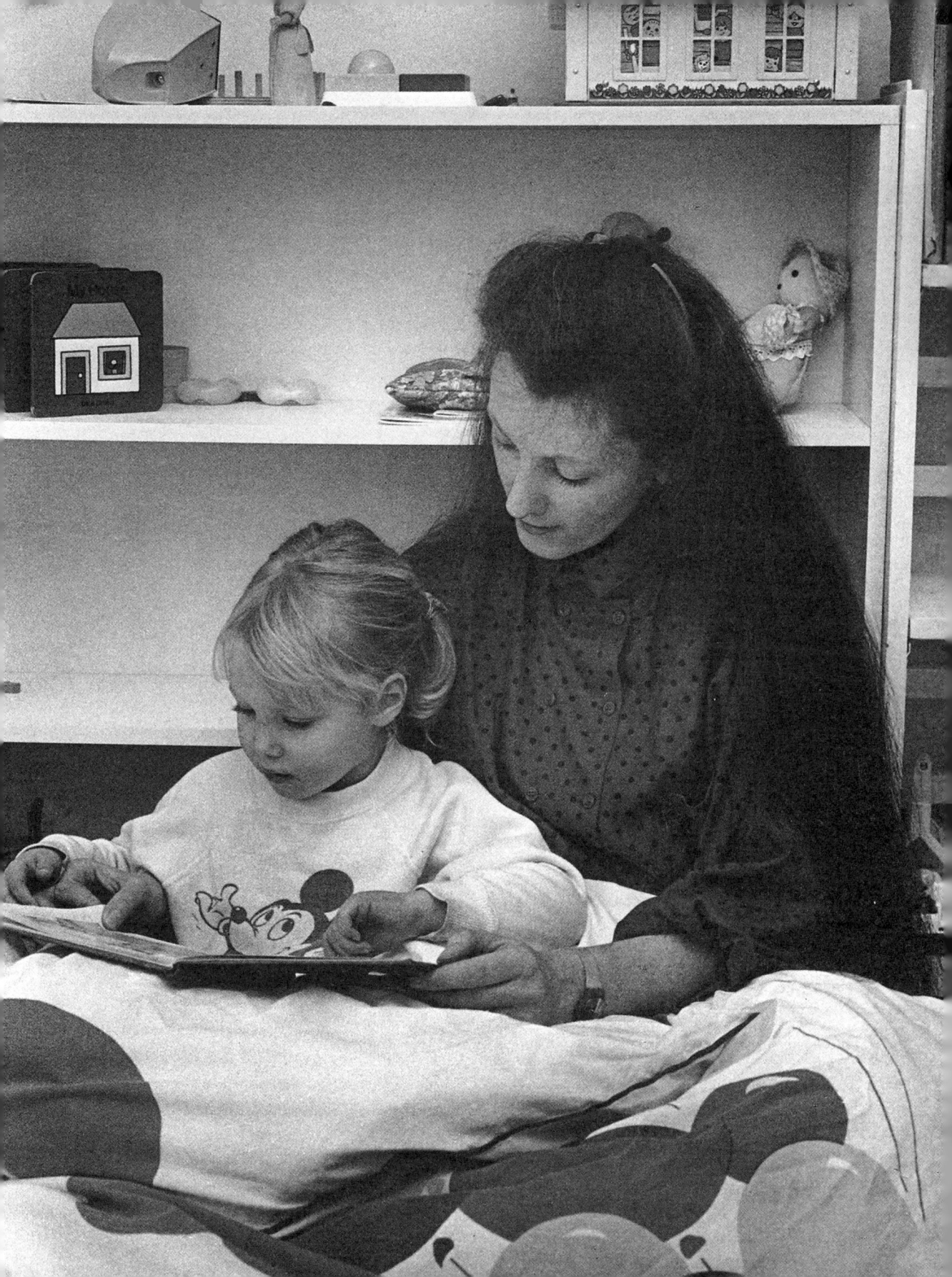

sick child, grandparents or older brothers and sisters may be able to help; if you are looking after an elderly parent, enlist as much support as possible from your brothers and sisters. Other members of the family can take their turn in caring, with perhaps one member of the family taking overall responsibility. This overall responsibility will include talking to the doctor or other health professionals, ensuring that medications and special treatments are given and generally co-ordinating and planning the sick person's care. Friends and neighbours may also be able to share the load: never refuse an offer of help, even if you really do not need help at that particular moment, as once someone has had an offer turned down they may not offer again.

It is also essential to have someone you can talk to – someone who really listens to what you are saying. You need to be able to talk freely, airing all your doubts, fears and feelings, to someone who cares for your welfare. Even if the listener is not able to help in practical ways, it will help you just to talk through a problem and you will probably find that you solve it yourself. This is one of the most positive ways of coping with any stress related to caring for someone at home.

Being honest with the person you are caring for is also important. People react very differently to illness. Some people who are sick for a long time are inclined to become self-centred and may make unkind or hurtful remarks. They may not mean to hurt you but it is better to tell them that they are upsetting you rather than keeping your feelings hidden, as this just breeds resentment. Other individuals may find it difficult to accept their dependence on others, which may lead to depression. They become discouraged or passively accept the illness and give up trying to get better; or they may even become openly hostile toward the caregiver. If you find this difficult to cope with, seek professional advice: there may be a recognized approach that will help to alleviate the problem.

Whatever your situation, never be afraid to admit to having problems or to ask for help when you feel that you can no longer manage at home. Talk to your doctor or health professional, explain how you feel and exactly what the problems are – after all they cannot help you unless they know your difficulties.

Looking after yourself

Caring for a sick person over a long period is hard work and requires stamina, so you must look after your own health. It is all too easy to become so involved with the invalid's needs that you forget your own. Anxiety and tiredness may reduce your appetite and encourage you to snatch snacks, instead of eating a well-balanced diet: it is important that you are well-nourished. You also need plenty of rest and sleep. Take advantage of any times that the sick person rests or sleeps to do so yourself. Try to get out into the fresh air and take some exercise, at least once a day. If you are tired and harassed, you will become prone to illness and infection, caught from visitors or the sickroom, and you will also become less able to cope. Take good care of yourself – it is in the sick person's best interests as well as your own.

Keep in touch with friends and, if you cannot get out to see them, invite them over to see you. Keep up with interests and hobbies, if you

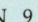

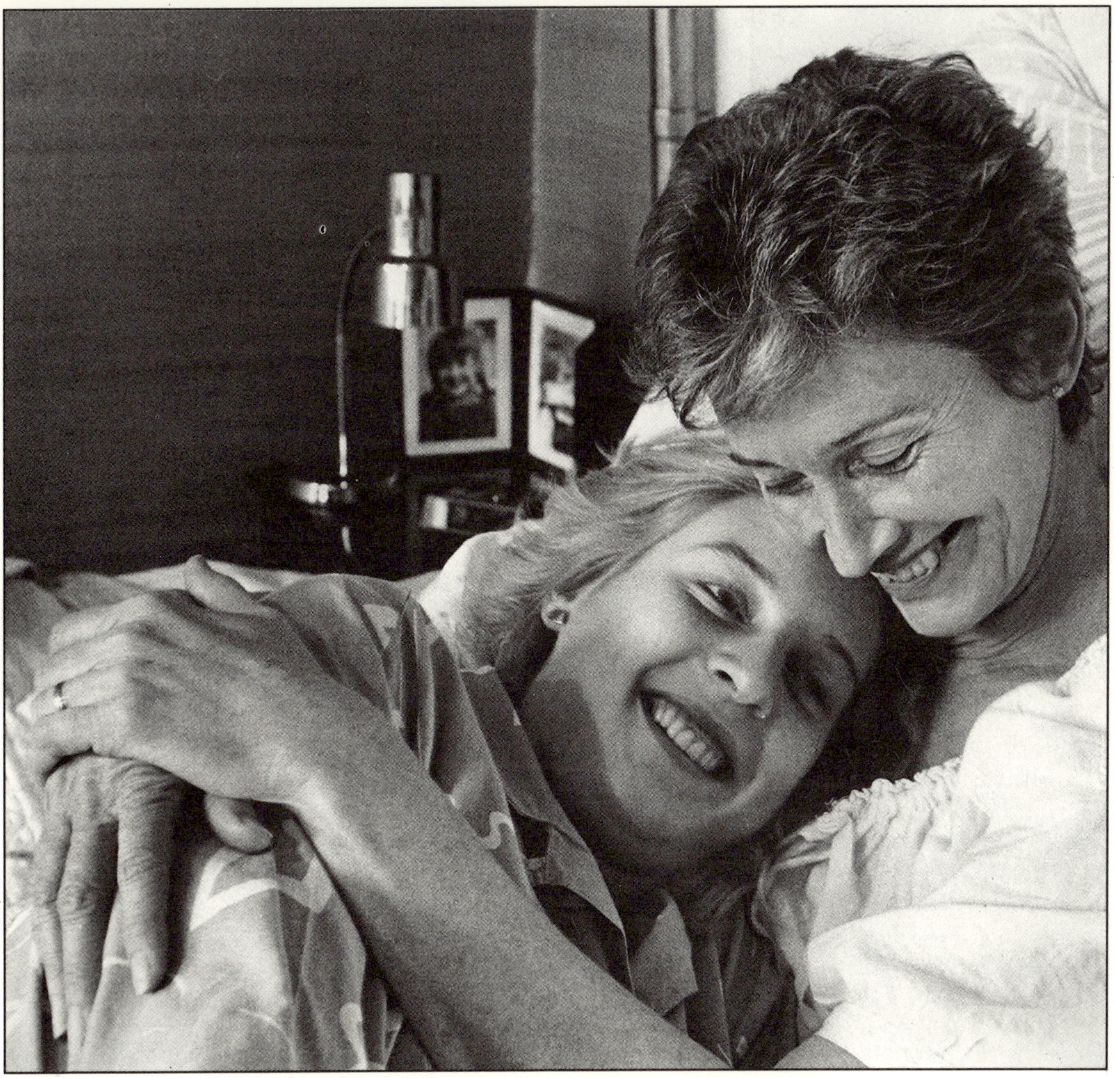

Affection and respect can flourish between you and the sick person only if you are not over-burdened.

can: this is particularly important if the sick person's illness is terminal, as you will need your own interests and in particular your friends and family later. It is also helpful for the sick person to be visited by friends and relations and to have an interest in a hobby or another activity that keeps his or her attention off the difficulties of being ill.

Encouraging independence

Helping the sick person to be as independent as possible is an essential part of home nursing. The temptation is to do too much for the sick person. For example, it is often quicker and easier to dress someone who is having difficulty using their hands and fingers, perhaps following a stroke. It may take a little longer to stand by while he or she dresses with only a small amount of assistance from you, but in the long run this enables the sick person to dress without your help, which is much better for everyone concerned.

So, unless the sick person needs to rest and to use as little energy as possible, it is in everyone's interests that he or she is active. If the sick person depends on others for every need, this can add to your problems by making him or her feel discouraged and depressed. This is why it is so important for the sick person to be involved in the planning of his or her care and the carrying out of that care, if at all possible. With some control over his or her life, the sick person's mental outlook is likely to be much better and this may lead to a speedier recovery. Children also benefit from being involved in their own care and from understanding the reasons for any treatment needed.

Preventing emotional problems

Sick people who are confined to bed and restricted in their general activities may become over-introspective, turning their attention inward so that they become morbid or over-concerned about their symptoms, perhaps imagining a few. To prevent this happening, encourage any sick person in your care to remain as active and outgoing as possible, with plenty of things to do and different people to talk to.

When a sick person is dependent on you for every need, this, combined with the fear aroused by the illness, sometimes results in a regression in behaviour, meaning that the invalid starts to behave less like an adult and more like a child. He or she may become over-dependent on you, demanding constant attention and doing little or nothing independently, which makes your caring job much harder. Again, encouraging independence helps to prevent problems.

If the sick person becomes irritable, irrational and behaves like a spoilt child, gentle but persistent attempts to correct this behaviour and reassurance that you are happy to look after her may reduce the fear there may be at the root of this type of behaviour.

The invalid may become over-anxious, frightened and need constant reassurance. It is quite likely that he or she will react to illness in the same way that he or she has reacted to other stressful situations in the past. The more that you reassure and allay any fears, the less change there will be in the invalid's normal behaviour. Reassurance means giving constructive encouragement, not a pat on the head and a dismissive 'there, there'. Let the sick person talk about his or her fears and pick out the points where you can help. There are positive aspects to all illness, even terminal illnesses, which you can point out.

Planning your day

When assessing what sort of care the sick person needs, bear in mind that there is no need to inflict your standards of hygiene or activities of daily living on someone just because he or she is ill. For example, if the sick person likes to have a bath in the evening there is no reason to insist that he or she baths in the middle of the morning, unless you are unable to give a bath in the evening. If this is so, discuss the problem with the sick person and come to a compromise. As a general rule, as long as the sick person's normal routine does not endanger his or her health, and the doctor is happy about it, there is no need to change it. Discuss and plan any care that is needed with the person who is to receive the care so that he or she knows exactly what care will be given and when. There is no need to stick religiously to a rigid routine: be flexible for your own sake and for the sick person's. Remember that the sick person's needs will change if his or her condition improves or worsens.

A daily flexible routine which suits you, the rest of the household and the sick person, helps the invalid to feel secure. It also ensures that you have some time for yourself and other members of the family. The following routine is intended only as a suggestion.

8.00 am Offer urinal, bedpan or commode or help to the toilet. Wash hands, face and teeth in bed. Sit the sick person up in bed.

8.30 am Breakfast.

9.30 am Bedbath, bath or shower. Help the sick person to sit in a chair out of bed. Make the bed.

10.30 am Coffee (perhaps family or friends can help, if necessary).

12.30 pm Offer urinal, bedpan or commode or help to the toilet. Wash the invalid's hands.

1.00 pm Lunch (again, family or friends may help by coming to sit with the sick person).

2.00 pm Offer urinal, bedpan or commode or help to the toilet. Wash the invalid's hands. Help him or her to bed for a rest. Tidy the bed.

4.00 pm Tea (as coffee and lunch).

6.00 pm Offer urinal, bedpan or commode or help to the toilet. Tidy the bed. Wash the invalid's hands and face.

7.00 pm Supper (as coffee and lunch).

9.00 pm Hot drink. Offer urinal, bedpan or commode or help to the toilet. Tidy the bed. Wash the sick person's hands, face and teeth.

10.00 pm Settle the invalid for the night.

The essential ingredient for success in home nursing is that you, the caregiver, are able to remain cheerful and positive in outlook. Planning your time, learning the practical techniques that will save you time and effort, and having the information you need will help you to feel competent and in control. But to remain cheerful, it is essential that you get the support you need, both the practical help which gives you time for yourself and the caring listening that enables you to care for the sick person without feeling drained yourself. With the right support and information, you can deal well with any difficulties or stresses that arise, and can have complete confidence in your ability to cope.

This book is intended to complement the care of your doctor and other health professionals, and is in no way intended to be a do-it-yourself guide to medicine. If you or someone in your care is unwell, seek medical advice.

The Sickroom

Caring for a sick person always involves some reorganization of your daily life. If the illness is likely to be serious or prolonged, it is worth thinking carefully about the sickroom – planning in advance can save you endless small journeys and repeated irritations. Both the choice of the room and the layout of the furniture are important. You may also need to borrow, buy, hire or improvise equipment.

Which room should you choose?

In the case of a short-term illness, it is probably better to look after the sick person in his or her own bedroom. After all, within a few days the invalid should be able to get up, so it is not usually worth rearranging the house.

In the case of a long-term illness, you may need to think of reorganizing your home. This can be difficult if you have others in the family to consider. Lively young children or teenagers studying for exams, for example, are just as much in need of your care and attention as the sick person, so you will find it easier to manage if you plan the sickroom so that normal family life can continue as far as possible.

It is also essential to think about your own welfare, whether you have a family to support you or are coping on your own. You will be a much better and more efficient caregiver if there is a quiet place away from the sickroom where you can relax, read, watch television or entertain a friend in privacy.

The sick person's needs

Whichever room you choose, it is important that the sick person has peace and quiet. Make sure that you can ensure privacy for any nursing care needed.

Ideally in the case of a long-term illness, you should choose a room as near to the bathroom and toilet as possible. If the sick person is able to get up, it is less tiring if the bathroom is close by. If the invalid uses a bedpan or urinal, a nearby bathroom saves you wasting precious energy on carrying water, bedpans, urinals and any other equipment. There is also a danger of spreading infection when carrying used bedpans and urinals, so the shorter the distance you have to carry them the better.

Remember that you will also need water for washing the invalid. Even if the sickroom cannot be close to the bathroom, you may be able to use a room near a water supply, perhaps near the kitchen.

If you live in a large house, especially one with several floors, you may decide that the sickroom should be near the kitchen or living room, so that the invalid feels less isolated from family life and so that you have less far to go between the sickroom and the rest of the family. If you are looking after someone who needs to use a wheelchair, it may be essential that the sickroom is on the ground floor. However, this may

A sickroom that reflects the personality of the sick person is far more appealing than one that is so clean and tidy that it looks like a hospital room.

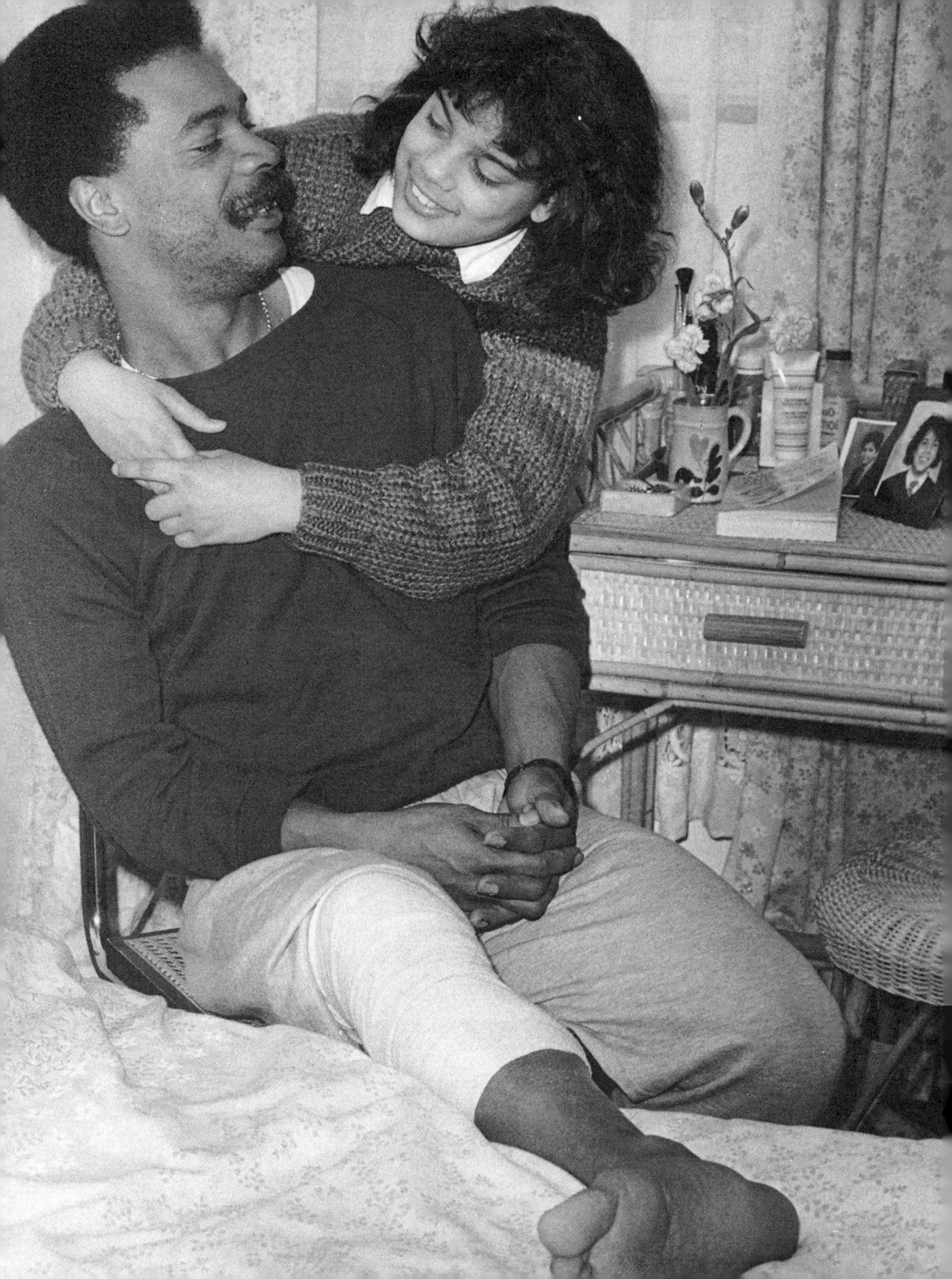

cause difficulties when the sick person needs peace if the rest of the family is noisy and lively. If you are looking after a child, you may want to move the child onto a sofa or a pile of cushions in the living room during the day to be close to you. Each situation is different and you will have to weigh up the advantages and disadvantages of the possible sickrooms available in the light of your family's needs and the layout of the house.

The room

In the case of a short-term illness, the room will often be the sick person's own and arranged in a way he or she has chosen. There may be quite a lot you can do to make the room cheerful: one easy way to do this is to add flowers and pot plants. There is no need to create extra work for yourself by removing them at night, as there is no truth in the old belief that they use up precious oxygen.

In the case of the chronically ill, the invalid may be confined to the sickroom for some years and it is essential that it is furnished in as imaginative and inspiring a way as possible, while retaining a restful and pleasant atmosphere. Books, newspapers and magazines help to pass the time and, along with television and radio, provide entertainment for the sick person, as well as encouraging an active interest in the outside world. However attractive the immediate surroundings, visiting friends and relatives will provide a welcome change and providing comfortable chairs will encourage them to stay and talk. Personal belongings, such as photographs of children and grandchildren, are comforting and familiar and a constant reminder of those who are dear to the invalid. A clock will help the sick person to keep track of time, and a small handbell by the bed is important so that he or she can call for help. A good bedside light is also essential.

While the sickroom should look like home, it is also important for the sick person's morale that the room is tidy, so make sure there is a wastebasket, preferably lined with a plastic bin-liner, for used tissues and other small items of rubbish.

Temperature and humidity

The room must be kept warm, particularly if the person occupying it is young or elderly. It is especially important that the sick person does not feel cold when being bathed or when you are carrying out any procedure that involves removing the bedclothes, so windows should be closed at these times. At all other times, the room should be airy and well ventilated. If the room is centrally heated, the air often becomes too dry and the sick person may complain of a dry mouth and nose, sore throat and headaches. The best way to help moisten the air is to buy a humidifier, or you can simply place a bowl of water near each radiator and replace the water as it evaporates.

Arranging the furniture

The room should be as uncluttered as possible to allow you to move around freely. If the bed is up against the wall, pull it further into the room so that you can walk up and down either side of the bed without bumping against the wall, bed or other furniture. If you cannot move the

Planning a sickroom
In both a small and a large bedroom, the sickbed will probably become the focus of the room. Make sure that the bed is not in a draught but that there is a good circulation of air.

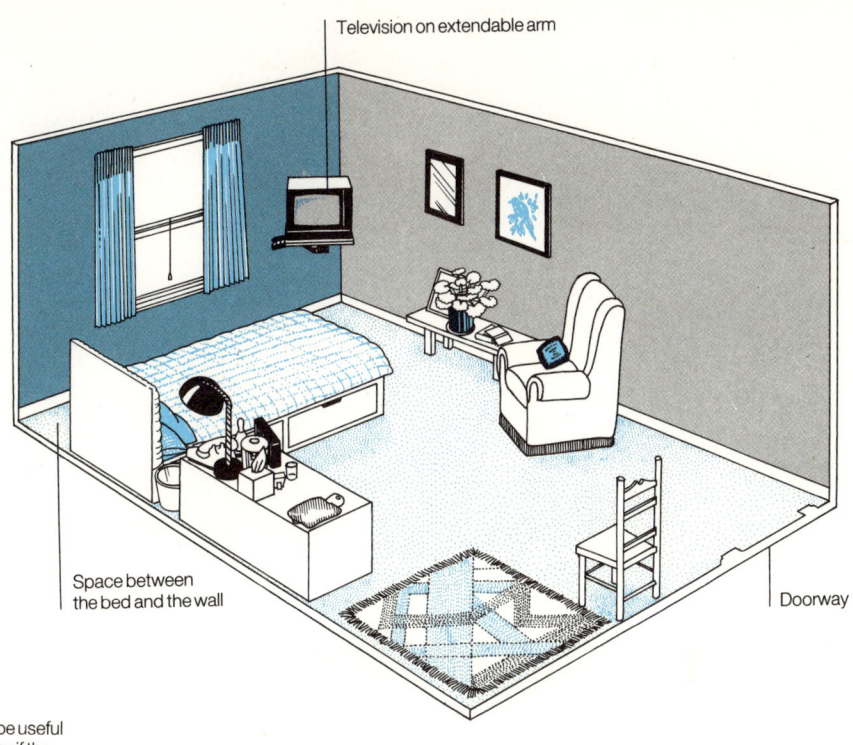

Television on extendable arm

Space between the bed and the wall

Doorway

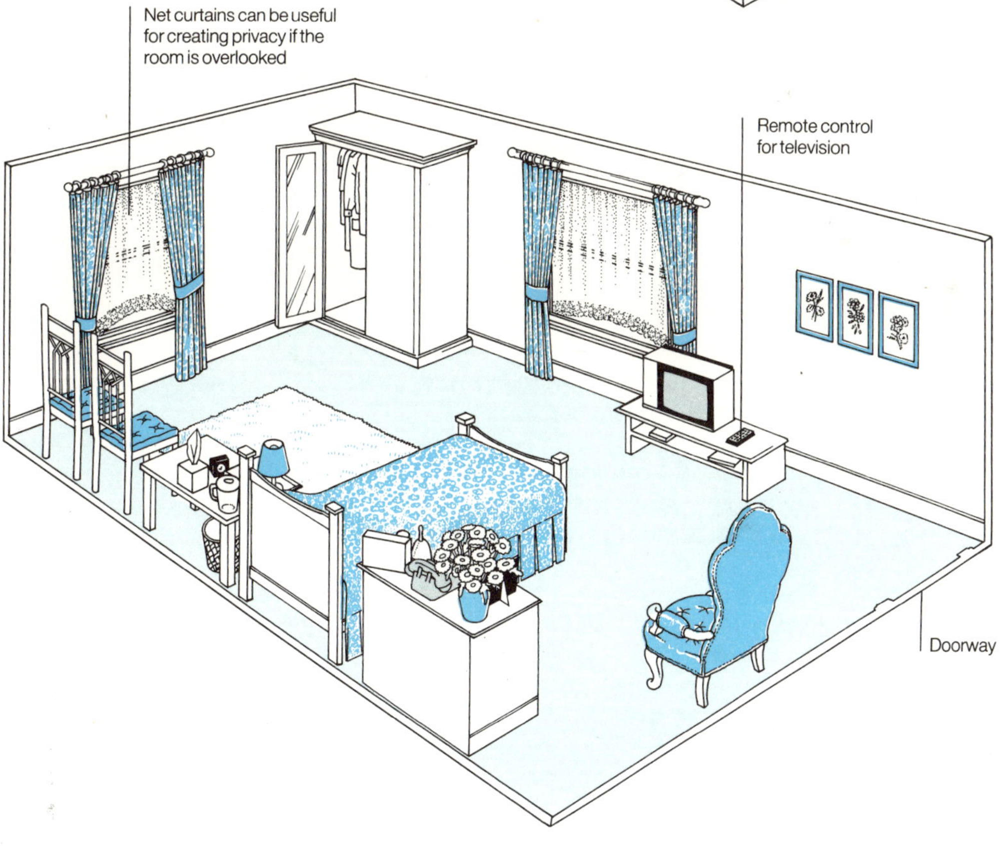

Net curtains can be useful for creating privacy if the room is overlooked

Remote control for television

Doorway

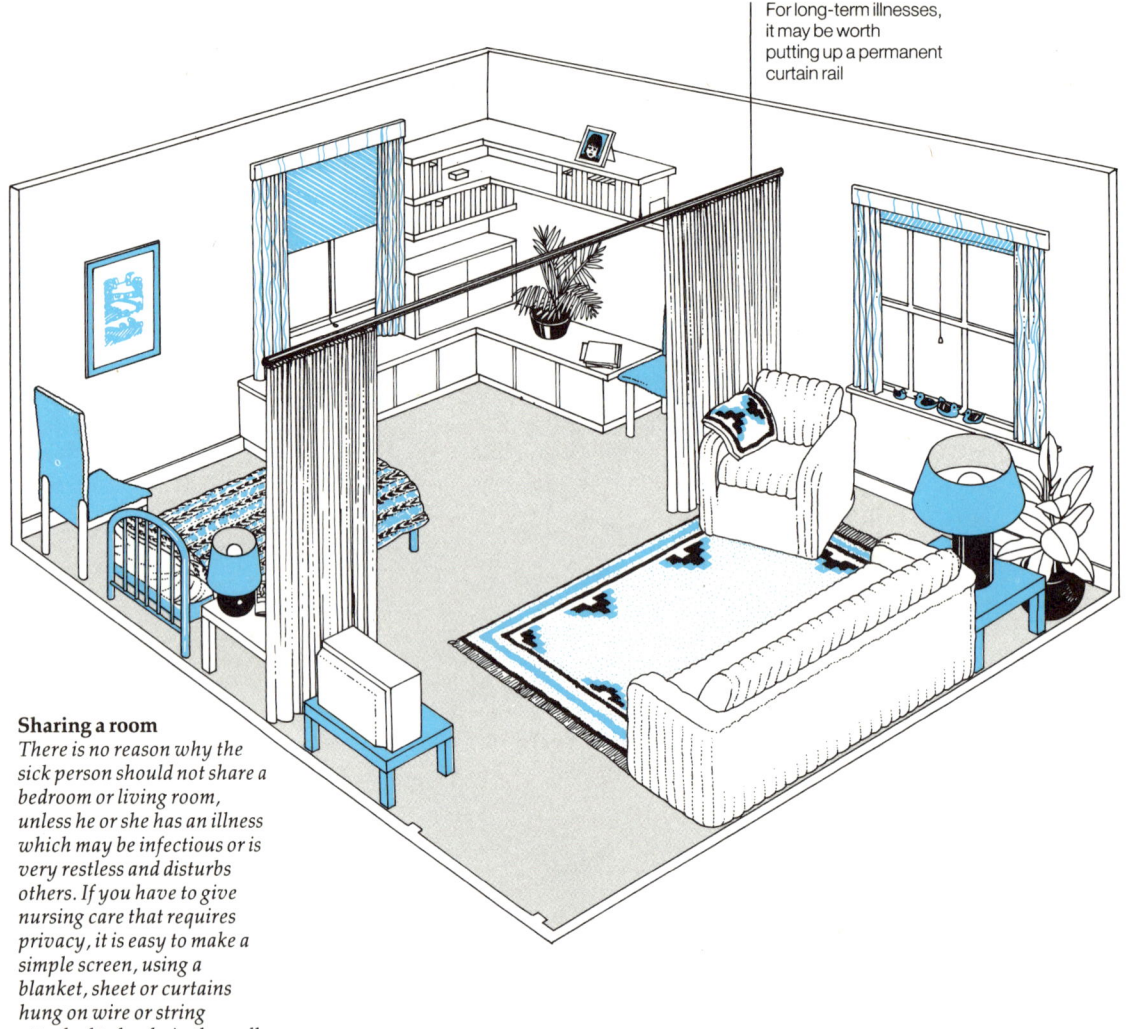

For long-term illnesses, it may be worth putting up a permanent curtain rail

Sharing a room
There is no reason why the sick person should not share a bedroom or living room, unless he or she has an illness which may be infectious or is very restless and disturbs others. If you have to give nursing care that requires privacy, it is easy to make a simple screen, using a blanket, sheet or curtains hung on wire or string attached to hooks in the wall.

bed permanently out from the wall, make sure it is possible to pull it out when necessary.

A couple of upright chairs are useful for bedmaking, as well as for visitors, and a comfortable armchair is important for an invalid who can get out of bed. The invalid will want a bedside table and an extra table provides a surface for any equipment that you may need.

Equipment for the sickroom

Having the right equipment makes looking after a sick person very much easier. Which items of equipment you need depends on the type and length of the illness that you are coping with. The checklist that follows is intended to suggest ideas – you are unlikely to need everything on the list.

It is important that the sick person has his or her own face flannel, towel, brush and comb, and other personal equipment – and that this is kept for the invalid's use alone, to avoid transmitting infections.

CHECKLIST OF EQUIPMENT

Washing equipment

Tray — Keep washing equipment together on the tray, stored in the bathroom: this makes it easier to carry to the bedside

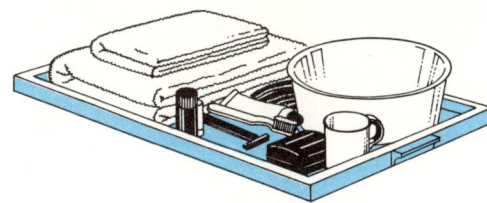

Washing bowl

Soap — Use a gentle soap that will not dry the skin, such as baby soap

Face flannel

Body flannel

Two large towels

Face towel

Tooth mug

Toothbrush and toothpaste — Use a soft brush

Dental floss

Small bowl or basin — For spitting into

Denture container

Denture cream or tablets

Denture brush

Mouthwash — Helps rid the mouth of unpleasant tastes that often occur with ill health or medication

Covered bottle or jug of water — The cover prevents dust or insects falling into the water

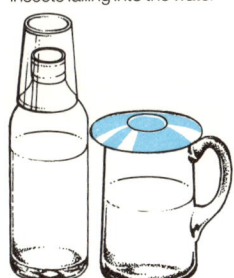

Petroleum jelly or lip salve

Deodorant

Talcum or dusting powder

Cream or body lotion

Make-up

Shaving equipment

Nail file

Nail scissors

Nail brush

Hair brush and comb

Shampoo and dry shampoo

Hairdryer

Tissues

Disposable wipes (see page 58)

Cotton-wool

Large kitchen roll — To cover bedpans and urinals

Large plastic bags — For disposal of rubbish

Plastic sheeting in various sizes

Sticky tape — For sealing refuse bags

Safety pins

Plastic disposable gloves

Bedclothes

Two pairs of sheets or two bottom sheets and two duvet covers — One set on the bed, one set in the wash. Bed linen should be made of cotton or a cotton blend as it can then be washed at high temperatures, which helps to prevent the spread of infection

Four pillows (minimum)

Eight pillowcases

Two extra sheets for drawsheets (see page 27)

Blankets or a duvet — Use whichever the invalid prefers. Cellular blankets are both light and warm

Protective plastic covers for the mattress and pillows — If soiling is likely. Do not give plastic-covered pillows to a baby

Bedcover — Preferably washable and not so slippery that it will slide off the bed

Nightclothes

Pyjamas or nightdresses — You may need several sets. They should be in light cotton or a cotton blend and should be loose fitting

Slippers

Dressing gown

Bedsocks, cardigans or shawls — Be careful not to over-wrap someone with a fever

Other equipment

Thermometer

Watch with a second-hand

Notebook and pencil

Dirty linen basket, or large plastic bag

Antiseptic — For cleaning thermometers. Keep this in the bathroom, out of reach of children

Door silencer (see page 20)

Bedpan, urinal and commode (see pages 68-70)

Long-handled brush for cleaning

Vomit bowl — Any plastic bowl or bucket

Deodorant or air-freshener — Using sprays may embarrass the patient: solid blocks or bottles are better

A pair of cotsides (see page 18)

Firm mattress

Bedtable (see page 18)

Backrest (see page 18)

Incontinence pads (see page 71)

Monkey pole or pull rope (see page 50) — To help an invalid pull him- or herself up in bed, if necessary

Bedcradle or foot support (see page 56) — Keeps the weight of the bedclothes off the legs

Footstool — For comfort when the sick person is out of bed

Sheepskin (see page 80) — Helps to prevent pressure sores if the invalid is elderly or confined to bed for long

The sickbed

If you are looking after someone who is unable to get out of bed and needs help to move about, the bed must be at the correct height or you will soon hurt your back. When you are standing beside the bed you should be able to rest your hands on the mattress with your arms straight and shoulders relaxed. You may be able to hire a higher bed.

If, on the other hand, your patient is able to get out of bed unaided or with a little help from you, do not raise the level of the bed as he or she may fall.

The mattress

The important point about a mattress is that it should be firm and should not dip in the middle, as this is very uncomfortable and also makes lifting the sick person and using bedpans much more difficult.

To make the mattress firm and flat, place a board under it. A surf board, the flat side of a large wooden tray or any large piece of wood about 1 cm to 5 cm thick (½ in to 2 in) would do.

Cotsides

In hospital these are used to prevent the patient falling out of bed. They are also very useful if you are turning an invalid on your own as they prevent the invalid falling out of bed and he or she can pull on the cotsides to help you. You can buy or hire cotsides, which clip onto the head or the side of the bed.

Backrests

A backrest helps to support an invalid in a comfortable position when he or she is sitting up in bed and helps to prevent backache and general discomfort.

Bedtables

A bedtable is a very useful piece of equipment. It provides a stable surface for eating a meal or writing, for example. You can also put a washing bowl on a bedtable so that the sick person can wash in bed more easily.

The ideal bed
Especially if you are looking after someone with a long-term illness, make sure that the bed is the right height, with a firm mattress, a backrest, a bedtable and cotsides.

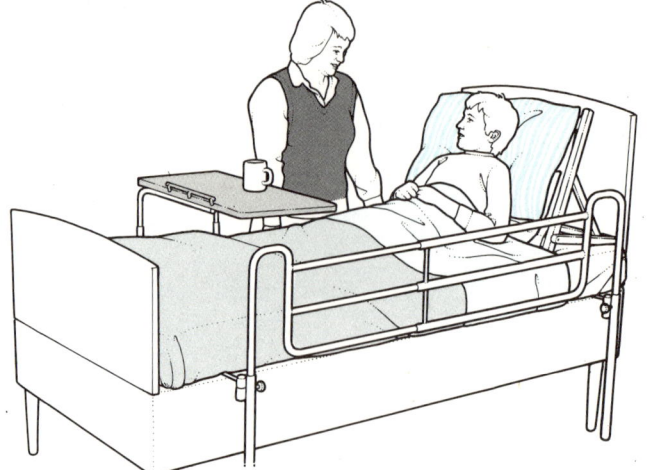

Improvised equipment

If you are caring for someone with a long-term illness or disability, you are likely to need specialized equipment. You may live in an area where it is easy to hire equipment from a hospital or voluntary organization. But if you do not have access to the equipment you need, there are many items that can be made at home. The improvised equipment suggested here and in the chapter on **Day-to-day Care** is neither expensive nor complicated to make, and may contribute a great deal to the sick person's comfort and good spirits.

RAISING THE HEIGHT OF THE BED

Bed blocks made of wood
You can raise the height of the bed using wooden blocks under the legs. Each block should have a base approximately 20 cm by 20 cm (8 in by 8 in) and each block should have a dip, about 9 cm (3½ in) deep, in the centre to prevent the bed legs slipping. The height of the block will depend on how far you want to raise the bed: for safety, the blocks should be no higher than 30 cm (12 in). Remove any castors before you put the bed onto the blocks.

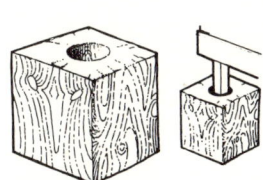

Raising a bed using four upright chairs
Four strong, upright chairs of the same height can be used to raise a bed, too, but you must be able to tie the chairs securely to the bed frame. This is usually a less satisfactory option as it makes attending to the sick person and changing bedclothes more difficult.

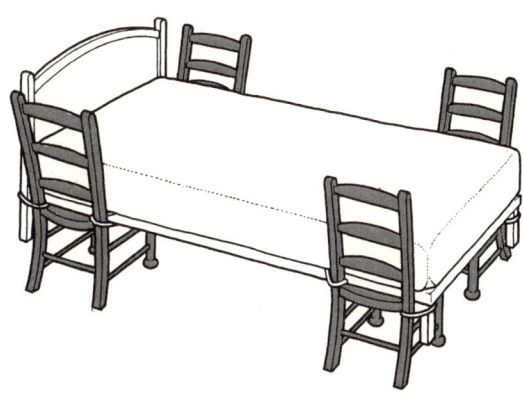

MAKING A BACKREST

Using a cardboard box
You need a large strong box, about 60 cm by 60 cm wide by 46 cm deep (24 in by 24 in by 18 in), with cover flaps.
1 *Cut down both sides of the front of the box and let the front fall forward.*
2 *Score along the dotted line: do not cut. Repeat on the opposite side of the box.*
3 *Bend the sides along the scored lines. Bring forward the cover flap on the back of the box and fold it over the sides.*
4 *Bring up the front part of the box and fold the excess over the back. Secure all the ends with wide, strong sticky tape or string. Cover with a pillow.*

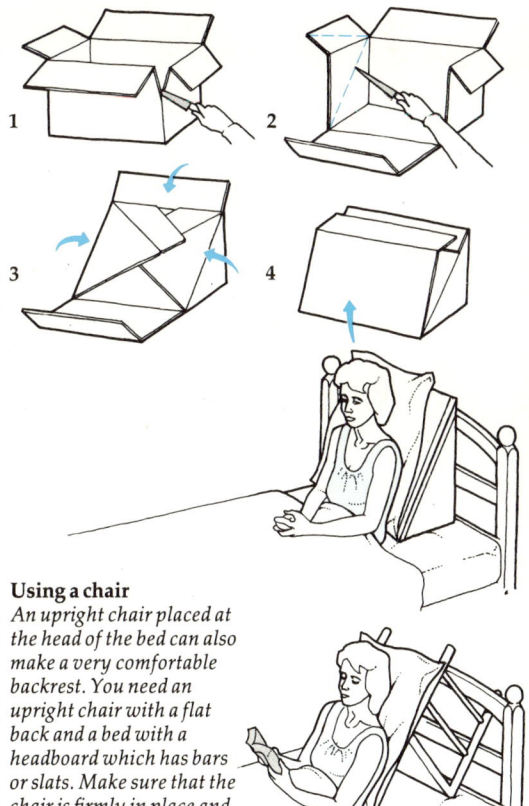

Using a chair
An upright chair placed at the head of the bed can also make a very comfortable backrest. You need an upright chair with a flat back and a bed with a headboard which has bars or slats. Make sure that the chair is firmly in place and cover the back with a pillow or two.

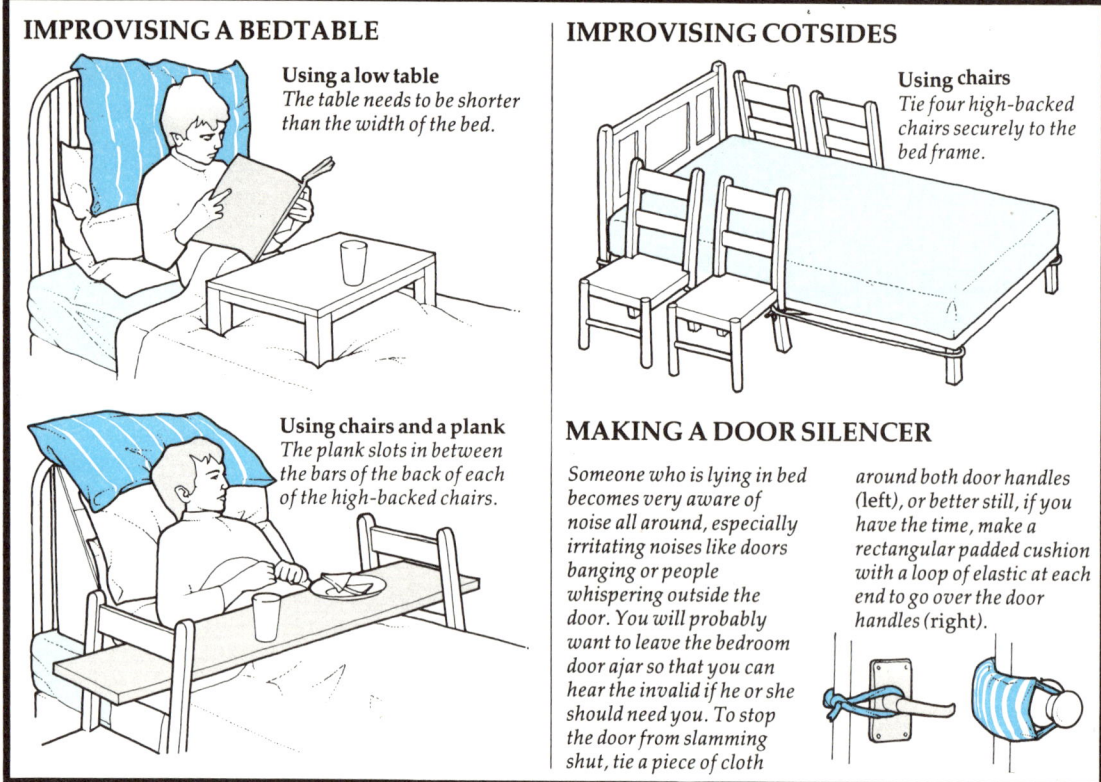

IMPROVISING A BEDTABLE

Using a low table
The table needs to be shorter than the width of the bed.

Using chairs and a plank
The plank slots in between the bars of the back of each of the high-backed chairs.

IMPROVISING COTSIDES

Using chairs
Tie four high-backed chairs securely to the bed frame.

MAKING A DOOR SILENCER

Someone who is lying in bed becomes very aware of noise all around, especially irritating noises like doors banging or people whispering outside the door. You will probably want to leave the bedroom door ajar so that you can hear the invalid if he or she should need you. To stop the door from slamming shut, tie a piece of cloth around both door handles (left), or better still, if you have the time, make a rectangular padded cushion with a loop of elastic at each end to go over the door handles (right).

Cleaning the sickroom

It is important to keep the sickroom clean, partly to minimize the spread of infection from bacteria in the room, and partly because it is much more pleasant to be in a room which not only looks clean and tidy but also smells fresh and clean. This does not mean that you have to clean out the room thoroughly every day: do only what is necessary at a time that suits you, the sick person and the rest of the household.

If you can, clean the room while the sick person is not there – perhaps while he or she has a bath or shower or sits in the living room, for example. If the invalid cannot get out of bed, it is important to work as quietly as possible to avoid disturbance. It is usually best to clean the room after the sick person has had a wash and the bed has been made, and any dust from bedmaking has had time to settle; but be flexible – if he or she needs a rest, the cleaning can wait until later.

☐ Open the windows to give the room a good airing, but make sure that the sick person is not in a draught.

☐ Tidy up; empty wastebaskets and reline them with plastic bags. Faded flowers should be removed, old newspapers thrown out, and used cups and glasses cleared away. Put all the waste into a strong plastic bag, ready for disposal.

☐ Vacuum thoroughly, especially under the bed. However, the noise of a vacuum cleaner may be very irritating to a sick person. If so, you could use a carpet sweeper or a brush instead.

☐ Damp dust to avoid dust rising into the air and spreading infection. Use a dust cloth dampened with oil or furniture polish or, for washable surfaces, a cloth soaked in water and household cleaner and wrung out.

☐ Occasionally you may wish to polish other surfaces, but avoid using polish with a strong scent or aerosol sprays as these may cause irritation.

☐ Leave the windows open for a while if the room is unoccupied, then partially close them and make sure the room is warm before the sick person returns to bed. If the sick person is in the room and the weather is cold, close the windows after cleaning and warm up the room. Unless the weather is icy, open the windows a little again once the room has warmed up.

☐ Make a final check that everything is tidy. Make sure that curtains are pulled back neatly and that any pictures are hanging straight when you have finished dusting, for example. These may be small points, but a sick person, confined to bed, can easily be irritated by a picture askew or a misplaced chair because he or she cannot set them right and may not like to ask you.

The sick person can do a little of the work as soon as he or she is able – perhaps arranging flowers by the bedside or dusting the furniture. He or she may also enjoy helping you with some small household jobs – maybe mending, cleaning silver or tidying a drawer – which can be done without strain or exhaustion. A convalescent soon becomes bored with reading or watching television and usually likes to feel useful and part of the household.

Removing stains

Stains and spills are much more likely if you are nursing someone in bed. Even if the invalid is not very ill, meals eaten from trays are more likely to be spilled, and if the sick person is helpless, incontinent or likely to vomit, stains are even more common. You will probably decide to live with some degree of staining, on sheets for example, but if an accident involves a precious garment, bedcover or carpet, you may well want to do your best to remove the stain as well as to clean up the mess. The table below tells you what to do in these instances.

SUBSTANCES SPILLED AND ACTION TO BE TAKEN

Milk	Soak up with a tea-towel or kitchen paper. Do not rub. Apply a solution of sodium bicarbonate. Clean with detergent or carpet shampoo.
Blood	Apply a salt solution before the blood dries, then clean with detergent or carpet shampoo. You may need to use a spot remover if the blood has dried hard.
Vomit	Clear away, and absorb moisture with a tea-towel or kitchen paper. Brush in a solution of sodium bicarbonate with a stiff brush. Clean with detergent or carpet shampoo.
Urine	Soak up excess moisture with a tea-towel or kitchen paper. Apply a little soda water, and soak up the moisture again. Clean with detergent or a carpet-cleaning solution especially designed for urine stains.
Faeces	Clear away, and soak up excess moisture. Clean with detergent or carpet cleaner.

Bedmaking

Bedmaking is a surprisingly important part of caring for someone who is confined to bed for some time. A badly made bed is uncomfortable to lie in, and wrinkles in the bottom sheet can eventually lead to pressure sores (see page 78). You will probably need to make the bed at least once a day, depending on the sick person's condition. So it is a good idea to learn how to do it quickly and effectively. The instructions for bedmaking in this chapter may seem discouragingly complicated at first. However, it is worth trying them out a few times, as making the bed effectively means that you are less likely to need to remake it every few hours. The methods set out here are much less tiring in the long run than a more haphazard approach.

Hints for bedmaking

□ Before you begin, try to ensure that the bed is at the correct height (see page 18). Move the furniture or the bed to give you free access to both sides of the bed, if necessary.

□ Change the sheets and pillowcases frequently as this helps the sick person to feel comfortable. Sheets that have not been changed for a long while are more likely to spread any infection.

□ Collect together everything you are likely to need before you begin.

□ Loosen the bedding all round the bed before starting to remove it.

□ Talk to the sick person and explain what you are doing as you work, to help maintain his or her dignity. Try to work quietly and confidently and to make sure that the invalid is as comfortable as possible throughout.

□ While changing the bed, handle all the bedclothes gently so that you do not create too much dust, and avoid too much contact with them by holding the linen away from your face and body. Do not allow bedclothes that you are going to re-use to touch the floor, as this increases the risk of spreading infection. Remove the coverings separately and fold them as you do so, to prevent them touching the floor and so that they are easier to put back if they are clean enough to use again.

□ Two chairs placed back-to-back at the end of the bed make a useful stand for bedclothes that you have just taken off the bed.

□ Remove soiled linen by bundling and rolling it up: this reduces the spread of infection. Generally, dirty linen can be put straight into the linen basket. Put heavily soiled linen into a separate plastic bag.

A well-made, comfortable bed is essential for the sick person's morale, and makes the sickroom a pleasant place for visitors.

□ The sheet under the sick person should be pulled tight and, if you can manage it, the corners mitred (see overleaf). This ensures that the sheet does not work itself loose and cause discomfort. Make sure that the sheet is tucked in tightly. A fitted sheet can make bedmaking easier.

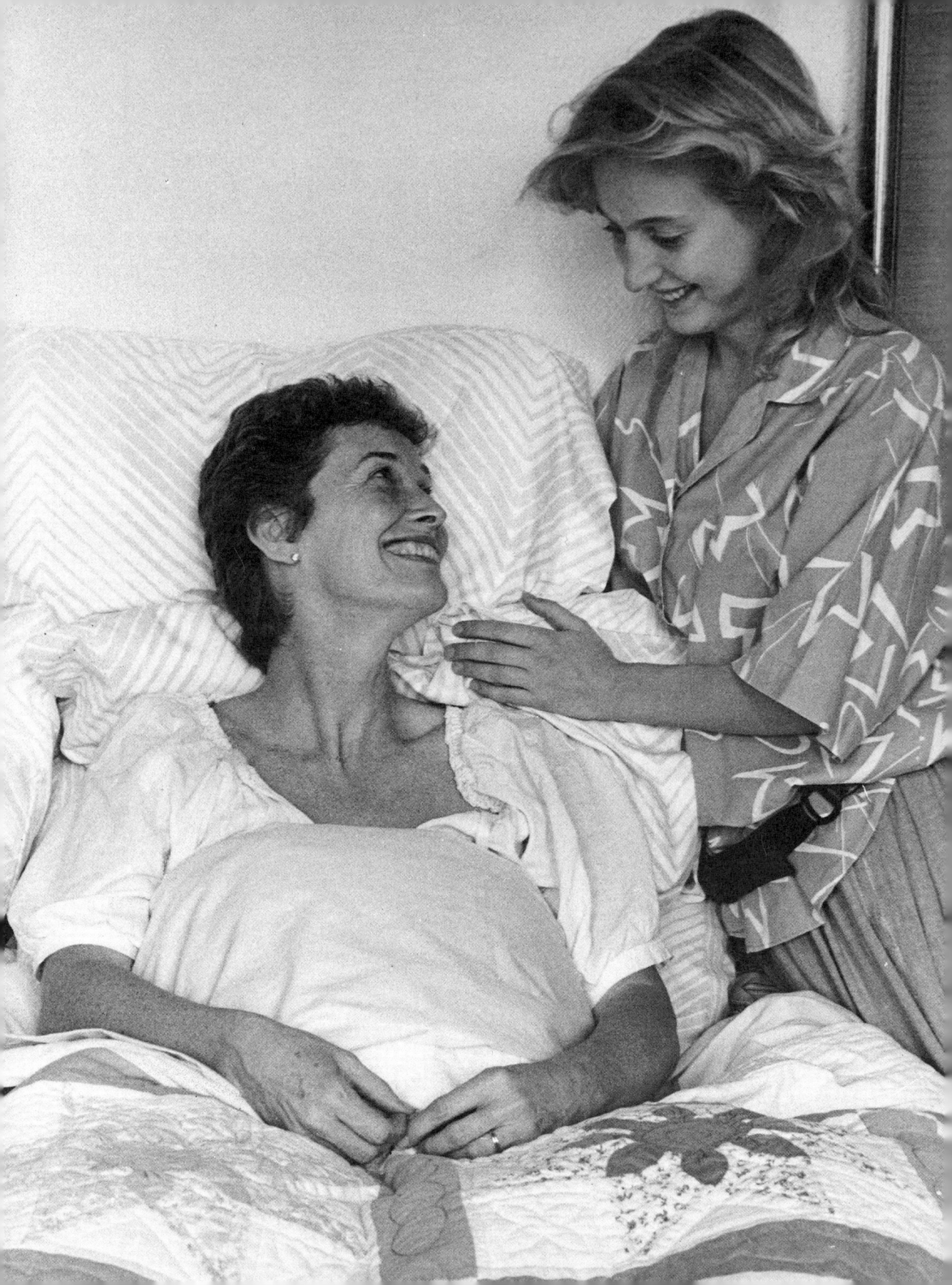

☐ When you have removed the bedclothes, check that the mattress cover is wrinkle-free and pull the mattress up to the top of the bed; if necessary, turn the mattress.

☐ Pleat the top sheet and blankets at the centre of the foot of the bed to allow the sick person freedom to move his or her feet about. There is no need to pleat the bedcover if it is not tucked in at the sides.

☐ The top sheet should be brought up high enough to cover the chest and shoulders but not tucked in so tightly that it restricts breathing and movement. There should be enough sheet at the top to turn over the blankets and bedcover.

☐ Blankets should not be doubled over the chest as this may restrict chest movements and breathing.

☐ If you are making a bed on your own, tuck in all the bottom bed linen on one side of the bed before tucking in the other side. You can also tuck in all the top covers on one side of the bed before tucking in the other side – this saves you effort, energy and time.

☐ When you have finished making the bed, wash your hands.

Making mitred corners
Tuck in the sheet at the bottom of the bed and leave the sides untucked. Lift the edge of the sheet, about 45 cm (18 in) from the corner of the bed. Tuck in the slack hanging loose near the corner of the bed. Fold down the rest of the sheet and tuck it in.

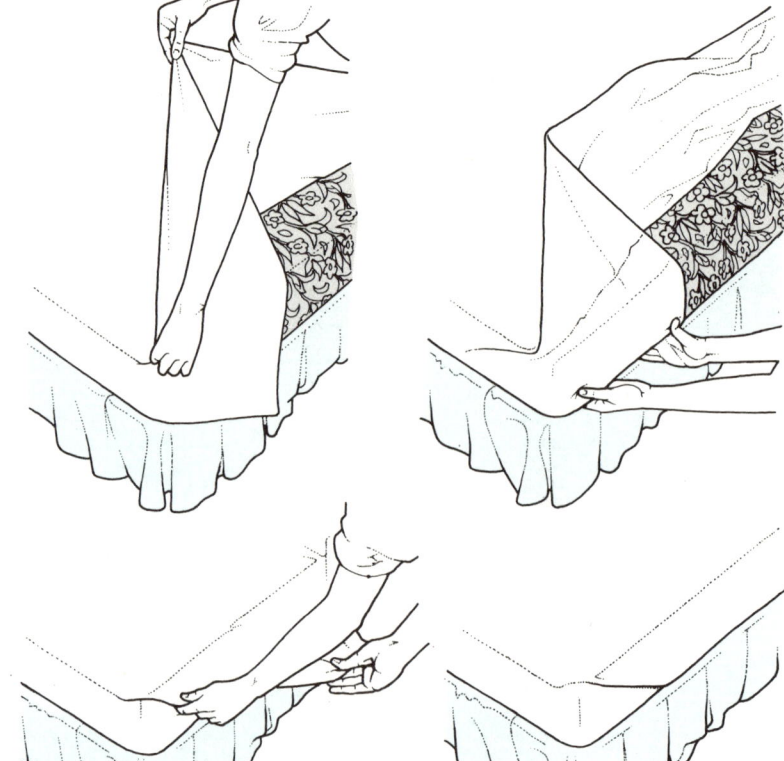

☐ An electric blanket that fits under the bottom sheet can be comforting, but is also a potential safety risk. As it should never be left on while the sick person is in bed, in case a drink is spilled, it has limited use for a sickbed, though you might use one while the sick person has a bath, for example. An electric overblanket has the same problems.

☐ An ordinary underblanket may help to keep the sick person comfortable and warm, but you must make sure that it does not become wrinkled. If the invalid is incontinent, an underblanket is not practical.

Pleating sheets or blankets
After you have laid the sheet or blanket over the bed, but before you tuck it in, lift the centre of it at the foot of the bed by about 30 cm (12 in). Fold the slack to one side so that it forms a pleat and tuck in the sheet or blanket under the mattress.

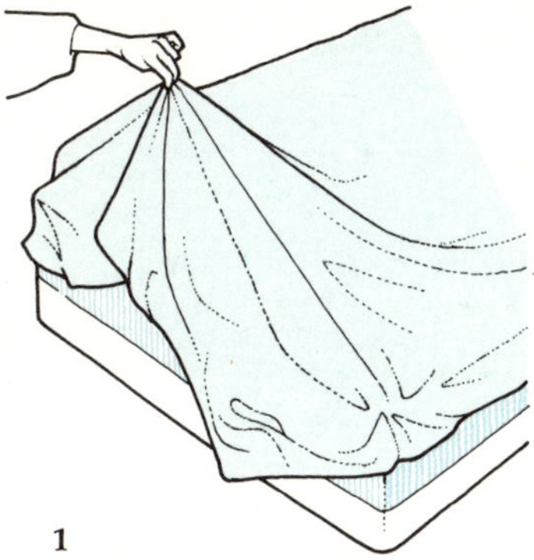

1

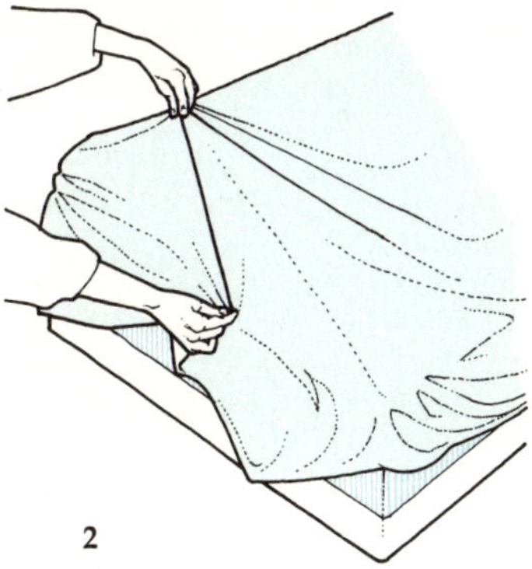

2

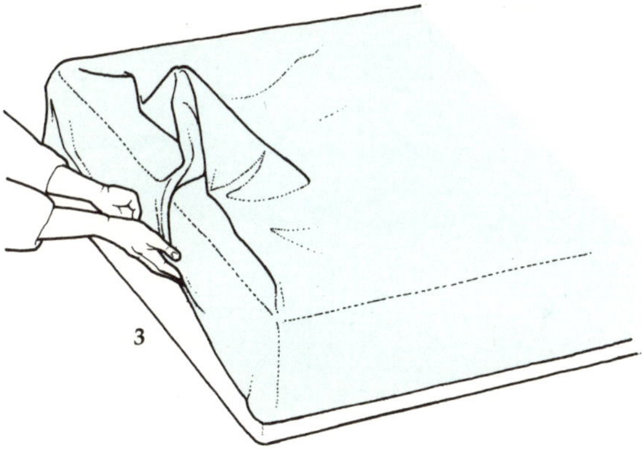

3

Folding a sheet or blanket on your own (below)
Fold the bottom half of the sheet or blanket up to the top of the bed, so that it is folded in half. Lift one side up and over the bed to fold it in half again.

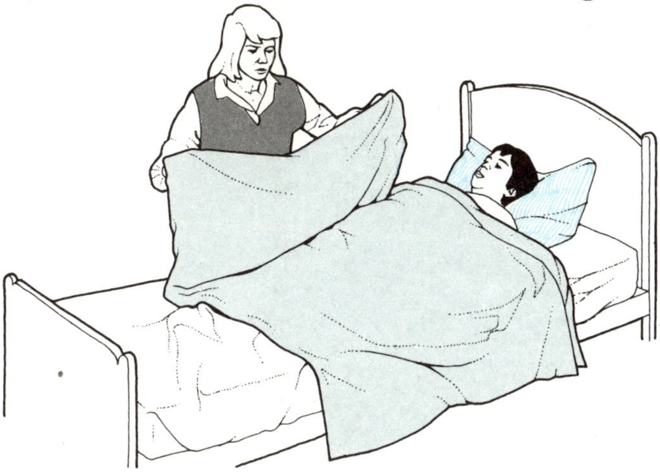

Replacing a pillowcase
Reach inside the pillowcase and, grasping the far corners, fit these onto the pillow. Gradually ease the pillow into the case.

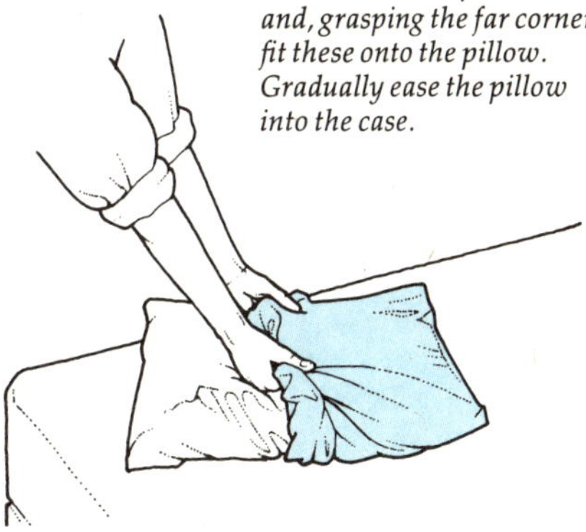

Bedmaking with duvets

If the sick person is prepared to use a duvet on the bed, bedmaking will be much easier. It is important that the duvet is large enough for the bed, so that the sick person can move freely in bed without feeling draughty. A down or down-mix duvet is warmer and lighter than a duvet made with synthetic fibres. If the invalid is incontinent, however, a duvet may not be suitable, as it may get soiled, and it is less easy to wash a duvet than sheets and blankets. However, a sheet between the duvet and the sick person may solve the problem.

Folding a duvet
If you need to remove the duvet to make the bed or for any other reason, fold it before lifting it from the bed. Fold a single or a double duvet into a third of its length by folding the bottom third up and the top third down. Lift it and rest it over the backs of two upright chairs placed back-to-back.

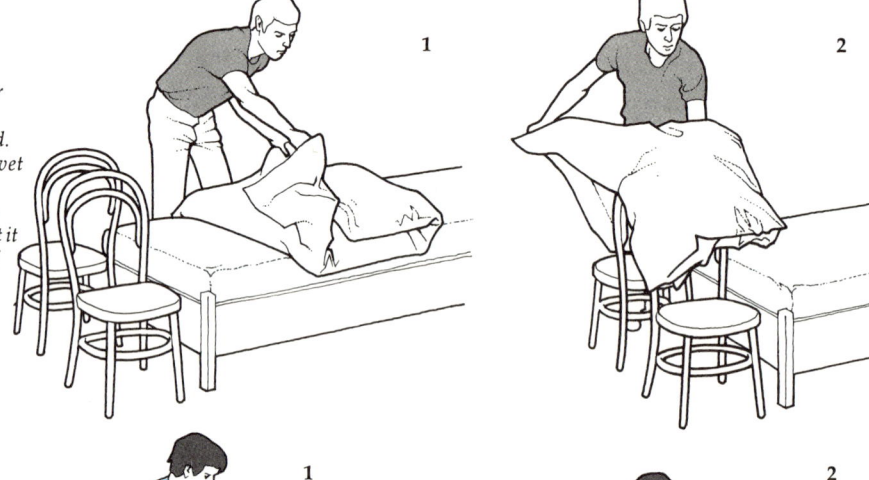

Replacing a duvet cover
Lay out the duvet over the bed and spread the new cover on top. Reach inside the duvet cover and grasp the far corners. Shake the cover down toward your hands, so that it forms gathers. Fit the corners you are holding onto the duvet and gradually ease the cover over the duvet. You may need to shake the duvet to redistribute the filling evenly.

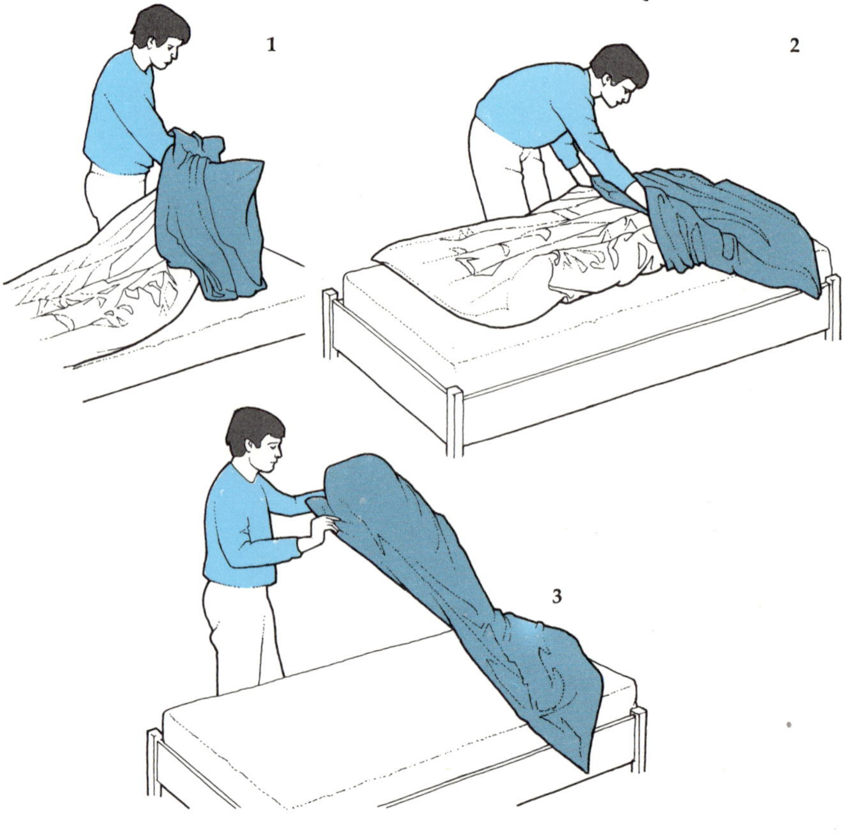

The drawsheet

If your patient is using bedpans, urinals or is incontinent, the mattress and bottom sheet will need extra protection in the form of some waterproof sheeting covered with a drawsheet. The waterproof sheeting made out of plastic or polythene needs to be about 60 cm (2 ft) wide, and long enough to tuck in either side of the bed.

As the name implies the drawsheet is a sheet which is drawn through over the bottom sheet. It should be placed under the sick person's buttocks.

Drawsheets can be made by folding an ordinary single sheet lengthwise. One side is tucked in as usual, but the other side, which is much longer, is folded and then tucked under the mattress. The long end can later be drawn through under the sick person with the minimum of disturbance, leaving a fresh cool part of the drawsheet to sit or lie on.

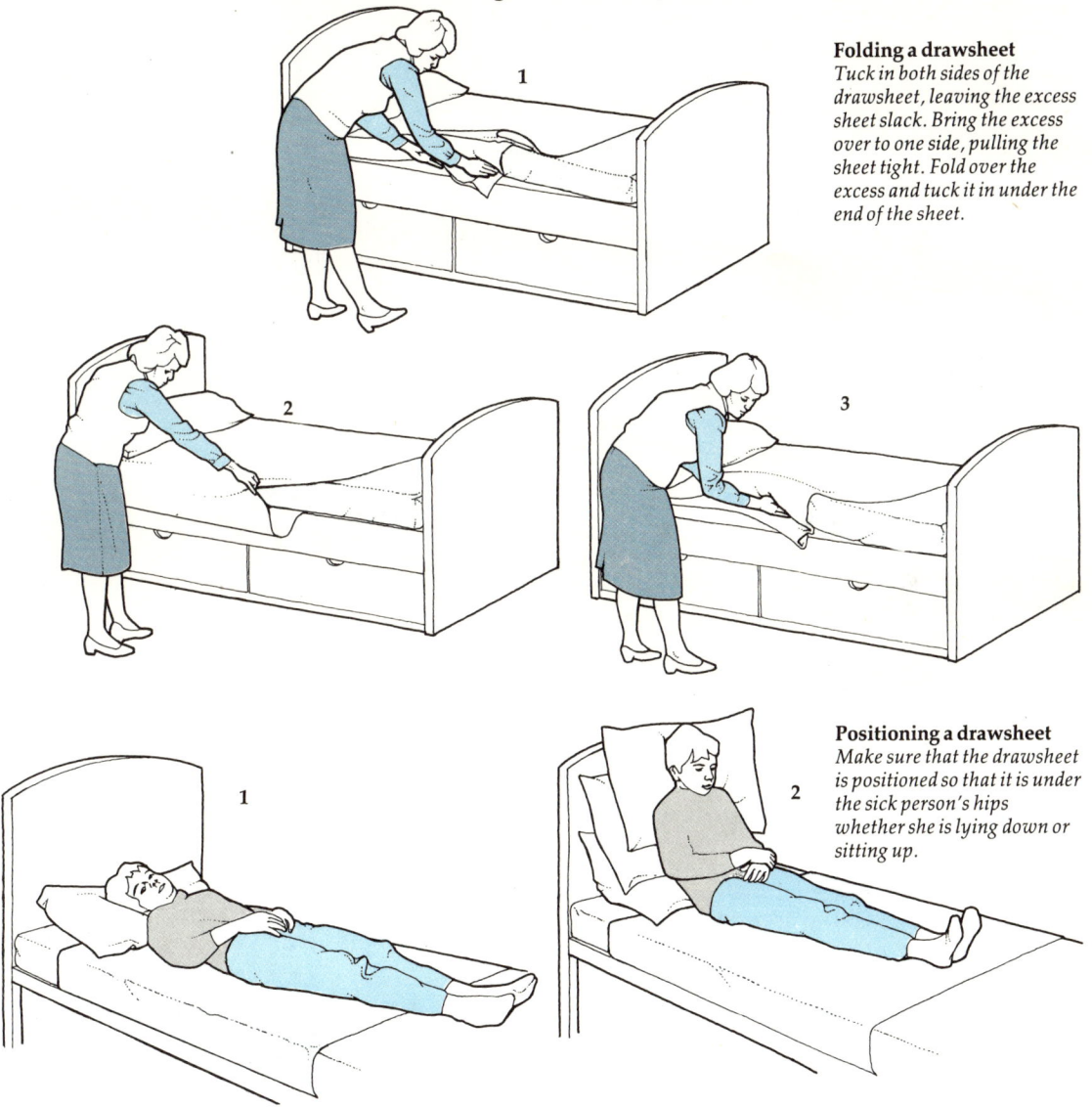

Folding a drawsheet
Tuck in both sides of the drawsheet, leaving the excess sheet slack. Bring the excess over to one side, pulling the sheet tight. Fold over the excess and tuck it in under the end of the sheet.

Positioning a drawsheet
Make sure that the drawsheet is positioned so that it is under the sick person's hips whether she is lying down or sitting up.

TWO PEOPLE MAKING AN OCCUPIED BED

Making an occupied bed involves more planning than making an unoccupied bed. It is much more difficult and tiring making a bed with the sick person still in it. So, if at all possible, get the invalid out of bed and into a comfortable chair before you begin. If you have to make a bed with a sick person in it, read through the chapter on **Lifting and Moving** before you start. It is easier if there is somebody else available to help you.

▶ This procedure is not suitable for someone who is breathless or uncomfortable lying flat.

Collect together
● Two chairs
● Clean linen, if required
● Dirty linen basket or plastic bag
● Separate plastic bag for heavily soiled linen, if necessary

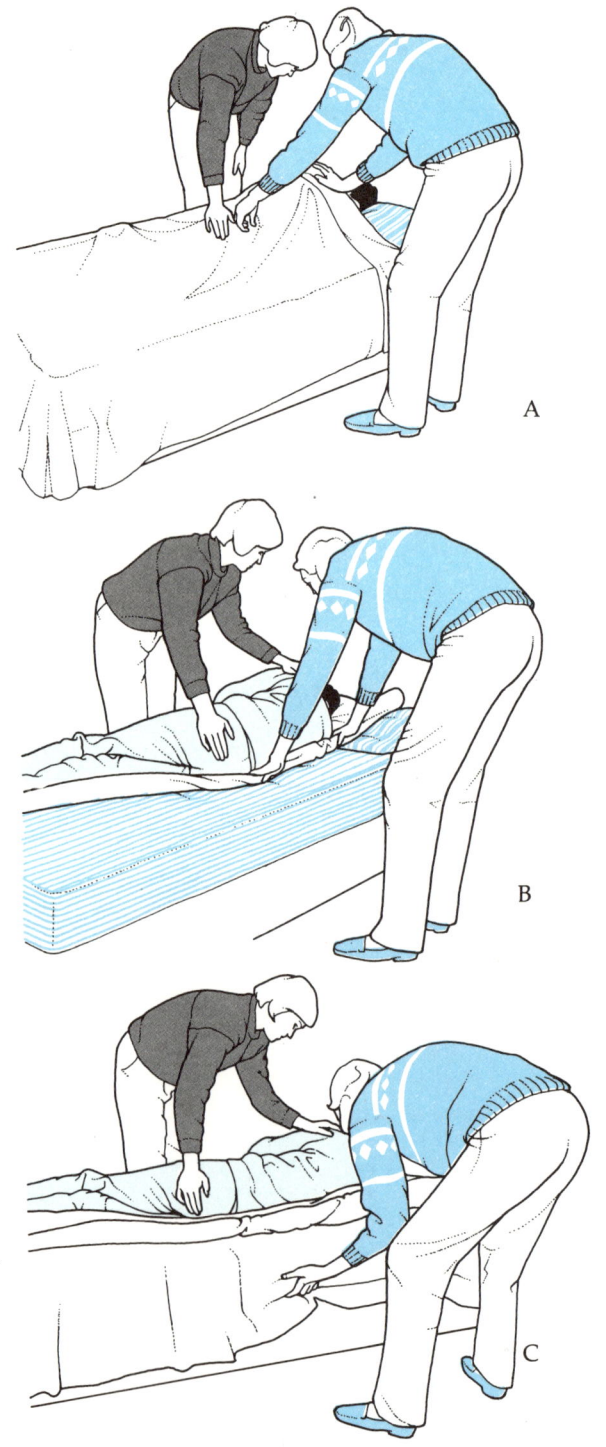

A

Preparation

1 Place the chairs back-to-back at the foot of the bed.

2 Loosen all bedclothes.

3 Remove all the pillows except one. Remove the pillowcases and discard into the linen basket. Place the pillows on the chairs.

Removing the bedcovers

4 Remove the bedcover, blankets and top sheet separately. Fold the top third of each cover to the centre and then the bottom third to the centre. Both people lift the covers over the backs of the chairs. Put the dirty linen into the basket or plastic bag. Fold a duvet in the same way.
▶ Leave the sick person covered with one sheet, and a blanket if the room is cold.

5 Turn him onto his side on one side of the bed. Make sure that his head is resting on the pillow and that his limbs are well supported (A).

6 Hold him securely, as he is near the edge of the bed, while the other person rolls each item of the bottom bed linen separately toward the centre of the bed (B). If you are not putting on a clean sheet, make sure there are no crumbs or debris in the bed.

B

C

Replacing the bottom bed linen

7 Straighten the mattress cover.

8 Place the clean sheet, half rolled-up lengthways, against the roll of dirty linen. Tuck in half the sheet and mitre the corners (C).

9 If you are using a plastic sheet, unroll it over half the bed and tuck it in. If you are using a drawsheet and it needs replacing, place the clean, half rolled-up sheet against the roll of dirty linen and tuck in the remaining half (D). If the drawsheet is clean, pull through and tuck in.

10 Move the pillow to the other side of the bed and roll the sick person over the linen and onto the other side.

11 Pull through and remove the dirty linen. Straighten the mattress cover. If the sheets are clean and not being replaced straighten them, mitre the corners and tuck in. Pull through the drawsheet and plastic sheeting and tuck in.

12 If you are replacing bed linen, unroll the clean sheet across the bed. Tuck in and mitre the corners of the bottom sheet. Unroll and tuck in the plastic sheeting and drawsheet (E).

13 Roll the sick person onto his back in the middle of the bed. Get him into a comfortable position. Replace the pillowcases as necessary, and replace the pillows (F).

Replacing the top bed linen

14 Remove the sheet or blanket covering the sick person, if you are using one. Change the top sheet as necessary. Make up the bed, pleating the sheet and blankets, and mitring the corners of the sheet. Fold the top sheet over the bedcover. If you are using a duvet, change the cover and replace the duvet.

15 Make sure that the sick person is comfortable.

Finally

Clear away all equipment and replace any furniture that you moved. Wash your hands.

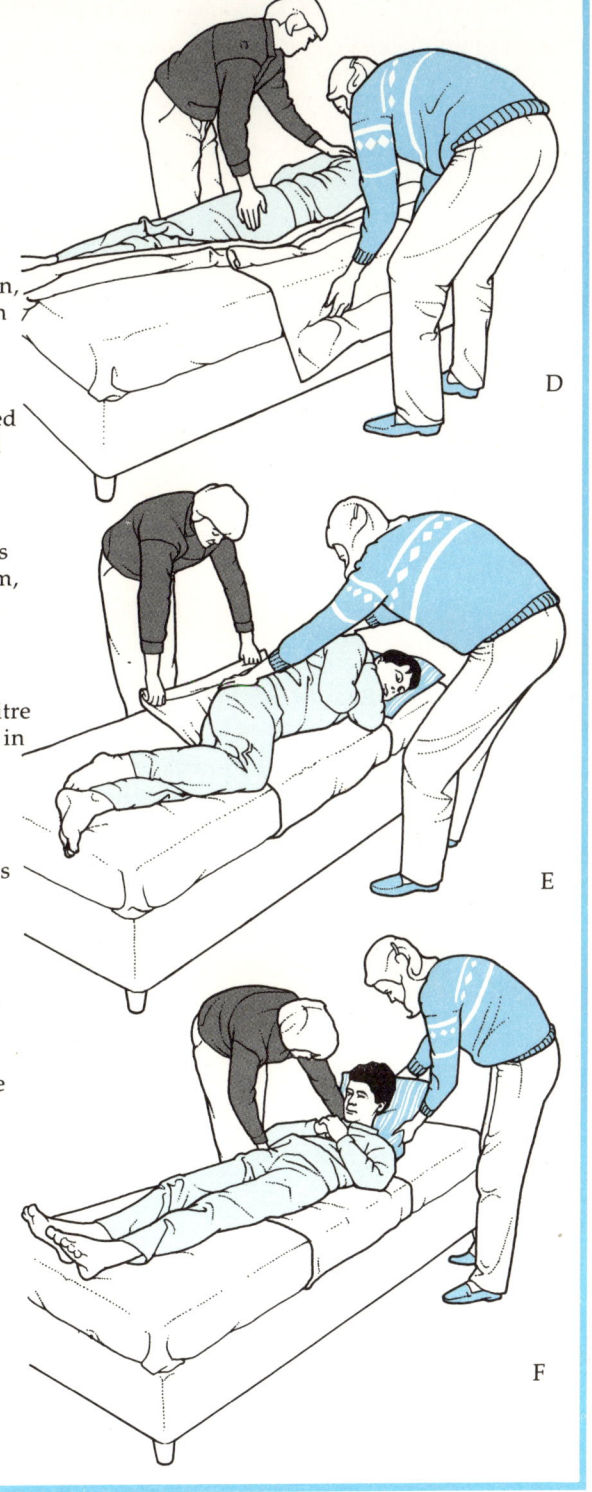

D

E

F

ONE PERSON MAKING AN OCCUPIED BED

It is possible to make an occupied bed on your own, but it requires some forethought. Make sure that the sick person cannot fall out of bed while you are working.

▶ This procedure is not suitable for someone who is breathless or uncomfortable lying flat.

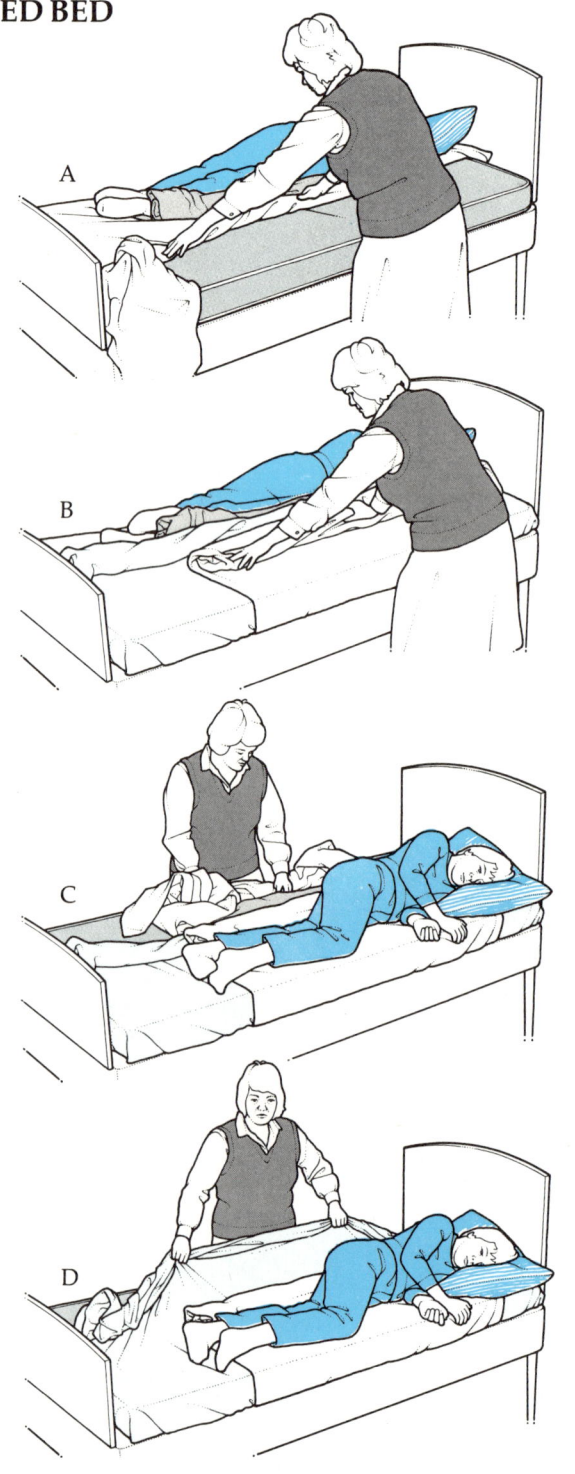

A

B

C

D

Collect together
- Two chairs
- Clean linen, if required
- Dirty linen basket or plastic bag
- Separate plastic bag for heavily soiled linen, if necessary

Preparation

1 Place the chairs back-to-back at the foot of the bed.

2 Loosen all bedclothes on one side of the bed, then the other.

3 Remove all but one pillow.

4 Remove the pillowcases and discard into the linen basket. Place the pillows on the chairs.

Removing the bedcovers

5 Remove each covering separately. Fold the covers in half by pulling the bottom up to the head of the bed. Lift the two corners nearest you to the centre (see page 25). Lay each cover over the chairs. Fold a duvet into thirds (see page 26).
▶ Leave the sick person covered with one sheet, and a blanket if the room is cold.

6 Put the dirty linen into the linen basket or plastic bag.

7 Move the remaining pillow to the far side of the bed, making sure that the sick person's head is still on the pillow. Turn the sick person on to her side. Push her away from you, at the same time asking her to help by pulling herself over onto her side. If she is likely to roll out of bed, make an improvised cotside (see page 20).

8 Roll each item of the bottom bed linen separately toward the centre of the bed, up against the sick person's back (A). If you are not putting on a clean sheet, make sure there are no crumbs or debris in the bed.

Replacing the bottom bed linen

9 Straighten the mattress cover.

10 Place the clean sheet, half rolled-up lengthways, against the roll of dirty linen. Tuck in half the sheet and mitre the corners.

11 If you are using a plastic sheet, unroll it over half the bed and tuck it in. If you are using a drawsheet and it needs replacing, place the clean, half rolled-up drawsheet against the roll of dirty linen and tuck in the remaining half (B). If the drawsheet is clean, pull through and tuck in.

12 Roll the sick person onto her back over the roll of bed linen toward you. Move the pillow slightly toward you. Roll the sick person onto her side so that her head rests on the pillow.

13 Go round to the other side of the bed, pull through and remove the dirty linen (C). Straighten the mattress cover. If the sheets are clean and not being replaced straighten them, mitre the corners and tuck in. Pull through the drawsheet and plastic sheeting and tuck in.

14 If you are replacing the bed linen, unroll the clean sheet (D), tuck in and mitre the corners. Unroll and tuck in the plastic sheeting and drawsheet.

15 Roll the sick person onto her back. Replace pillowcases as necessary. Replace the pillows and make the sick person comfortable.

Replacing the top bed linen

16 Remove the sheet or blanket covering the sick person, if you are using one. Change the top sheet as necessary. Make up the bed, pleating the sheet and blankets, and mitring the corners of the sheet. Fold the top sheet over the bedcover. If you are using a duvet, change the cover and replace the duvet.

17 Make sure that the sick person is comfortable.

Finally

Clear away all equipment, and replace any furniture that you moved. Wash your hands.

If the sick person cannot lie down flat

You may be looking after someone who is neither able to lie down flat nor to get out of bed. In this case, you can modify the procedure described for making a bed occupied by a sick person who can lie down.

Instead of rolling the sick person over onto one side, lift him or her to sit on the end of the bed with his or her legs over the side (A). Support the invalid's feet on a footstool or a chair if the bed is high off the ground. You can then unmake and remake the top half of the bed. Roll all the linen down to the middle of the bed. Then make up the top half of the bed. Move the sick person back up to the head of the bed to sit up in a comfortable position while you remove the dirty linen and remake the bottom half of the bed.

If you are working on your own, use pillows to support the sick person as he or she sits at the end of the bed. If the invalid cannot move unaided and you cannot lift him or her, you may be able to use a hoist (see page 52). Alternatively you can turn the sick person from one side to the other, propped up comfortably with pillows.

If you can ask someone else to help you, this will make your task much easier. Your helper can support the sick person while you remove the dirty linen and remake the bed (B).

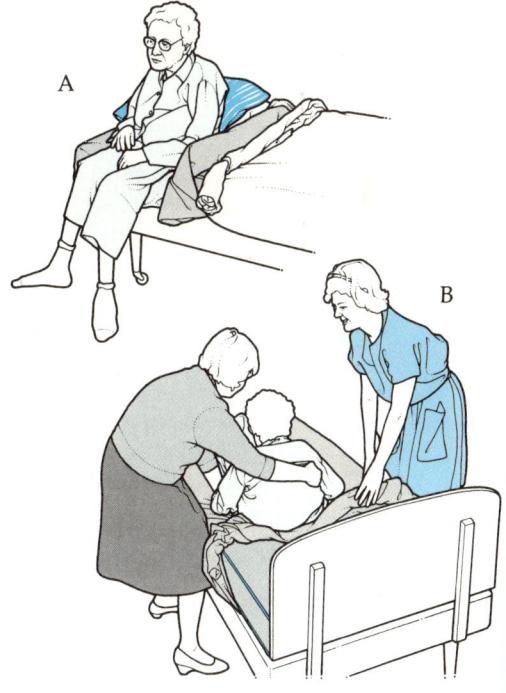

Lifting and Moving

Learning how to lift and move a sick person is a very important part of home nursing, especially if the invalid you are looking after is unable to stand up and move unaided, or finds it difficult. If the sick person is suffering from a long-term illness, getting him or her up and into another room with the rest of the family, or even out into the garden, will provide a welcome change of scene and can act as a wonderful boost to morale.

There is no need to be alarmed at the prospect of lifting someone; with time and practice, you are likely to find that you can do it. However, it *is* worth being careful: never try out a new lift on a sick person until you are confident you are doing it correctly, and stop at once if you feel out of control or if you or the sick person feel any discomfort. Ask for a demonstration from a physiotherapist or other health professional. If you need assistance and friends and relatives are available and willing to help, it is well worth sparing the time to show them how to lift correctly. In some cases the sick person may be able to help you and should be encouraged to do so. Various aids to lifting and moving are also available and can be helpful.

Important points to remember

☐ It is very important that you learn to lift correctly in order to avoid injuring yourself as well as the sick person.

☐ Practise each procedure on a friend a couple of times and only once you are confident you are doing it correctly, should you try it out on the sick person.

☐ Do not take risks. If the sick person is too heavy for you to lift or move, or if you are at all worried, ask for help.

☐ Unless it is absolutely unavoidable, do not lift a completely helpless adult out of bed by yourself, as this is the riskiest type of move; always get help if you can.

☐ Find out from the sick person or the doctor how he or she is used to being lifted and moved around. For certain conditions, some lifts may be inadvisable.

☐ Explain clearly to the sick person what you are going to do and what he or she can do to help. Speak calmly and confidently. Remember that an invalid may be confused and weak and unable to take in all your instructions at once, so explain a little at a time as you go along.

☐ Before getting an invalid out of bed, it is important that you talk to the doctor and get his advice and approval.

Time spent in the open air can be invigorating and enjoyable for a convalescent or someone with a long-term illness. Make sure that the invalid does not get too hot or cold.

☐ When lifting with the assistance of a helper, or on your own with a sick person who is able to help, co-ordinate your movements to prevent any jarring. Try counting one, two, three and on the command 'lift', lifting together in one movement.

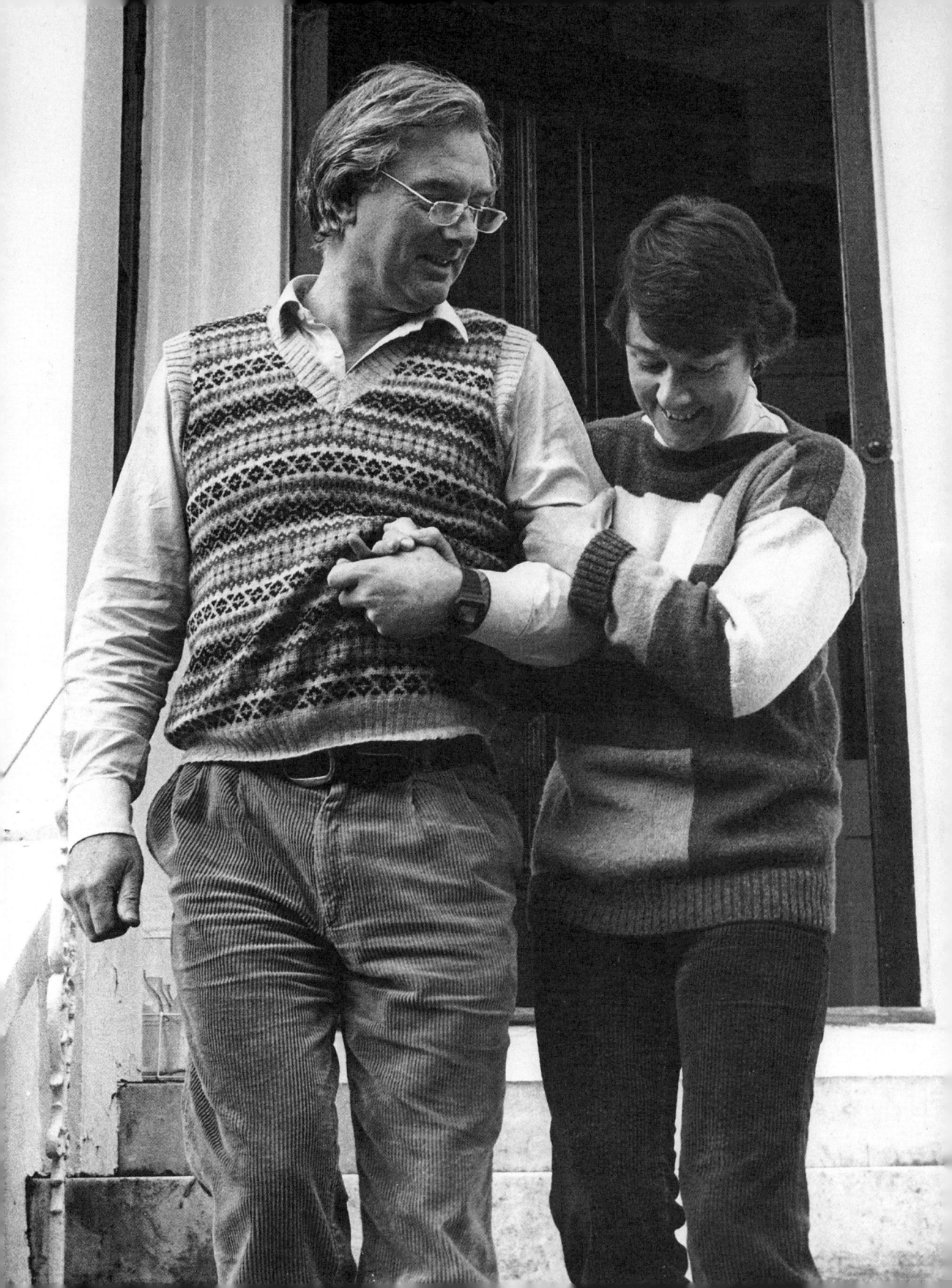

Before you begin

☐ Move any obstacles, such as bedside tables, out of the way so that you have enough space to move around in.

☐ Adjust the bed to the correct height, if necessary (see page 18).

☐ You will find lifting and moving easier if you wear clothes that are not tight and comfortable, low-heeled shoes.

☐ Collect together everything you need before you begin the move.

☐ Make sure that the sick person will be warm enough and has privacy before you begin.

☐ If you are turning someone in bed, find out if the sick person is comfortable and able to breathe lying down; if not, leave him or her sitting upright, propped up on several pillows, and turn in a sitting position.

Protecting your back

Make use of the following advice before attempting any lift or move, otherwise you risk injuring your back.

☐ Stand straight but not stiff, with your head erect and chin tucked in. This keeps your back straight and protects your joints and ligaments.

☐ Bend your hips and knees slightly.

☐ Stand as close to the sick person as possible, with your feet apart to help you keep your balance and your toes pointed in the direction in which you intend to move.

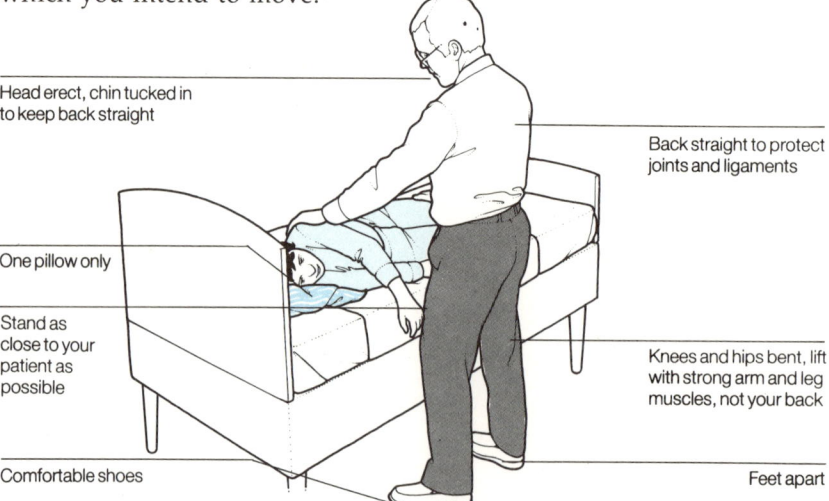

Head erect, chin tucked in to keep back straight

Back straight to protect joints and ligaments

One pillow only

Stand as close to your patient as possible

Knees and hips bent, lift with strong arm and leg muscles, not your back

Comfortable shoes

Feet apart

Try this position yourself a couple of times and you will soon find that it becomes automatic. It is the correct way to stand because you are using your strong leg and thigh muscles to lift the sick person and carrying the weight as near to the centre of your body as possible.

Turning

You may need to turn a sick person while you are making the bed or washing him or her. If the sick person cannot move at all, you may need to turn him or her frequently to avoid bedsores.

TWO PEOPLE TURNING A SICK PERSON WHO IS UNABLE TO HELP

It is always better for both the sick person and the caregiver if a helpless person is moved by two people.

To turn him onto his left side

1 Stand one on either side of the bed.

2 Fold back the bedclothes to the end of the bed.

3 Lay the sick person on his back in the centre of the bed. If he is facing the right-hand side, roll him gently onto his back.

4 Remove all but one pillow.

5 Move the remaining pillow nearer to the side of the bed.

6 Place his right arm across his chest, his left arm by his side and his right leg over his left (A).

7 The caregiver stands on the left of the bed and gently pulls the sick person toward her, supporting the sick person with one hand on his buttocks and the other over his shoulders. The helper on the other side gently pushes the sick person onto his side (B).

8 Both you and your helper grasp wrists under the sick person's buttocks and under his thighs and lift his pelvis into the centre of the bed.

9 Place some pillows behind the sick person's back if he needs supporting in this position, and replace the pillows and bedcovers, making sure he is warm and comfortable (C).

To turn the sick person onto his other side, read left for right as you go through the procedure.

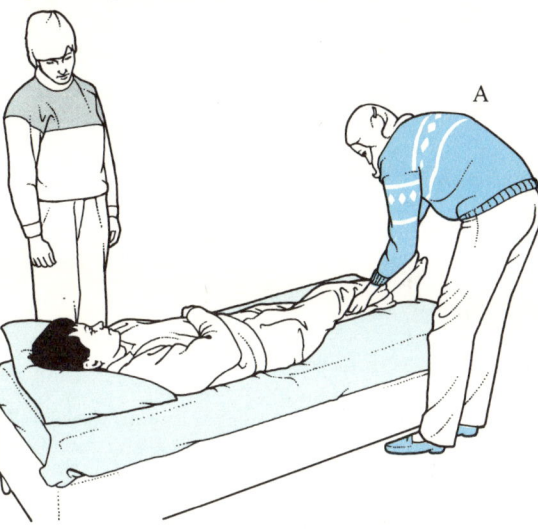

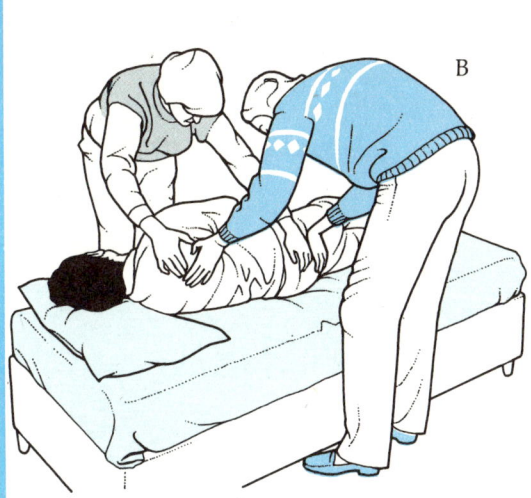

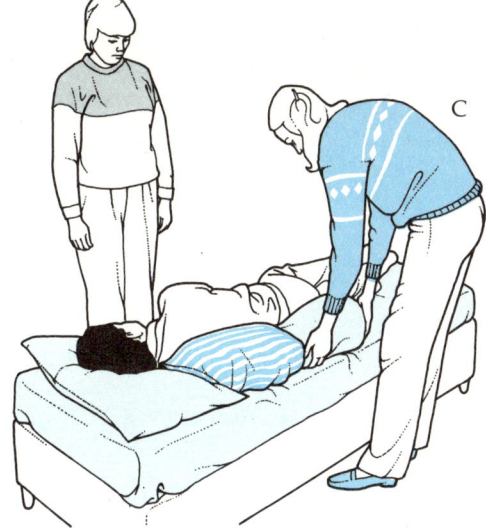

TURNING A SICK PERSON WHO IS ABLE TO HELP, ON YOUR OWN

If another person is available to help you, he or she can assist with moving the patient's pelvis into the centre of the bed, as on page 35.

To turn her onto her left side

1 Fold back the bedclothes to the end of the bed.

2 Help the sick person to lie on her back in the centre of the bed.

3 Remove all but one pillow.

4 Move the remaining pillow nearer to the left-hand side of the bed.

5 Stand on the left-hand side of the bed. Place the sick person's right arm across her chest, with her left hand, palm upward, comfortably on the pillow, ready to support her head when you turn her onto her side. Place her right leg over her left (A).

6 Ask her to grasp your right forearm with her right hand and on a count of three to pull herself toward you as you pull her toward you with both hands (B). Reassure her that she will not fall out of bed but will simply roll against you.

7 Go round to the other side of the bed and lift her pelvis into the centre of the bed (C).

8 Replace the pillows and bedcovers, and make sure she is warm and comfortable.

To turn the sick person onto her other side, read left for right as you go through the procedure.

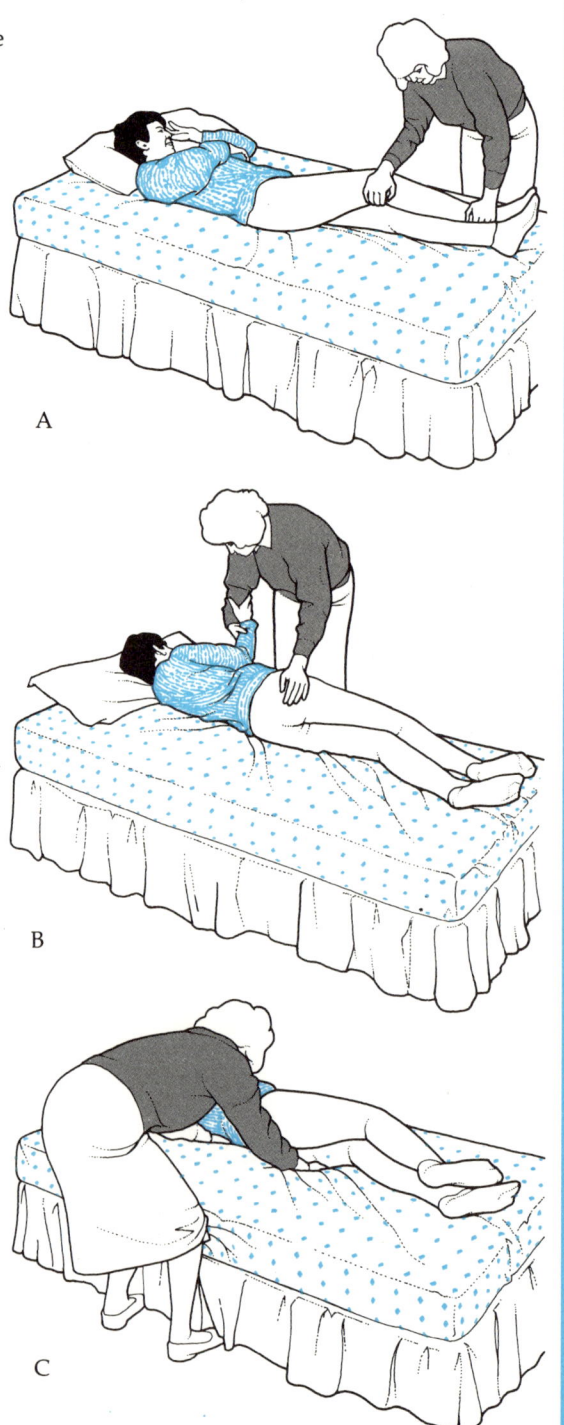

A

B

C

TURNING A SICK PERSON WHO IS UNABLE TO HELP, ON YOUR OWN

It is possible to turn a sick person on your own if the bed is made up with a drawsheet.

To turn him onto his left side

1 Fold the bedclothes down to the end of the bed and make sure the sick person is lying in the centre of the drawsheet.

2 Lay the sick person on his back in the centre of the bed. If he is facing the right-hand side, roll him gently onto his back.

3 Remove all but one pillow.

4 Untuck the drawsheet on the right-hand side.

5 Go round to the other side of the bed and move the remaining pillow nearer to the left-hand side of the bed.

6 Place his right arm across his chest, his left arm by his side and his right leg over his left.

7 Take the right-hand side of the drawsheet and roll it up toward him.

8 With the roll of drawsheet held firmly in both hands, pull the sick person toward you (A). If you are worried that he might fall out of bed, use cotsides or improvise with high-backed chairs (see page 20).

9 Go round to the right-hand side of the bed and, placing one arm under his thigh and the other under his hip joint, gently lift his pelvis into the centre of the bed.

10 Tuck in the drawsheet (B).

11 Place some pillows behind his back if he needs supporting in this position.

12 Replace the pillows and bedclothes, and make sure he is warm and comfortable.

To turn the sick person onto his other side, read left for right as you go through the procedure.

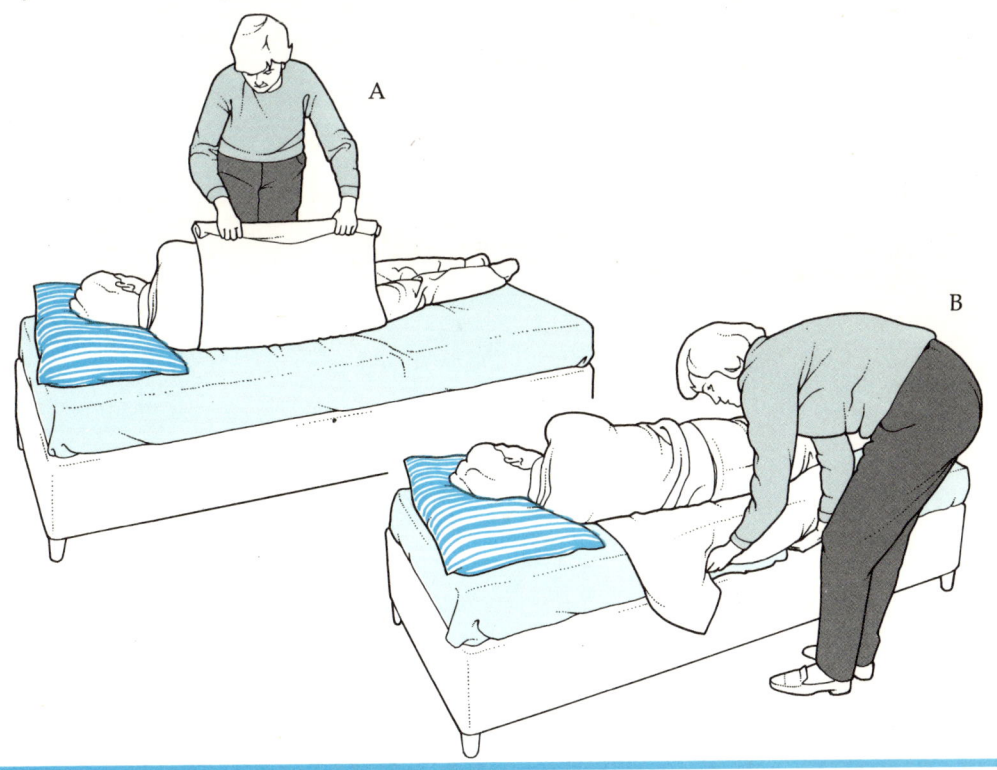

A

B

Lifting

In this section, six different lifts are described in detail, each of which enables you to move a sick person safely. There is no need to read the section right through: just concentrate on the lift which will enable you to make the required move. If the sick person is lying down flat in bed, you may want to get him or her up and sitting in a chair. This would involve three lifts (**1**, **2** and **3**). Once you have read through the instructions and are quite clear about what you want to do, tell the sick person and explain what he or she can do to help.

---

1 HELPING A SICK PERSON INTO A SITTING POSITION IN BED

A sick person will need to be lifted into a sitting position several times during the day so that he or she can eat, read or watch television in comfort.

Always make sure that the invalid is comfortably supported with pillows and backrest once you have completed the move.

**Underarm lift –
two people**
1 You and your helper each pass an arm under the sick person's armpits and ask the sick person to grasp your elbows or shoulders.
2 Lift together – shifting your weight onto your leg nearest the bed head and steadying the sick person with your free hand.

**Underarm lift –
one person**
Ask the sick person to reach under your arm and grasp your shoulder, while you hold her upper arm or shoulder. Ask her to pull down on your shoulder with one hand and to push with her other arm and foot, as you lift, pulling her toward you.

**Holding the bed –
one person**
Place one arm across the sick person's shoulders and with your other hand grasp the side of the bed. To lift, pull on your hand and shift your weight onto your foot nearest the bed end, as the sick person lifts her head forward and pushes her hands down her thighs.

**Lifting a helpless
invalid – one person**
If the sick person is unable to help, use the lift in the diagram below left but support her head against your shoulder. As you lift her forward, take the weight off the upper part of her body onto yours.

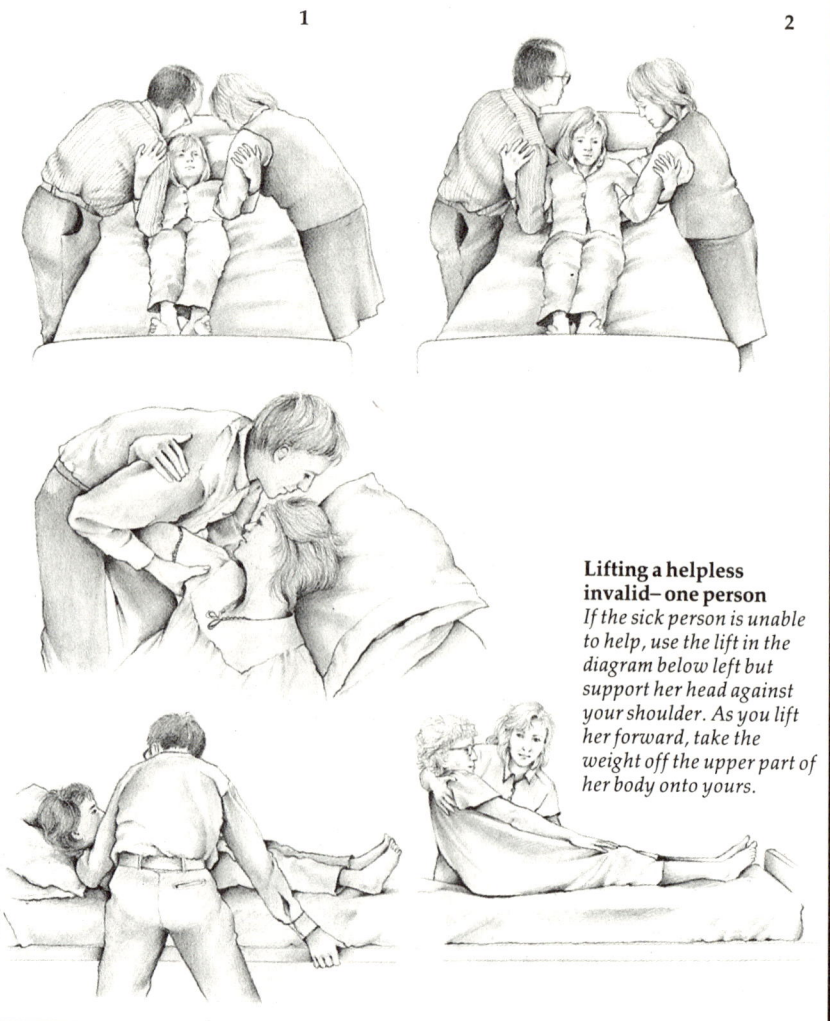

1

2

2 MOVING A SICK PERSON UP THE BED

The instructions that follow are for moving a sick person up the bed, but these lifts can also be used for moving an invalid down or to one side of a bed. The orthodox lift described below can be used if a sick person is complaining of pain in the chest or shoulder areas, or is so ill that he or she is unable to help you. It is a method which should only be used to lift a light patient on a narrow bed of the correct height, otherwise both you and your helper will have difficulty keeping your backs straight. A similar lift using a drawsheet can be carried out on a low bed and is a useful alternative if the patient is complaining of pain in the back region.

The shoulder or Australian lift shown over the page considerably reduces the amount of strain put on the back of the person who is doing the lifting and is really the best lift to use, providing the sick person is able to help you. Once again the bed should be at the correct height, unless variations of the lift are used which are specifically designed for a low bed.

☐ The sick person should always be lifted clear of the bed and not dragged along the bedclothes as this will damage the skin and may cause pressure sores to develop.

☐ Both lifts involve lifting the patient clear of the bed, so it is a good idea to ask for a demonstration from a physiotherapist or other health professional at your local hospital.

Finger or wrist grip
If two people are lifting a sick person, this often involves grasping or gripping each other's fingers or wrists to secure a firm grip. Make sure that your nails are short or they will dig into your helper's hand.

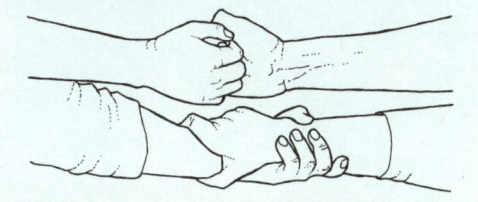

From the front

From the back

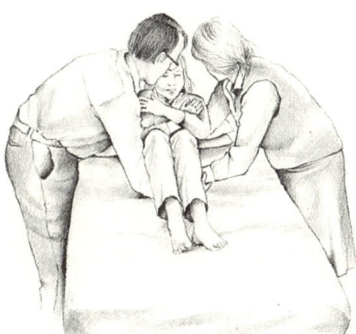

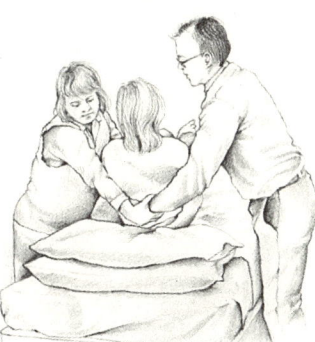

The orthodox lift – two people
Ask the sick person to fold her arms across her chest and to bend her knees. You and your helper grasp wrists under her thighs and stand with your legs apart, knees bent, feet pointed outward, backs straight and heads lifted. Grip hands behind her back. Lift together – straightening your legs and shifting your weight onto your foot nearest the bed head.

Using a drawsheet – two people
1 *Untuck the drawsheet on both sides. Ask the sick person to fold her arms across her chest. You and your helper each grasp the drawsheet beside the sick person's thighs and behind her buttocks so that you are supporting her back against your forearms.*
2 *Lift together – pulling up on the drawsheet and shifting your weight onto your foot nearest the bed head.*

1

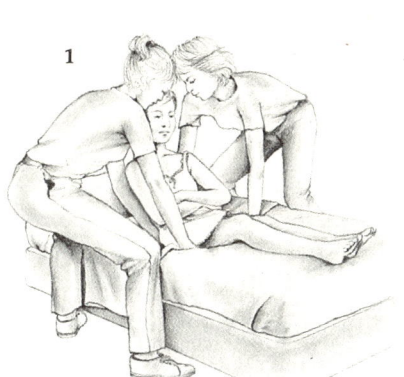

2

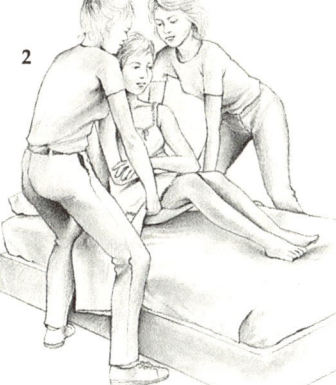

MOVING A SICK PERSON UP THE BED

The shoulder or Australian lift – two people

You and your helper both place a shoulder under the sick person's armpits and grasp wrists or fingers *under her thighs. Stand level with the patient's hips. Keep your hand nearest the bed head flat on the bed and your foot nearest the bed head pointed in the direction of* *the intended move. With heads lifted, both lift together, pushing up into the sick person's armpits and shifting your weight onto your leg and hand nearest the bed head.*

From the front

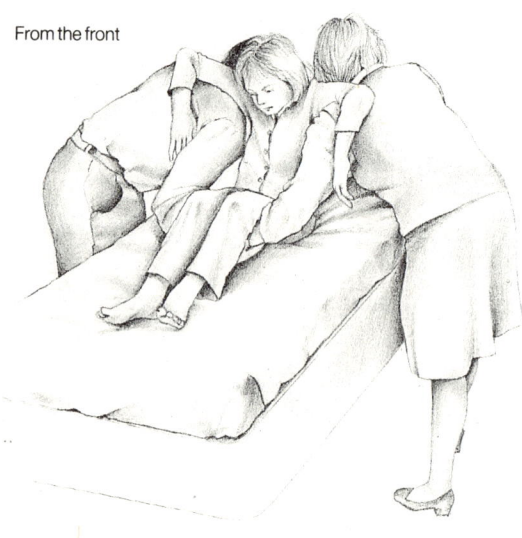

From the back

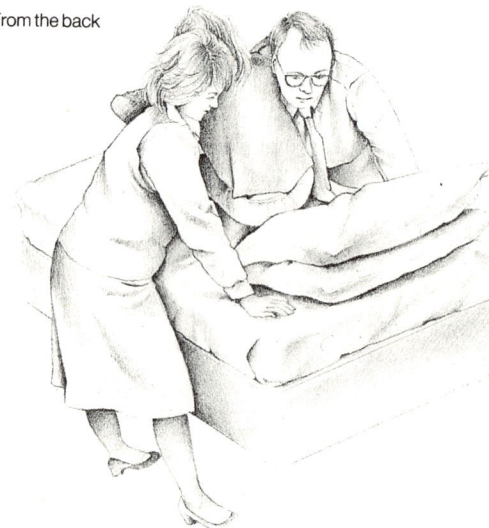

On a low bed – two people

You and your helper each kneel with one leg on the bed, level with the sick person's hips. Grasp wrists under her thighs and place *your other hand flat on the bed. Lift together – pushing up into the sick person's armpits, carrying your body forward and shifting part of your weight onto your outside arm and hand.*

On a low double bed – two people

Move the sick person to the side of the bed. Kneel on the bed with one leg, while your helper kneels on the bed with both legs. Lift together – pushing up into the sick *person's armpits, carrying your body forward and shifting part of your weight onto your outside arm and hand. If the sick person cannot be moved to the side of the bed, both kneel on the bed and lift.*

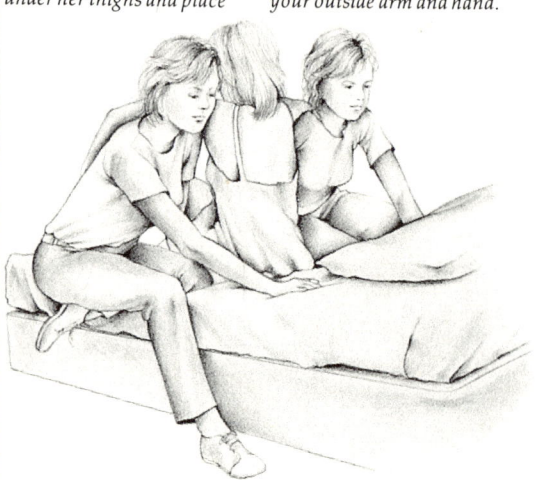

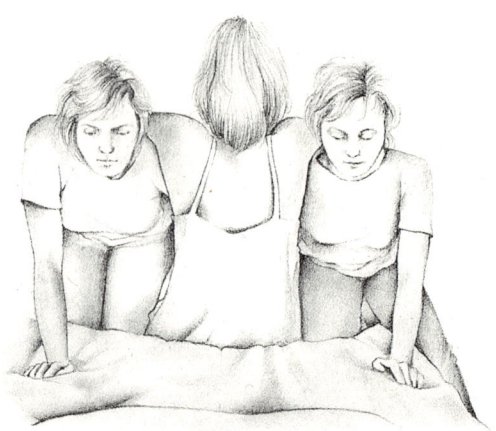

Shoulder lift – one person

Ask the sick person to put one arm over your shoulder and to bend his outer knee.

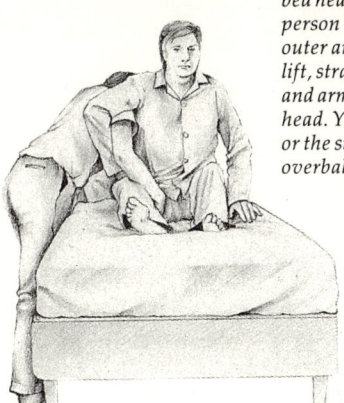

Tuck his forearm between your chest and upper arm, grasp hold of his thigh and bend your knee nearest the bed head. Ask the sick person to push down on his outer arm and heels as you lift, straightening your leg and arm nearest the bed head. You must lift together or the sick person may overbalance.

Underarm lift – one person

Ask the sick person to grasp the back of your shoulder with one hand and to keep her other hand flat on the bed, and to have her knees bent and heels down. With one arm, reach under her arm and grasp her shoulder. Lift up and back as the sick person pushes down with

her heels and hand and pulls on your shoulder, keeping her chin on her chest.

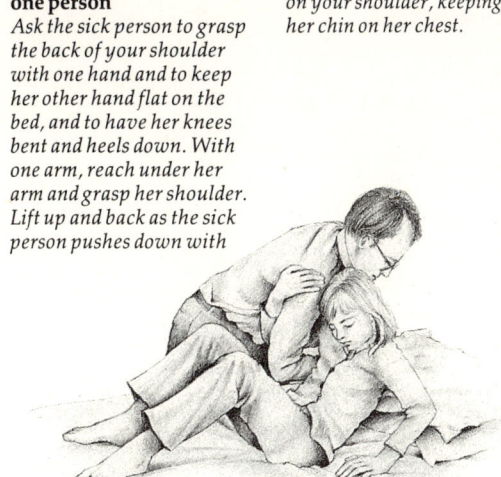

Lifting a helpless invalid – when the lifter is tall

Remove your shoes, then remove all the pillows. Kneel on the bed, with your head slightly to one side over the sick person's shoulder and grasp her arms as shown, right. Straighten your own and the sick person's back before lifting. Ask her to bend her knees and push on her heels as you lift, if she is able to.

Then straighten your hips and lift her toward you. You may need to do several small lifts to achieve the full move.

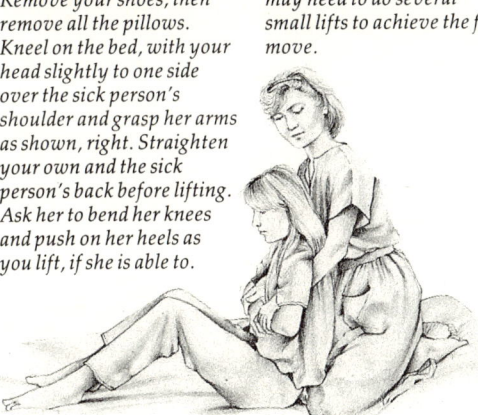

Position of hands when lifting

Tell the sick person to grasp her right wrist with her left hand.

Grasp her forearms with your hands. If the sick person is unable to grasp her wrist, grasp hold of her forearms near the elbows.

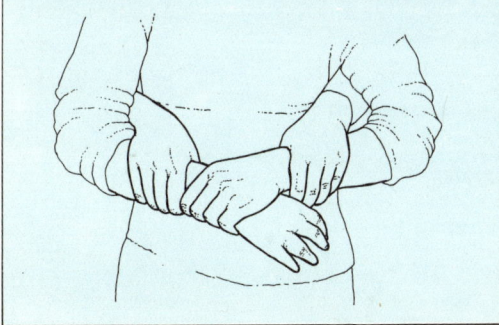

Lifting a helpless invalid – when the lifter is short

1 Place your feet apart, slightly behind and to the side of the sick person's buttocks. Bend your hips and knees and point your feet slightly outward. Place your head over the sick person's shoulder and grasp her arms as shown above. Straighten your own and

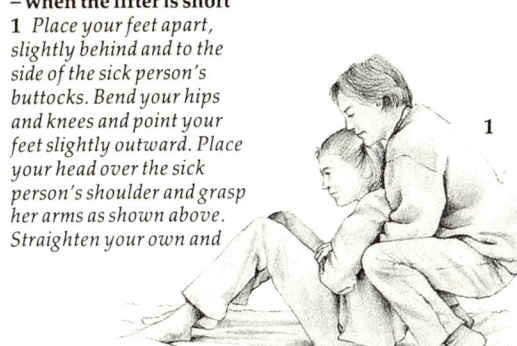

the sick person's back before lifting and ask her to bend her knees and push on her heels as you lift, if she is able to.

2 Straighten your hips and knees and lift her toward you. Do not try to swing her back too far in one lift as you may fall forward on top of her; it is safer to use several small lifts.

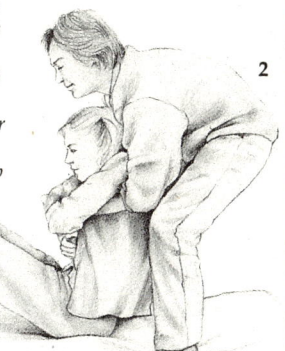

3 MOVING A SICK PERSON FROM A BED TO A CHAIR

Getting a sick person up and out of bed not only makes him or her feel better but also reduces the likelihood of some problems, such as deep vein thrombosis, kidney stones, pressure sores and loss of muscle tone leading to general weakness.

☐ Prepare the chair that the sick person is to sit in, making sure that it cannot slip backward by placing it against a wall or heavy piece of furniture near the bed.

☐ Make sure the sick person is wearing socks or tights and shoes to prevent him or her slipping when you help him or her to stand. Belts and waist ties should be fastened so that nothing falls or hangs down to trip you or the sick person up.

☐ If the bed is too high for the sick person to step down from safely, place a low wide stool beside the bed, making sure that it will not slip.

Rather than attempting to lift a really helpless sick person on your own, it will be safer to wait until he or she has regained some strength and independence. Alternatively, you can make use of a hoist. If necessary, the lift on page 45 can be used to move a helpless person from a bed to a chair or commode.

The lifts described below can also be used to move a sick person from a wheelchair to a bed, chair or toilet. Remember to remove the sides of the wheelchair, if they are detachable, beforehand.

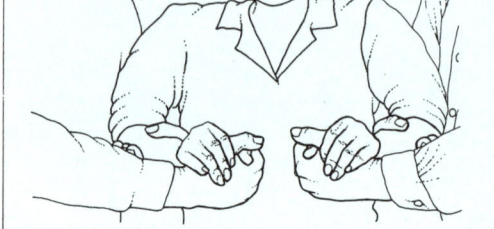

Hand grasp
Stand close to the sick person. Each place one arm between the sick person's body and forearm so that *your hand is supporting her elbow and forearm. Ask her to grasp hold of the thumb and back of your other hand.*

Moving someone who can stand – two people
1 Both you and your helper stand facing each other, with your feet angled to prevent the sick person slipping forward when she stands. Stand close to her, with your knees bent and backs straight. Hold one of her hands and support her under the armpit with your other hand as you raise her to her feet. Ask her to straighten her knees and stretch up as her feet touch the floor.

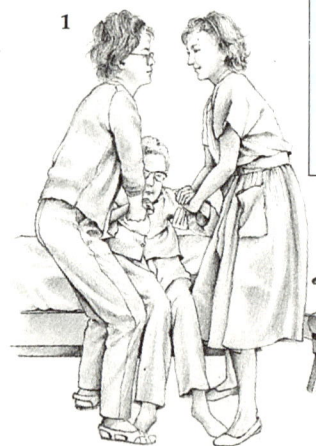

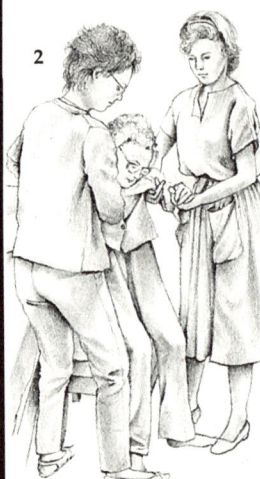

2 If the sick person is unable to walk, place the chair at a right angle to the bed and help her to turn; or else help the sick person to walk to the chair. Ask her to feel for the chair seat with the back of her legs.

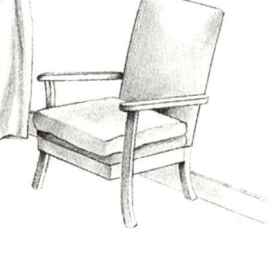

3 If the chair is placed firmly against a wall, you can continue supporting the sick person with both hands; if not, move your hand from the sick person's armpit to the back of the chair to keep it steady. Each place one foot in front of the sick person's feet to prevent them slipping. Ask the sick person to bend her knees and hips. Transfer your weight onto your foot nearest the back of the chair as you lower her gently into the chair.

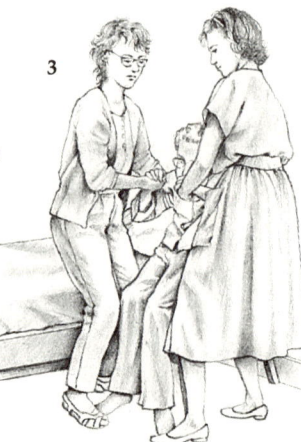

Moving someone who cannot stand – two people

1 Place the chair at a right angle to the bed. Help the sick person to the side of the bed. Ask her or help her to place her arms over your shoulders. You and your helper push up into her armpits, and grasp wrists under her thighs, keeping your weight on your leg nearest the bed. Lift together – straightening your hips and knees.

2 Lift the sick person up off the bed and carry her toward the chair.

3 Bend your knees and lower the sick person gently into the chair, steadying the chair with your free hand as you do so.

Back to bed again

1 Help the sick person to the edge of the chair. Both you and your helper crouch near the floor. Grasp wrists under the sick person's thighs and place your free hand on the chair seat.

2 Keep your backs straight, push up into the sick person's armpits, and, using your leg muscles, lift together.

3 Support the sick person's back or buttocks with your free hand.

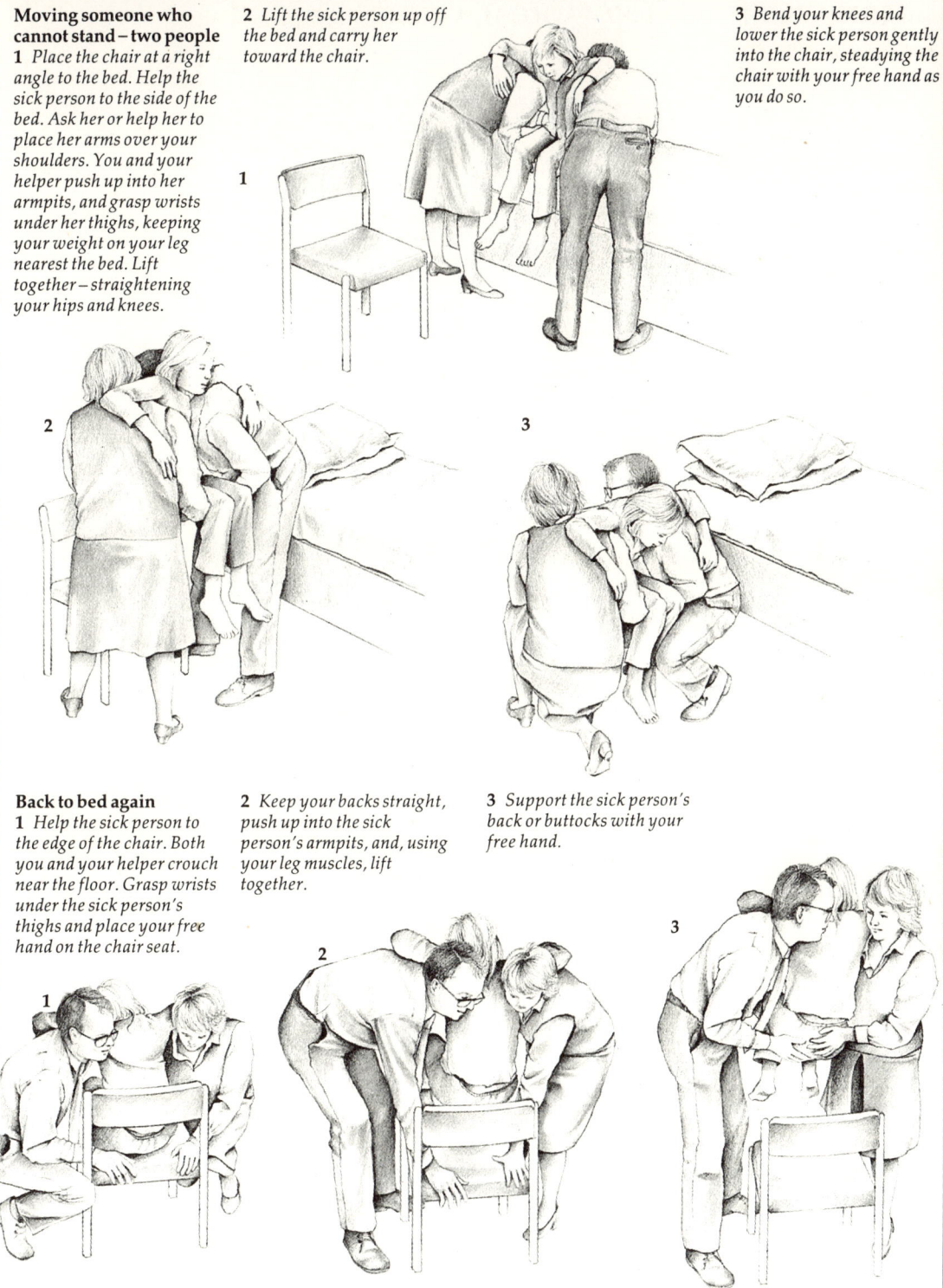

MOVING A SICK PERSON FROM A BED TO A CHAIR

Moving someone who can stand – one person

1 Place the chair at a right angle to the bed. Help the sick person to the edge of the bed and lift her into a sitting position with her legs hanging over the edge of the bed. Ask her to place her hands on your shoulders, with her weight held forward and her head over your shoulder. Put your arms under her arms and place your hands on her upper back. Stand close to the edge of the bed with knees bent and one foot placed well in front of the other between the sick person's knees.

2 Ask the sick person to keep her weight forward. Lift, shifting your weight onto your back foot at the same time as you push upward with your hands.

3 Continue to push upward with your hands. Shift your feet to a sideways position and at the same time turn the sick person so that the backs of her legs are touching the chair. Ask her to tell you when she can feel the chair.

4 With a straight back, place one foot well in front of the other between the sick person's knees with your knee bent.

5 Shift your weight onto your front leg and, by bending your front knee, lower the sick person into the chair as she bends her knees.

Back to bed
To help her back to bed, just follow the above instructions in reverse order.

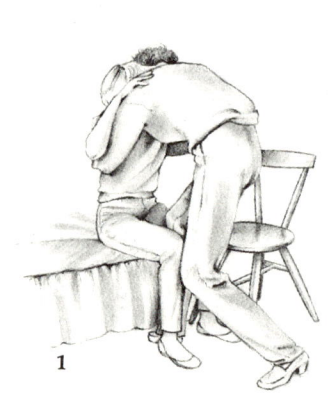

1

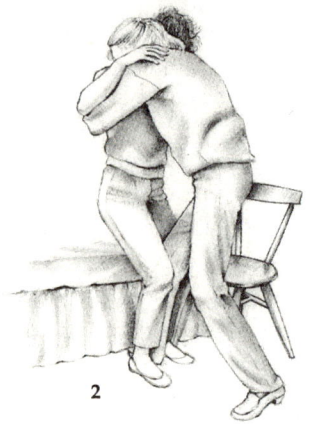

2

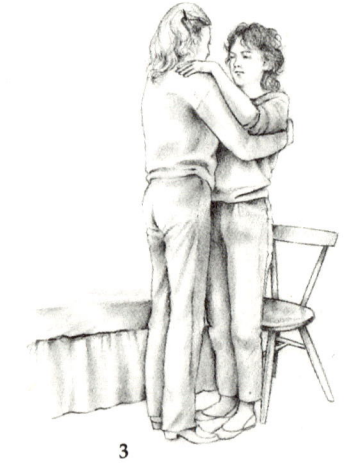

3

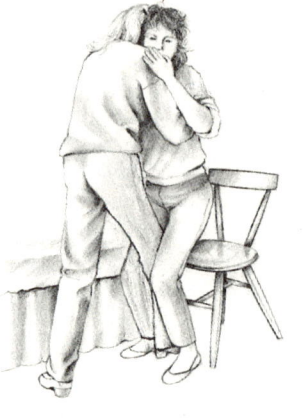

4

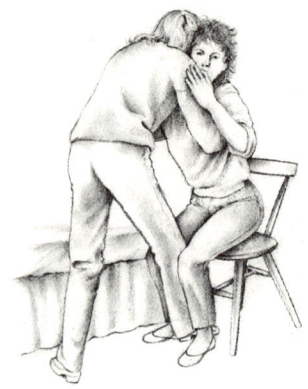

5

Moving someone who cannot stand – one person

1 Use a chair without arms. The distance between the bed and the chair must be the same as the length of the sick person's thighs to ensure that you can swing her from one to the other safely. Make sure the sick person is wearing shoes. Rock her gently from side to side to bring her to the edge of the bed and place her feet on the floor.

2 Place one foot in front of her feet with your knee against her knees, and your other leg against the side of the bed. Turn and face her. Grasp hold of both her elbows and pull her forward so that her nearest shoulder is supported against your side and her head is tucked under your arm. Do not exert any pressure on her neck.

3 To lift, transfer your weight onto your back leg.

4 Swing her round by shifting your weight onto your other leg. Lower her onto the chair.

Back to bed

To get the sick person back into bed, follow the above instructions in reverse order.

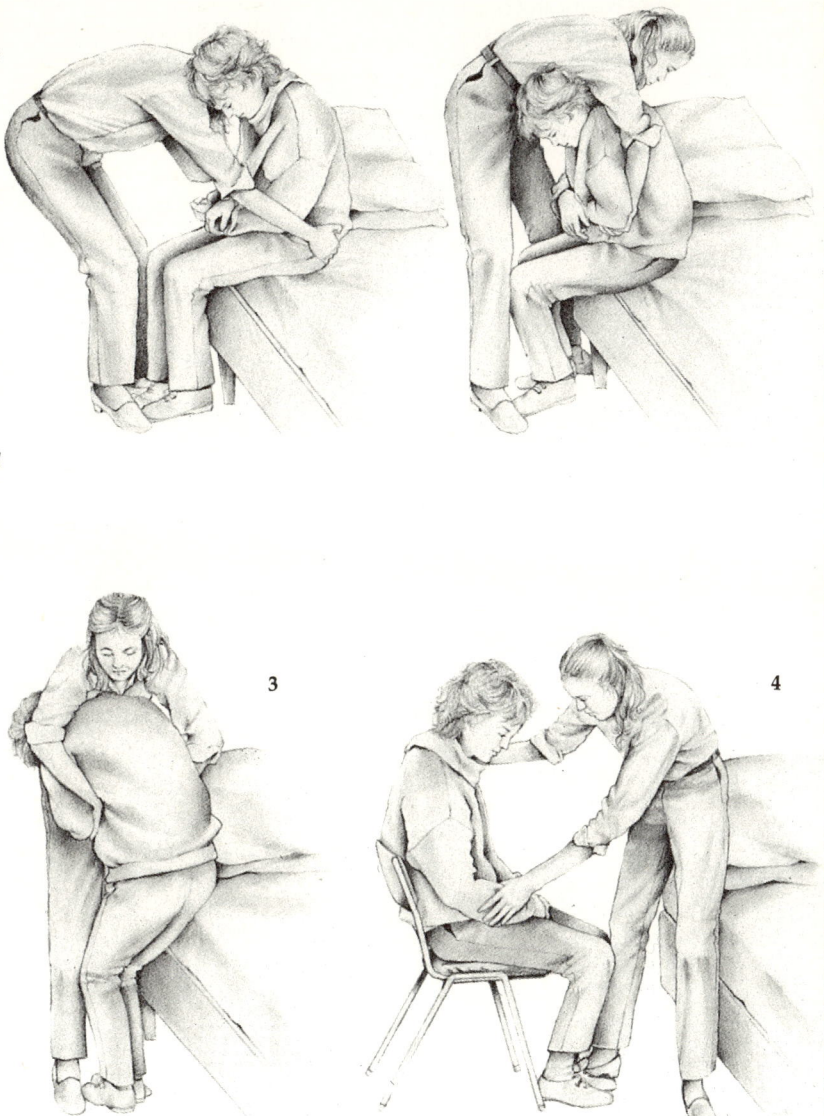

4 LIFTING A SICK PERSON UP INTO A CHAIR

A sick person should always be sitting well back in a chair both for security and comfort. If left sitting for a long while, he or she may well slip forward and will need to be lifted back.

If you are short you will need to stand on a low footstool to avoid hurting your back when you lean over to lift him or her. Make sure the stool is secure, sturdy and wide.

Underarm lift – two people
You and your helper stand on opposite sides of the chair, with your feet angled to prevent the sick person's feet slipping when she stands. Each place one hand under her arm and grasp the back of her shoulder. Place the other hand on the back of the chair. Hold the chair steady or place it against a wall. Lift together, up and back, straightening your knees.

Underarm lift – one person
Stand with your feet apart, one foot angled to stop the sick person's feet slipping when she stands. Place one hand under her arm and grasp the back of her shoulder and ask her to grasp the back of your shoulder. Hold the chair steady with your other hand or place it against a wall. Ask her to push on the arm of the chair with one hand, to pull on your shoulder with the other hand and to push away from your foot with her foot. At the same time, lift up and back, straightening your knees.

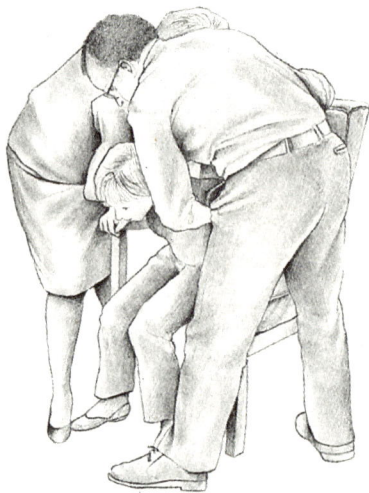

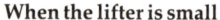

When the lifter is tall
Ask the sick person to grasp her right wrist with her left hand if she is able. With one foot forward, back straight and knees bent, reach under her arms and grasp her forearms, lowering your head over her shoulder. Straighten your back. Lift the sick person up off the seat and swing her back into the chair.

When the lifter is small
Place the stool so that you can stand on it with one foot slightly in front of the other. Ask the sick person to grasp her right wrist with her left hand if she is able. With a straight back and bent knees, reach under her arms and grasp her forearms, lowering your head over her shoulder. Straighten your back. Lift the sick person up off the seat and swing her back into the chair.

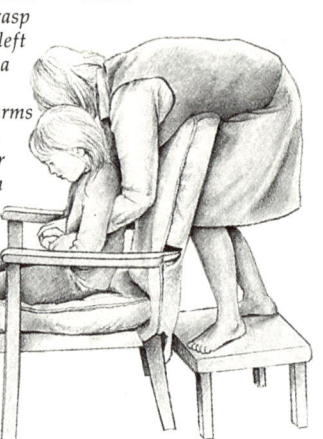

5 FROM SITTING TO STANDING

Helping a sick person to stand is an important first stage in the struggle to walk again. The sick person must be wearing socks or tights and shoes to prevent him or her slipping, and any belts should be fastened so that nothing falls or hangs down to trip him or her up.

Underarm lift – two people

1 Both you and your helper stand close to the sick person on either side of the chair, supporting her under each arm. Place your other hand on the back of the chair and have your feet angled to prevent the sick person's feet slipping when she stands. Lift together – shifting your weight onto your back foot, as the sick person pushes up on the arms of the chair.

2 Bring your arm forward from the back of the chair so that it is supporting the sick person's elbow and forearm, and ask her to grasp hold of the back of your other hand.

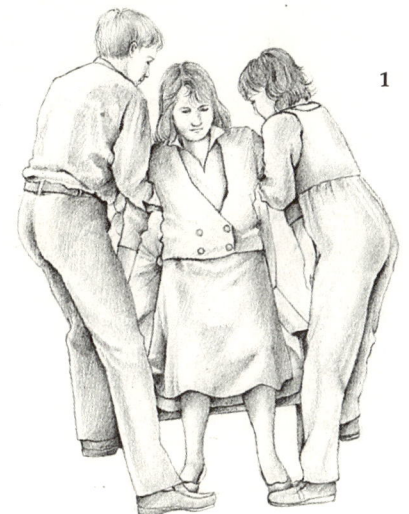

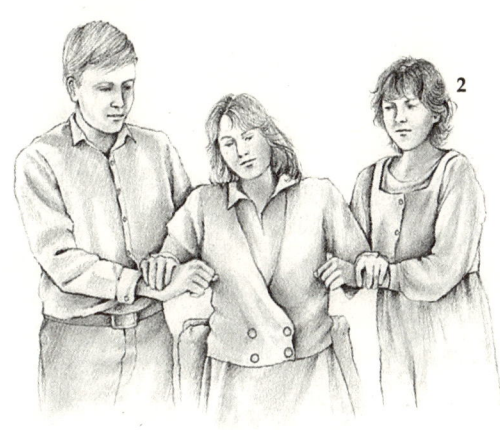

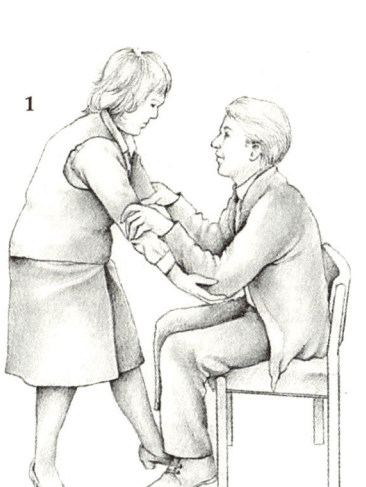

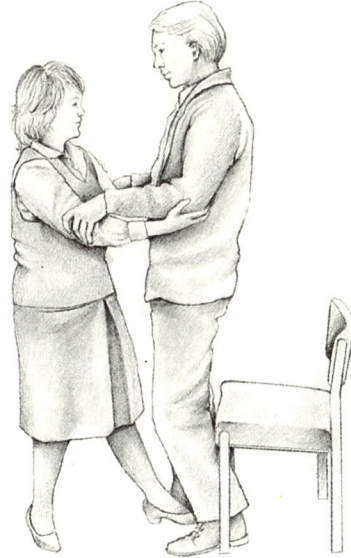

Elbow grip – one person

1 Stand with your legs apart, knees slightly bent and one foot placed in front of the other between the sick person's feet. Keep your forearms flexed and take hold of the sick person's elbows. Ask the sick person to place his forearms on yours and to grasp hold of your arms at the level of your elbow.

2 Warn the sick person to bring this head and trunk forward before straightening his hips and knees. To stand, push up on the sick person's elbows and straighten up as he presses down on your forearms.

Wheelchairs

It is important to be aware of how the person feels about using a wheelchair. There may be misunderstandings: for example, the invalid may believe that he or she will always be confined to a wheelchair when this is not the case. So check with the doctor and find out exactly what the position is so you are better able to discuss it.

On the other hand, if the sick person is to be confined to a wheelchair, he or she will need a great deal of support from you, both physically and emotionally, in adjusting to a new way of life. You may be able to help with practical details, such as finding out about motorized wheelchairs.

Using a wheelchair

☐ Make sure the person is sitting securely and well back in the chair. He or she may need a harness for safety.

☐ Place the invalid's feet on the footplate. If there are any footstraps or loops, make sure they are securely tied.

☐ If you are using a blanket over the sick person's knees, make sure it is tucked in at the sides and under his or her feet, so that no loose ends drag along the ground or get caught under the wheels.

☐ When you wheel the chair along, make sure the sick person's elbows do not stick out as they may get knocked.

☐ When you go through a doorway, always turn the chair round and pull it through backward. Similarly, when negotiating a step, turn the wheelchair round and lower the back wheels down the step first.

☐ When going up a step, tip the wheelchair back with your foot, using the specially provided footpiece, and put the front wheels on the step before lifting up the back wheels.

☐ Always put the brakes on when the chair is standing still and remember to release the brake before trying to move the chair.

☐ Never leave someone who is sitting in a wheelchair staring at a blank wall or with his or her back to interesting activity.

Maintenance of a wheelchair

☐ Check that the brakes are effective and the tyres fully inflated, where applicable.

☐ Check that all the nuts and screws are tightened up.

☐ Grease the small wheels according to the manufacturer's instructions. *Never* oil the hinges or clamps which control the folding footrests.

☐ Pay attention to the ballbearings in the large wheels. These should be checked every year or as often as recommended by the manufacturer.

☐ Clean the upholstery regularly with a damp cloth, and the metal parts with a soft cloth. Keep the wheels, hubcaps and footrests clean.

☐ To fold a wheelchair, place the footrests in an upright position and pull the seat canvas up by the centre; to open, press down on the side supports of the seat with both hands.

6 HELPING A SICK PERSON FROM A CAR INTO A WHEELCHAIR

Careful preparation will make this an easier and safer move.

☐ Remove the armrest nearest to the car.

☐ Remove the footplates or, if not removable, turn or lift them to one side.

☐ Make sure the small front wheels are turned in under the wheelchair.

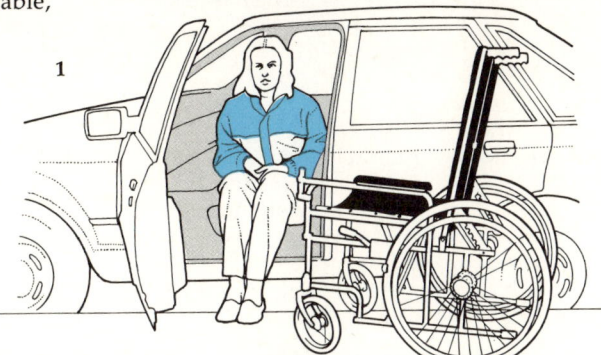

From a car to a wheelchair

1 *Place the wheelchair alongside the car and just behind the seat the sick person is sitting in, so that you have enough room to swing her round onto the chair. Check that the brakes are on. Help the sick person to sit on the edge of the car seat with both feet close together on the ground.*

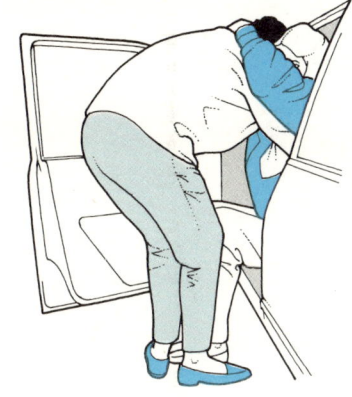

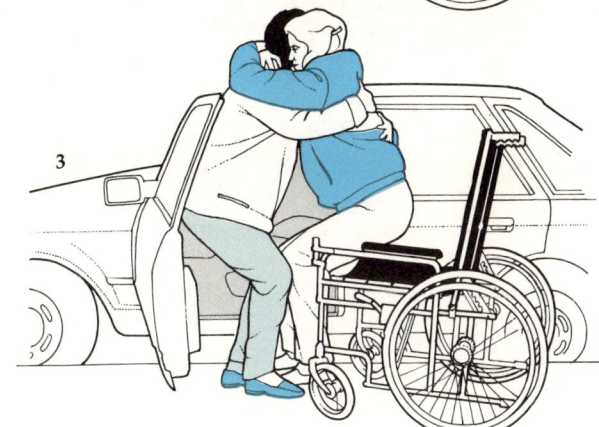

2 *Stand in front of her with one foot slightly forward and the other knee against her knees. Bend your knees and ask the sick person to put her arms across your shoulders. Put your hands on her back.*

3 *To lift, stand up, bringing your knees in front of hers. Swing the sick person round until you are facing the wheelchair. Make sure that the sick person is leaning forward, with the upper part of her body against yours as you lower her into the chair, continuing to control her hip and knee movement with your knees.*

4 *Make sure the sick person is comfortable and sitting well back in the chair.*

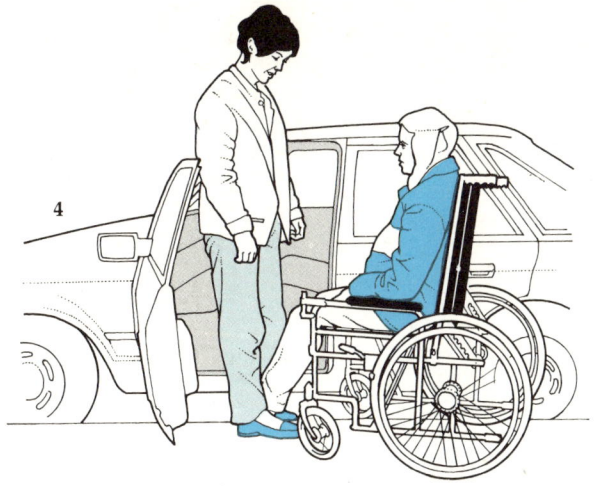

HELPING A SICK PERSON TO REGAIN INDEPENDENCE

It is important to encourage as much independence as possible as the sick person can come to rely on you and lose confidence in his or her own ability to cope. Dignity and self respect will be greatly restored if the sick person can learn to help him- or herself again and, once confidence has been regained, he or she will probably go from strength to strength.

TURNING

If the sick person has difficulty in moving and changing position in bed, he or she will very quickly become uncomfortable and may need to call frequently for your help; or he or she may just lie there in discomfort because of not wanting to disturb you. Either way it is better if the sick person can learn to help him- or herself. This can be achieved by using cotsides or improvising with one or two high-backed chairs.

Using cotsides
Tie the cotside or chair securely to the bed. The sick person should lie on his back with his knees flexed. He can then grasp the cotside or the back of the chair with his right arm, if turning to the left, and pull himself over.

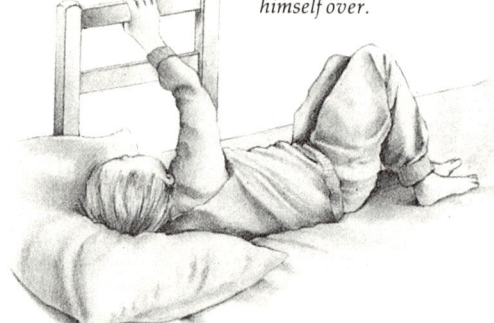

SITTING UP OR MOVING IN BED

The following improvised aids will enable the patient to sit up or move in bed independently.

Bed with a rail at the end
Attach a handle to one end of a strong piece of string or rope or any other material that does not stretch. Tie the other end to the rail at the foot of the bed, so that the invalid can pull herself up on the rope.

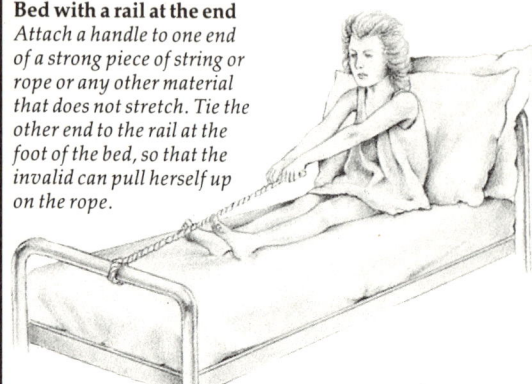

Bed without a rail
If the bed has no rail at the end, tie a strong piece of rope between the legs of the bed. Tie the piece of string with handle attached to the piece of rope between the legs of the bed.

Pull rope
A piece of sheeting or rope can be tied to the head of the bed to help the sick person pull herself up in bed.

A monkey pole
The sick person can reach up and grasp the monkey pole to pull herself up into a sitting position.

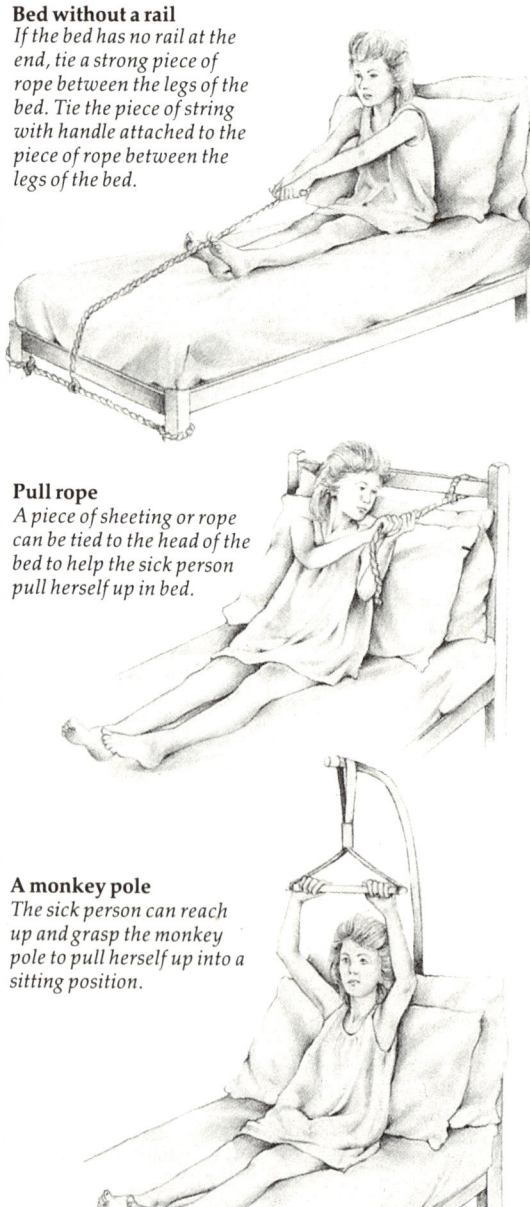

MOVING IN A CHAIR

The sick person may like to be left in privacy to read or write a letter while sitting in a chair, so it is a good idea if he or she can learn to move forward and backward in the chair without having to call for your help.

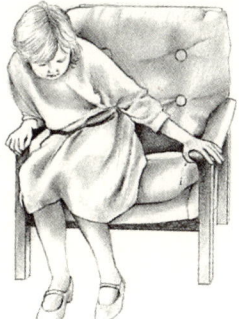

Using the chair-arms
The sick person pushes or pulls on the arms of the chair, lifting her buttocks as she does so and either moving them forward or backward.

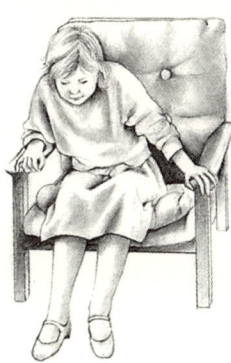

MOVING FROM A WHEELCHAIR TO A COMMODE

This method is equally effective for moving from a wheelchair to a toilet or from a bed to a chair or commode.

Using a plank
Place the wheelchair beside the commode. Place a substantial piece of wood securely between the two *seats. Remove one arm of the wheelchair and of the commode. Make sure the wheelchair brake is on. Tell the sick person to move across from one seat to the other using her arms. Make sure the piece of wood does not tip up when she sits on it.*

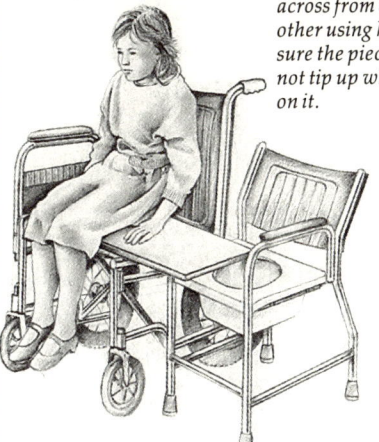

STANDING AND LEARNING TO WALK AGAIN

Encourage the sick person to do as much as possible and, as strength is regained, gradually reduce the amount of help you are giving. For instance, encourage him or her to walk to a chair, or toilet, with you gently supporting on one side only; or encourage use of a walking frame (see page 53).

When the sick person first begins to walk, he or she should start with very short distances, which should be gradually increased as strength is regained. It is important to agree on a realistic distance and then both work toward this goal. Making progress and achieving what he or she set out to do, no matter how small the step, will help boost the sick person's morale. It is also very rewarding for you to see the person you are caring for make some progress, however small. Constant encouragement and reassurance are necessary to give the sick person the confidence he or she needs to walk again.

Walking with a sick person
Stand close to the sick person. Place your arm between the sick person's body and forearm so that your hand is supporting her elbow and forearm. Ask her to grasp hold of the thumb and back of your other hand.

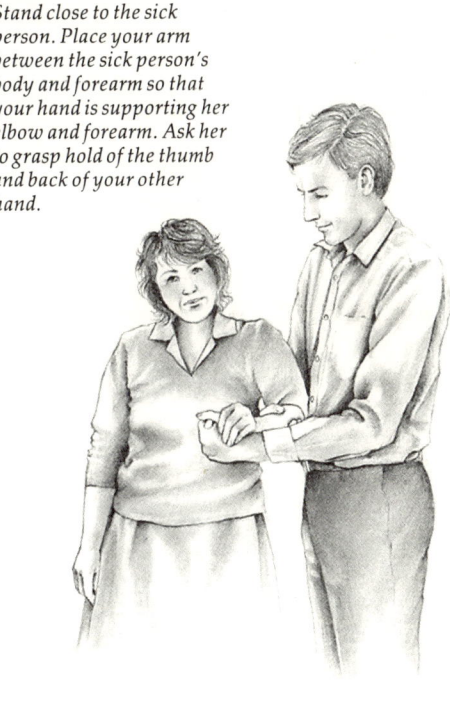

Hoists

There are a variety of hoists on the market and the type of hoist you need will depend on the size and disability of the sick person you are caring for, the size of the room in which the hoist is to be used and the capability of the people who are to operate it. If you think a hoist would be appropriate, ask your doctor or chemist for advice. The firms that make them also offer expert advice.

The caregiver and any helpers must be trained in the use of a hoist and should be absolutely confident in the handling of it before using it on a sick person. Hoists are extremely useful for lifting and moving a sick person who is heavy or disabled. However, some people are very frightened at the idea of being lifted up and moved from one place to another in a sling or on a seat. It is therefore important to act in as confident and reassuring a way as possible so as to gain the sick person's confidence.

Sling type (left)
Specially designed for use in the home, this hoist has to be operated by the caregiver and can be used to transport a severely disabled person from room to room or from bed to toilet.

The stairlift (far left)
This electrical hoist is ideal for use by the elderly and those with an illness or handicap which prevents them from climbing the stairs unaided. It is operated by the patient.

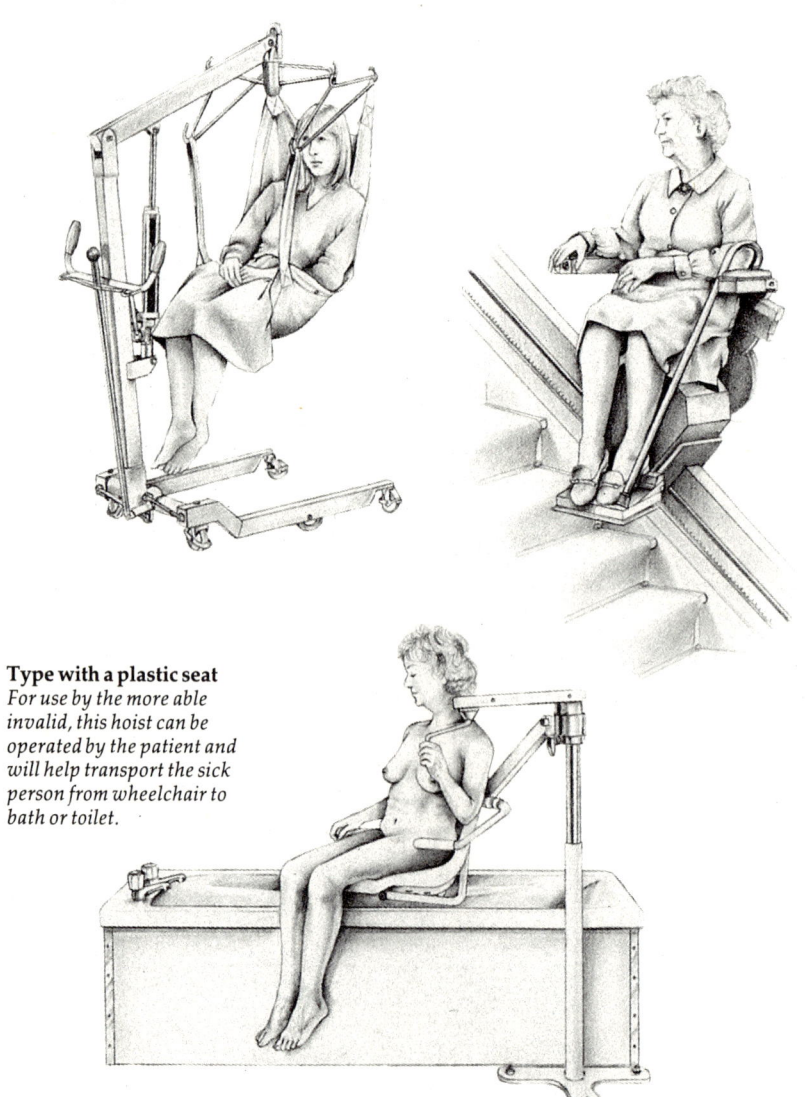

Type with a plastic seat
For use by the more able invalid, this hoist can be operated by the patient and will help transport the sick person from wheelchair to bath or toilet.

Walking frames

The frame should be chosen to suit the sick person's needs and must be the correct height and preferably height-adjustable. When standing upright inside the frame, the invalid should be able to straighten his or her arms while holding onto the hand grips. If the sick person cannot straighten his or her arms, the frame is too high; if he or she has to stoop, it is too low.

Walking with a standard adjustable walking frame
Before using the frame, the sick person must be given some tuition.

☐ The frame must be lifted clear of the floor.

☐ When the sick person lifts the frame you may have to support him or her at first until he or she is stronger and more practised.

☐ When lowering the frame to the floor, the sick person should straighten his or her arms and take the weight onto them.

☐ Leaning on the frame, the patient should bring one leg forward, straighten his or her back and then bring the other leg forward.

☐ Never allow an invalid to help him- or herself up to a standing position by pulling on a walking frame as it may topple toward the sick person and he or she will fall.

☐ If, for any reason, the sick person has difficulty lifting the frame clear of the floor, there are special frames available that have swivel joints and hinges or wheels fitted.

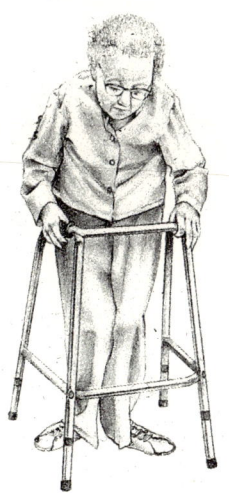 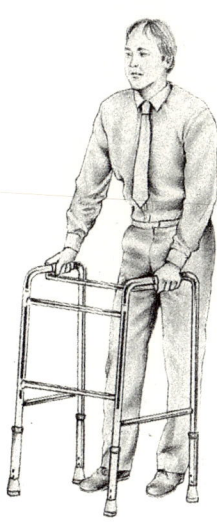 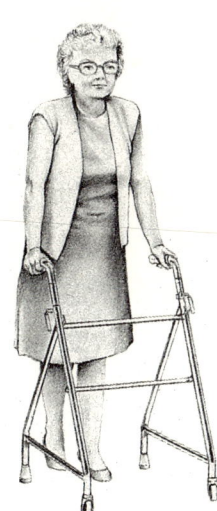

Standard walking frame – fixed height

Frame of adjustable height with swivel joints and hinges which move as the sick person walks

Frame with wheels

Day-to-day Care

Someone who is confined to bed will depend on your help for many everyday activities that we normally take for granted, such as washing, brushing teeth and going to the toilet. Some invalids need only minimal help – perhaps a steadying hand as they get into the bath – while others need virtually all their daily physical needs to be taken care of by someone else. A sick person also needs to be made comfortable: for someone who is mobile but confined to bed, this may be simply a matter of making sure that he or she has enough pillows and is neither too warm nor too cold. Someone who is unable to move about in bed, however, needs considerable help in keeping comfortable, including regular turning to prevent bedsores developing.

Maintaining a sick person's dignity

□ If you have a helper, the sick person may feel more at ease if you yourself deal with the more intimate procedures, such as washing or offering a bedpan. Your helper can speed up your work by collecting together equipment, clearing up and seeing that the sick person is comfortable.

□ You may find some procedures distasteful – giving a sick person a bedpan, for example. However, it is very important that you do not allow this distaste to show. After all, it is distressing enough for the sick person to feel dependent on you for help without feeling that you are embarrassed or disgusted.

□ Some people adopt a brisk or even joking manner when dealing with intimate procedures, which can be very irritating. Think how you would like to be treated if you were in the sick person's place – you would probably like your caregiver to be kind, helpful and gentle.

Comfort in bed

Discomfort may be caused by a wide range of factors, apart from illness itself. The invalid may be too cold or too warm, in a draught, or may need to go to the toilet; or the bed may need remaking. A firm mattress and sufficient back support are important: the chapter on **The Sickroom** gives advice on backrests and mattresses. Pillows can also be used to

Using pillows for support
If you have no backrest, you will need at least three pillows to give back support. You may also be able to buy a special triangular support pillow, which needs less adjustment.

Paying attention to the details of everyday care helps the sick person feel well cared for.

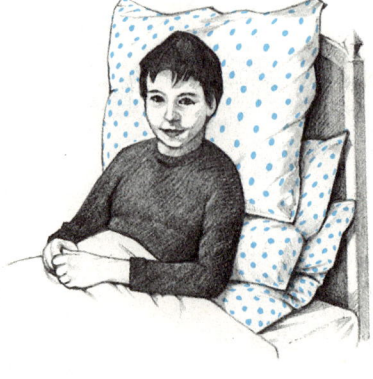
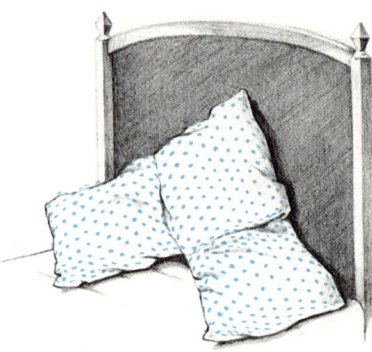

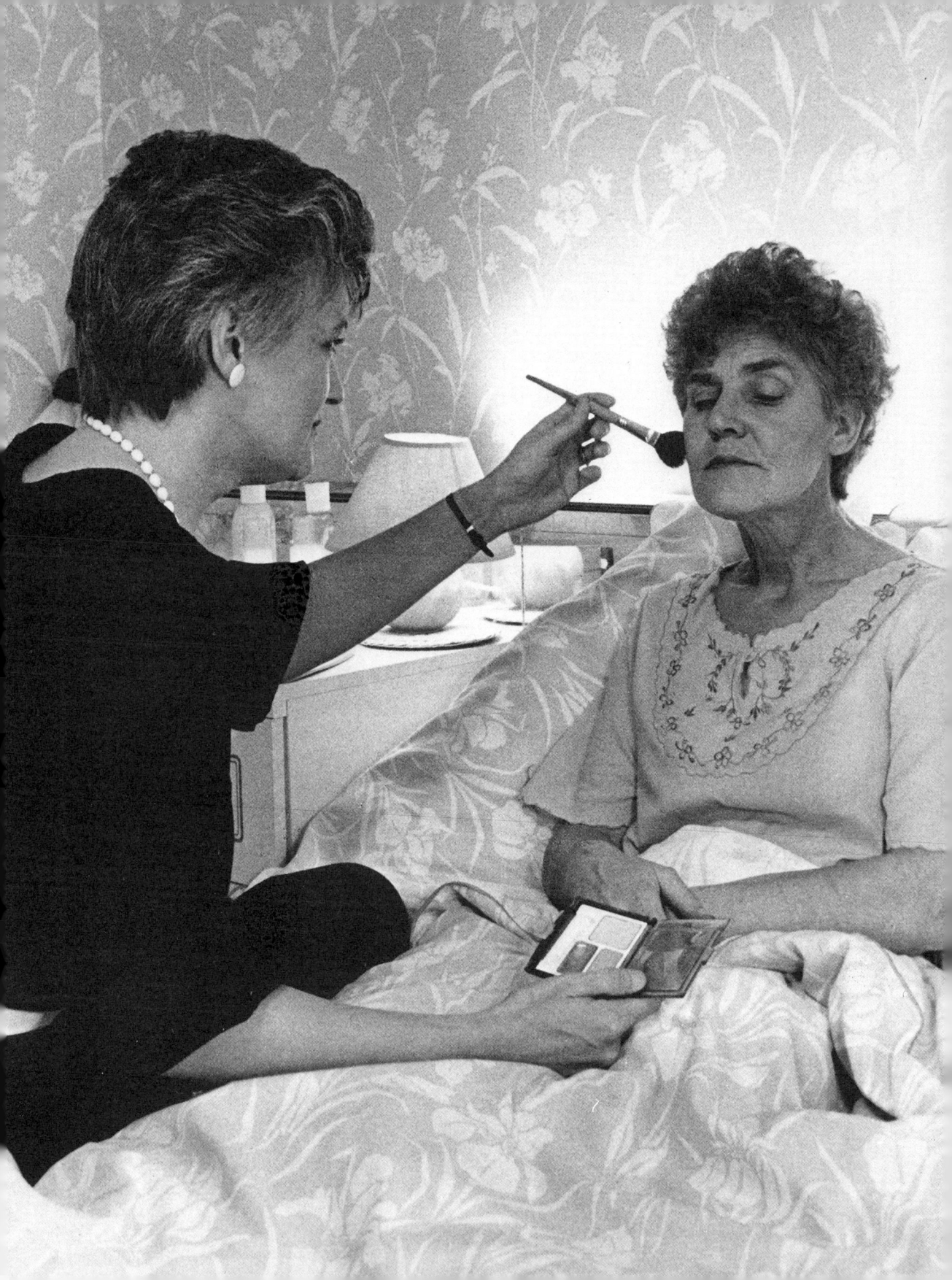

Using a footstool

A footstool is useful for supporting the sick person's legs when she is sitting out of bed in a chair. For comfort, the whole length of the leg should be supported. If you cannot buy a footstool, a coffee-table can be used to provide this full-length support. A pillow helps to make the footstool more comfortable.

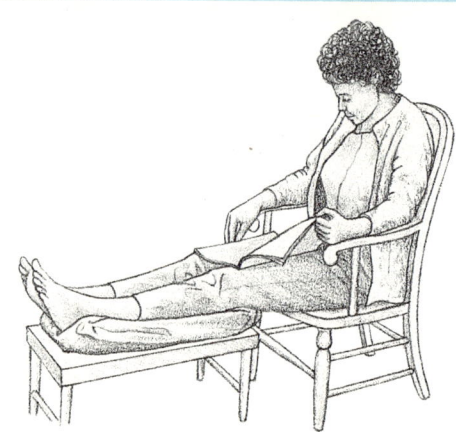

give effective back support, and their position can make a great difference to the sick person's comfort.

The sick person may be more comfortable sitting or even sleeping in an armchair, particularly if he or she is breathless. Make sure the patient is well supported with pillows and covered with blankets. A footstool is also important for comfort.

A hot-water bottle can be very comforting when you are ill in bed. The water in the bottle must not be more than 49°c (120°F) and the bottle must be completely safe: check that there are no leaks and that the rubber has not perished. If the bottle does not have a cover, wrap it in a towel. Do not give a hot-water bottle to a baby, as it may cause burns.

Bedcradles

A bedcradle is designed to keep the weight of the bedclothes off an invalid's feet and so enable legs to be moved about more freely. Lifting the bedclothes also helps to prevent foot drop: a condition caused by the weight of the bedclothes pushing the sick person's feet down, which can cause distortion of the feet and great difficulty in walking.

If you buy a bedcradle, slide one side under the mattress and drape the top sheet and covers over the top, tucking them in under the cradle.

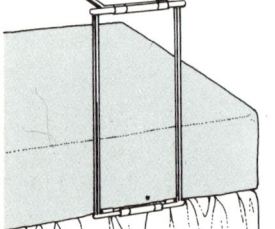

A manufactured bedcradle

IMPROVISING A BEDCRADLE

Using a low table
A low table that is shorter than the width of the bed can be used to hold up the bedclothes at the foot of the invalid's bed.

Using a cardboard box
Cut away one side of a large cardboard box and place it under the bedclothes, so that the invalid's feet are inside the box.

Foot supports
A block of wood at the foot of the bed also helps prevent foot drop.

Cleanliness

Ideally, a sick person confined to bed should be washed daily, unless the doctor advises against it. Cleanliness helps to keep a sick person's skin in good condition and a high standard of personal hygiene lessens the risk of infection entering the body. Washing also removes the waste products carried out of the body by sweating: some diseases may cause profuse sweating. Moreover, being washed daily, or more frequently if necessary, makes a sick person feel more comfortable and cared for.

Bathing may take the form of a bed bath, self-wash in bed, or an ordinary bath or shower. The sick person should also be given the opportunity to wash his or her hands and face at other times during the day. It is important that the patient is given a bowl of water, soap and towel after using a bedpan or going to the toilet.

Bed baths

A bed bath is given when someone is unable to get up and wash independently. The sick person may be very embarrassed at being bathed by you so try to give the appearance of being confident in what you are doing and avoid showing signs of embarrassment yourself.

☐ Offer a bedpan or urinal before you start washing (see page 68).

☐ Allow the sick person to carry out as much of the procedure as possible: this helps the patient to feel more independent.

☐ Make sure the sick person has privacy and is not exposed unnecessarily: this maintains his or her modesty, saves embarrassment and ensures warmth. Bed bathing needs to be done quickly and methodically so that the sick person does not get cold.

☐ The water must be changed if it becomes tepid or very soapy.

☐ Washing an area of the body is always followed by rinsing and thorough drying. Make sure that all the skin folds are clean and dry. Use talcum powder sparingly, if at all.

☐ Use a non-alcohol based hand or body lotion or cream to prevent skin dryness.

FILLING A HOT-WATER BOTTLE

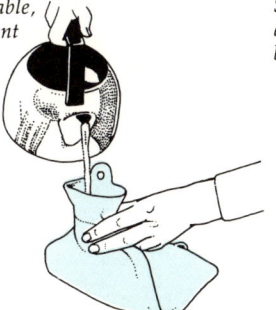
Sit the bottle on a table, with the top half bent up. Using hot (not boiling) water, fill the bottle, leaving some space at the top to allow the steam to escape.

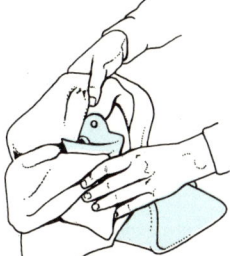
Screw in the stopper firmly and dry the mouth of the bottle.

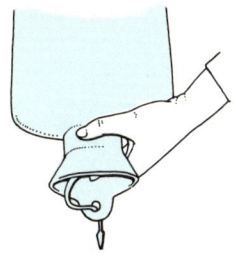
Turn the bottle upside down to check that there are no leaks.

GIVING A BED BATH

An invalid who cannot wash or get up needs to be bathed in bed.

▶ Read through the chapter on **Bedmaking,** especially the section on pages 30 to 31, before you begin.

Collect together
- A deep bowl for hand-hot water
- Soap
- A flannel for the face and one for the body
- A towel for the face and one for the body
- Shaving equipment, if required
- Make-up, if required
- Disposable wipes (special strong tissues: do not use pre-moistened ones) for genital care; or a special flannel, kept for this purpose only and washed frequently at a high temperature
- Plastic bag for soiled disposable wipes
- Nail brush
- Brush and comb
- Nail scissors or clippers
- Mouth-care equipment (see pages 65–67)
- Talcum powder and body lotion
- Clean linen
- Clean nightwear
- Two upright chairs
- Linen basket, or plastic bag for heavily soiled linen

Preparation

1 Explain the procedure and offer a bedpan or urinal.

2 Place the chairs back-to-back at the foot of the bed. Put the dirty linen basket nearby.

3 Make sure that the sick person has privacy and is not in a draught: close windows, doors and curtains, if necessary.

4 Get the sick person into the position that she finds most comfortable. For example, if she is breathless she should sit upright, well supported with pillows.

5 Fill the bowl three-quarters full with hand-hot water, about 40° to 44°c (105° to 110°F).

6 Strip the top bedclothes onto the chairs and leave the sick person covered with a sheet or blanket.

7 Undress her and cover her with the sheet or blanket again.

Washing

8 Spread the bath towel over her chest. Wash, rinse and dry her face, ears and neck with the face flannel (A). Wring out the flannel well and use the same sort of pressure you would use on yourself: there is nothing worse than a soaking wet flannel flopping about over your face and your body.

▶ Not everyone likes soap on his or her face, so ask before using it.

9 Wash, rinse and dry her hands and clean her fingernails, if she cannot do so herself.

10 Wash, rinse and dry each arm in turn, then her chest and abdomen, then each leg and

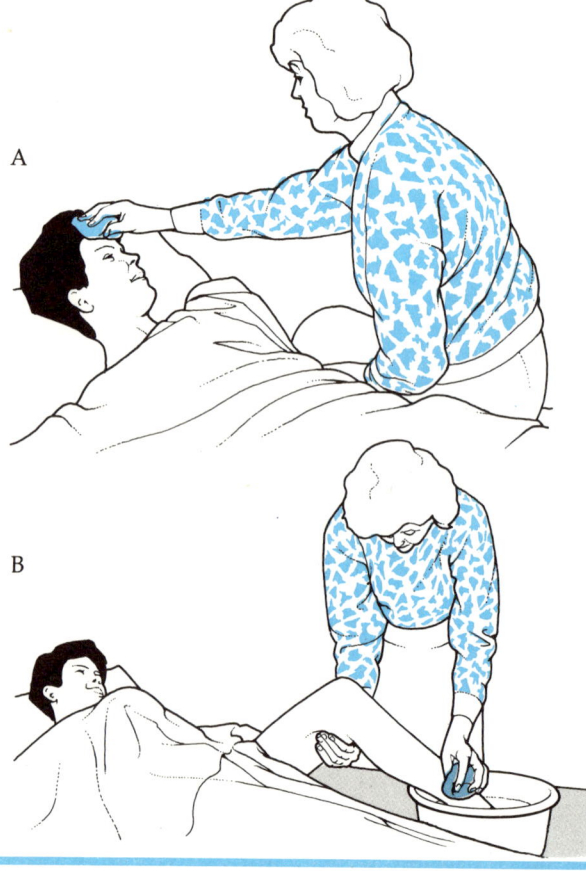

A

B

foot in turn (B). Uncover each area only as long as necessary. Place the large body towel under her limbs when washing and rinsing, then cover and dry thoroughly. Sprinkle on some talcum powder sparingly.

11 Fold the sheet or blanket up to waist level, leaving the chest and arms covered. Wash the genital area: use disposable wipes soaked in soap and water, discarding them into the plastic bag. Rinse and dry. Replace the sheet or blanket. The sick person will probably prefer to wash this area herself if she is able to.

12 Discard the water and refill. This prevents any infection in this area being taken to the next area to be washed.

13 Turn the sick person onto her side (see pages 36-37). If she is breathless she should sit upright and lean forward while you wash her back.

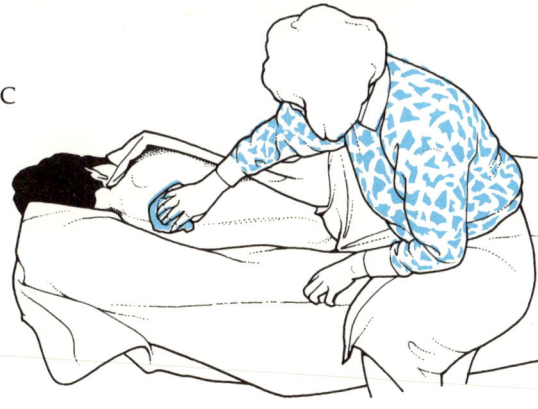

C

14 Place the large body towel under the sick person's back (if she has been incontinent, see page 72). Wash, rinse and dry her back (C).

15 Wash, rinse and dry her buttocks. Repeat for the anal region, using disposable wipes and discarding them into the plastic bag. Turn the sick person and wash the other side of her buttocks. If the sick person is breathless, prop her up on the pillows and gently turn her on her side to wash this area. She will probably prefer to wash herself if she can.

Bedmaking

16 While she is turned on her side, replace or tidy the bottom bed linen on one side of the bed. Turn her over and tidy the bottom bed linen on the other side. Remake the bed with clean linen, if necessary. If the sick person is able to get up, you can dress her and make the bed while she sits in a chair.

Grooming

17 Dress her or help her to dress herself.

18 If necessary, trim her fingernails over a disposable wipe and discard the wipe plus clippings into the plastic bag.

19 Toenails should be cut after soaking, when they are softer. Always cut straight across the top of the toenail and never poke the scissors into the corners. If the nails are too hard or thick for you to cut, or if the sick person is a diabetic, she should be seen by a chiropodist.

20 Wash your hands. Brush the invalid's teeth (see page 65). Brush or comb hair. Help the sick person put on her make-up if she feels like it (D). Help a man to shave.

Finally

Clear away and clean all equipment; wash your hands; replace the furniture and re-open any windows that you closed; and make sure the sick person is comfortable.

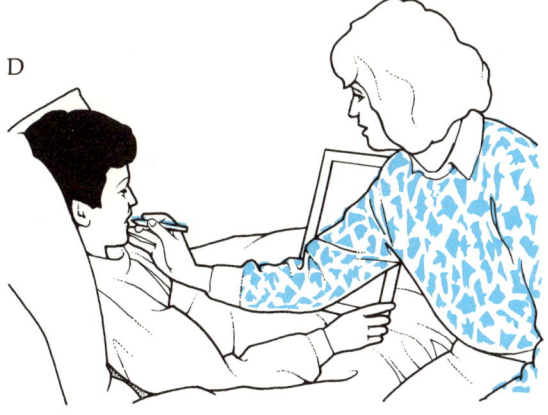

D

SELF-WASH IN BED

If the sick person is unable to get out of bed but is capable of washing him- or herself, the following procedure may be used.
▶ Read through the chapter on **Bedmaking**, especially the section on pages 30 to 31, before you begin.

Collect together
- A bedtable
- Washing equipment as on page 58

Preparation

1 Explain the procedure and offer a bedpan or urinal.

2 Collect all the washing equipment together. Place the dirty linen basket at the foot of the bed, together with the two chairs, back-to-back.

3 Make sure the sick person has privacy and is not in a draught.

4 Fill the bowl three-quarters full with hand-hot water, about 40° to 44°C (105° to 110°F).

5 Strip off the top bedclothes onto the chairs at the end of the bed, and leave the sick person covered by a sheet or blanket.

6 Undress him, if he needs help, and make sure he is covered with the sheet or blanket.

7 Put the bedtable across the bed, with all the washing equipment on it.

Washing

8 Leave everything within reach. Allow the sick person to wash in private. Ask him to wash his genitals last and to call you when he is ready to wash his back.

9 Change the water and move the washing bowl onto the bedside table. Move the bedtable away from the bed.

10 Ask him to turn onto his side. If he is breathless, wash his back while he sits upright and leans forward. Place the body towel under his back. Wash, rinse and dry his back. Repeat for the buttocks.

11 Turn him and wash the other side of his buttocks. Wash the anal region, using disposable wipes soaked in soap and water. Rinse and dry. If the sick person can manage to wash his own anal region, hand him the disposable wipes and put the plastic bag within his reach.

Bedmaking

12 While the sick person is turned on his side, replace and tidy the bottom linen on one side. Turn him over and tidy the bottom bed linen on the other side. Remake the bed with clean linen, if necessary.

13 Help the sick person dress, if necessary, and wash your hands.

Grooming

14 Replace the bedtable and place on it all the equipment required for mouth care (see pages 66-67). Put his brush and comb on the bedtable; help him with his hair if necessary. Put shaving equipment (or, for a woman, make-up) within reach, if required (see page 65).

Finally

Clear away and clean all equipment; wash your hands; replace the furniture and re-open any windows that you closed and make sure the sick person is comfortable.

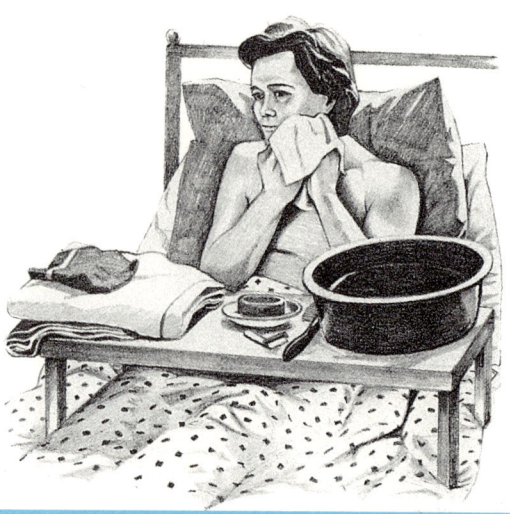

SELF-WASH SITTING IN A CHAIR

If the sick person is able to get out of bed and to stand with minimum support, but is unable to walk to the bathroom, or if you do not have a bath, the following procedure may be useful.
▶ Read through the chapter on **Bedmaking**, especially the section on pages 22 to 27, before you begin.

Collect together
- A low table
- Washing equipment as on page 58

Preparation

1 Explain the procedure and offer a bedpan, urinal, commode or sanichair, or help the sick person to the toilet.

2 Collect all the washing equipment together. Place the two chairs back-to-back at the end of the bed, together with the dirty linen basket.

3 Close the windows and ensure privacy. Make the sick person comfortable in a chair.

4 Fill the bowl three-quarters full with hand-hot water, about 40° to 44°c (105° to 110°F).

5 Put the washing equipment on a low table beside the sick person and put the clean nightwear within reach.

6 Help her undress to the waist, if she is not able to do so herself.

Washing

7 Leave the sick person to wash the top half of her body.

8 Wash her back while she is sitting in the chair. Wash, rinse and dry thoroughly.

9 Put on the top half of her nightwear and remove her pyjama trousers or tuck up her nightdress.

10 Leave her to wash her legs and then her genital area. Ask her to use the disposable wipes for her genital areas and to discard them into the plastic bag.

11 Change the water.

12 Wash her buttocks, if necessary supporting her in a standing position.

13 Hand her a wipe soaked in soap and water so that she can wash her own anal region. Then she can rinse and dry with disposable wipes which should be discarded into a plastic bag. She may need help with this.

Grooming

14 Clear away the washing things.

15 Place the equipment for oral hygiene (see pages 66-67) on the table so she can manage herself. For a man, place the equipment for facial shaving (see page 65) on the table. Offer to bring a woman her make-up. Place a brush and comb on the table. She may need help with her hair.

Bedmaking

16 Strip and remake the bed.

Finally

Clear away and clean all equipment; wash your hands; open any windows that you closed and replace the furniture; and make sure the sick person is comfortable.

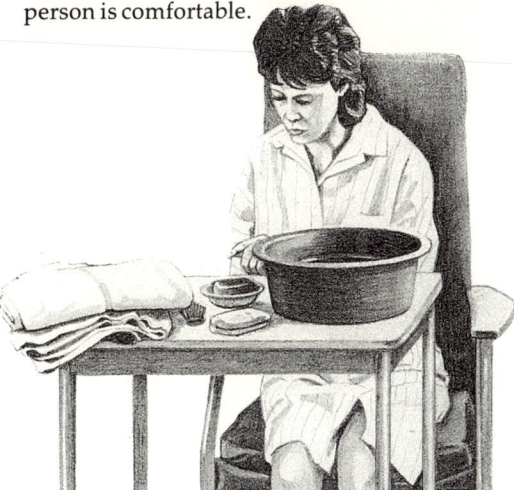

Bathing in the bathroom

Even if the sick person needs help with taking a bath, it is much easier for both of you if he or she can use the bathroom as usual. The patient may be worried about having a bath, particularly if he or she has recently undergone surgery and has a wound, but with a sympathetic and understanding approach you can allay any fears. The sick person will feel refreshed and much better after a bath.

An elderly person may not have had a bath for years for fear of slipping or of being unable to get out. He or she may prefer to wash at the sink and, if so, you should respect this choice.

☐ Close all the windows to prevent the sick person becoming chilled. Make sure that the bathroom is warm.

☐ Check that the bath is clean.

☐ Always run the cold water into the bath first. This prevents the bottom of the bath becoming hot enough to burn. It also reduces the amount of steam in the bathroom.

☐ Test the temperature of the water with your elbow: for an adult, it should feel comfortably hot, about 44° to 49°c (112° to 120°f); for a child, it should feel warm, about 38°c (100°f).

☐ Make sure that the hot tap cannot burn the sick person: wrap a flannel round the tap if necessary.

☐ Ask the sick person if he or she needs to use the toilet before getting into the bath.

☐ Help the invalid wash his or her face at the basin or with a flannel dipped in the bathwater before the bath begins.

☐ The sick person may need help undressing, washing his or her back, drying and dressing.

☐ If you are using a shower, a wooden or plastic chair placed under the shower may be useful.

☐ Leave the invalid alone if he or she is well enough: this will ensure privacy and helps the sick person feel more independent. Stay within earshot, so that if he or she does feel unwell or faint you can help. Do not let the sick person lock the door.

☐ After the bath, offer to help brush the person's hair, clean and trim his or her fingernails and toenails and brush his or her teeth.

☐ Finally, clean the bath or shower, bathmat and chair, if used. Clear away and clean all other equipment and wash your hands.

Help getting in and out of the bath

There are many aids, both manufactured and improvised, that you can use to help someone into the bath. A low stool may be used in the bath, to make the transition from standing to sitting and back again easier. A stool may also be helpful outside the bath, to act as a step. A non-slip bathmat is essential, especially if you are using a stool in the bath. Rails fitted to the wall may be useful. A plank across the bath can be used as a

Aids for the bath
There is a wide range of equipment that you can buy to help a sick person into and out of a bath.

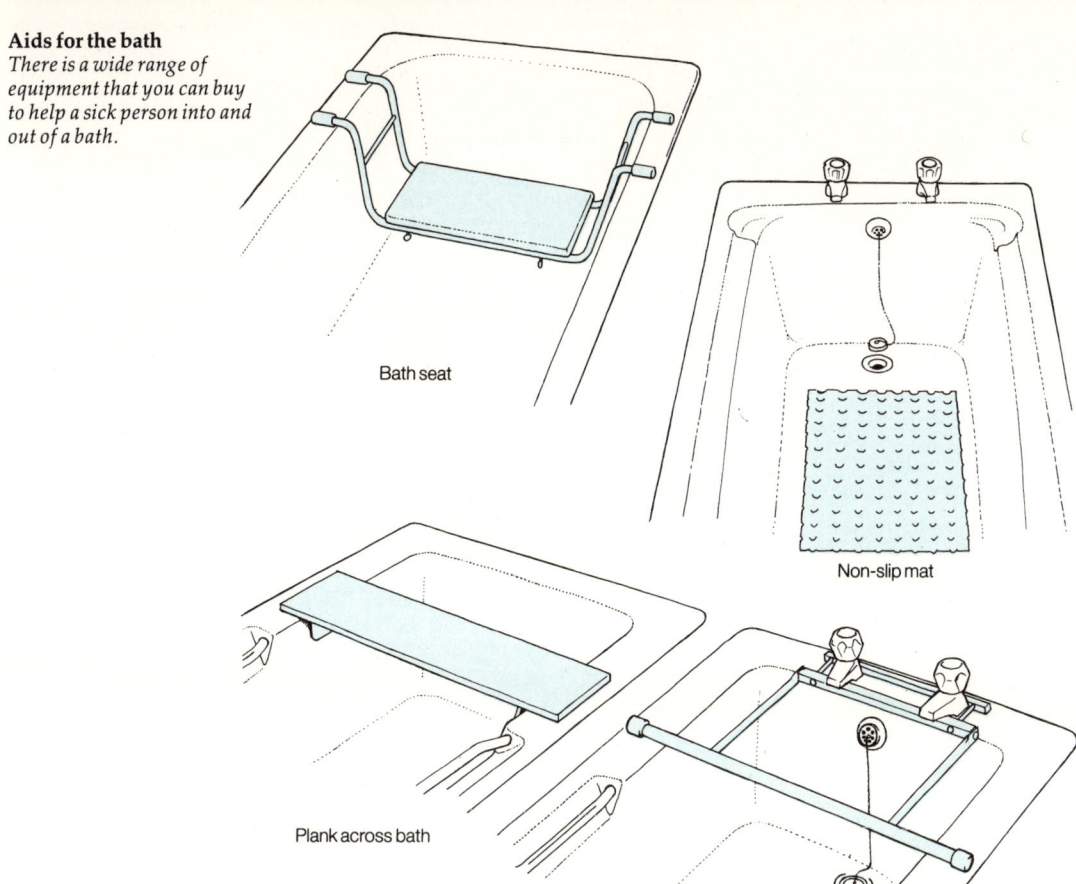

Bath seat

Non-slip mat

Plank across bath

Bath rail

seat, from which the sick person can swing his or her legs over the side of the bath.

If you are worried about getting someone into or out of the bath, consult your doctor.

Hair-washing

It is very helpful for a sick person's morale and well-being for his or her hair to be clean and attractive. There is nothing worse than lying in bed with hair that feels greasy and uncomfortable, knowing that you are not well enough, or able, to get up and wash it yourself. Hair should be shampooed as soon as, and preferably before, it becomes dirty or greasy. If the sick person is well enough, you may be able to wash his or her hair at the sink, basin or under the shower. If, however, the person is not well enough to get out of bed, but is well enough to have his or her hair washed (check this with the doctor), you can do so while he or she lies in bed. A dry shampoo, in either powder or spray form, can also be used as a short-term measure.

WASHING HAIR IN BED

Collect together
- A low chair or stool
- Two jugs of warm water, about 44°c (112°F)
- Shampoo
- Bucket for dirty water
- Small plastic sheet
- Large plastic sheet
- Pillow in a plastic case or wrapped in plastic
- Flannel
- Face towel
- Two bath towels
- Safety pin
- Hairdryer

Preparation

1 Close the windows.

2 Place the chair or stool at the bedside near the head of the bed. Cover the chair or stool with the small plastic sheet and put the bucket on the sheet.

3 Make the sick person comfortable with his head close to the edge of the bed. Support his shoulders on the plastic-covered pillow to ensure that his head is lower than his shoulders.

4 Wrap one bath towel around the patient's neck and pin it in position with the safety pin.

5 Roll three sides of the large plastic sheet to form sides against which the water will flow down into the bucket. Put the sheet under the sick person's head so his head is surrounded by the rolls and drop the end of the sheet into the bucket.

Washing

6 Give the sick person the flannel to put over his eyes and pour water over his head until the hair is wet all over. If he is nervous, pour a small amount of water over his head until he gets used to it, and pour gently to prevent splashing.

7 Apply the shampoo and gently massage it into the scalp. Do not hurry this: it is a very pleasant sensation for the sick person.

8 Rinse the hair.

9 If necessary, refill the water jugs and repeat shampoo, massage and rinsing until the hair is clean.

10 Squeeze the excess water out of the hair.

11 Dry the sick person's forehead with the face towel and wrap it around his head to absorb the wetness.

12 Lift his head, remove the rolled plastic and put it in the bucket.

13 Remove the pillow under his shoulders and place it under his head.

14 Remove the face towel and replace with a dry, clean bath towel. Gently rub the hair partially dry and leave the towel wrapped around the person's head.

Finally

Change any clothes or bedclothes that are wet or damp. Make sure the sick person is comfortable. Clear away and clean the washing equipment. Complete drying with a hairdryer.

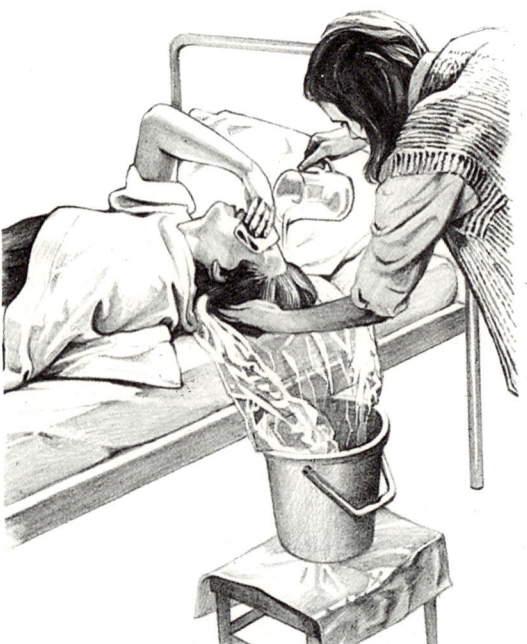

FACIAL SHAVING

You may have to shave a sick person if he is very ill or too weak to manage it alone. It is much easier to use an electric razor than a wet razor, if you have the choice.

Collect together
- A razor
- Shaving cream
- Two towels
- Paper towels
- Aftershave
- A bowl of hot water

1 Have a good light on the sick person's face. Sit him upright if his condition permits.

2 Spread a towel under his chin. Dip another towel in hot water, wring it out and place it over the patient's lower face and chin for a few minutes. This helps to soften the stubble.

3 Put some shaving cream on the palms of your hands and rub it over his face.

4 Stretch the skin tight to prevent you cutting it and shave downward in a long smooth movement.

5 Clean the razor on a paper towel, dip it in warm water and continue until the area is shaved.

6 Pat the sick person's face dry with the towel which was around his neck. Put on some aftershave, again using the palms of your hands.

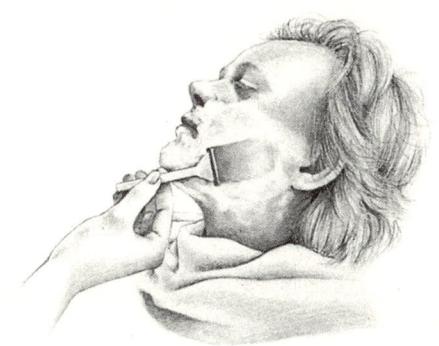

Care of the mouth and teeth

Keeping a sick person's mouth clean, moist and free from infection enables him or her to enjoy food and also prevents dental problems. The mouth may become dry because of illness, especially when the sick person has a high temperature, because of vomiting or other digestive upsets or simply because the invalid has not been taking adequate amounts of fluid. Encourage the sick person to:
- Eat a well-balanced diet (see the chapter on **Diet and Nutrition**)
- Drink plenty of fluids, unless these are restricted by the doctor
- Eat citrus fruits, unless this is against medical advice, as these stimulate the production of saliva which naturally cleans the mouth
- Breathe through the nose: mouth breathing leaves a dry mouth
- Clean his or her teeth and see the dentist regularly
- Have well-fitting dentures
- Avoid sweets, biscuits or other sugary foods. If the patient's mouth is dry, and he or she is on a diet with restricted fluids, sugar-free chewing gum may encourage the natural flow of saliva and help to keep the mouth moist

Signs of trouble

If the sick person's mouth is dry or in need of special care, he or she may have one or more of the following symptoms. With regular mouth care, all these problems can be avoided:
- Dry cracked lips
- A diminished appetite

○ A dry furred tongue and an unpleasant taste in the mouth
○ A bad smell from the mouth (halitosis)
○ Pieces of food stuck on the lips, tongue or teeth
○ A hoarse-sounding voice
○ Sores inside the cheeks and gums

Brushing teeth in bed

If the sick person is unable to get out of bed, but can brush his or her own teeth, you can help by bringing the equipment he or she needs to the bed. Apart from the toothbrush and toothpaste, the invalid will need a glass of water, a small bowl or dish to spit into, a towel and tissues to wipe the mouth. Put the equipment on the bedtable or bedside table and wrap the towel around the sick person's shoulders. You can help by squeezing the toothpaste onto the brush, and by holding the bowl while the sick person rinses his or her mouth. Afterwards, clear away and clean all the equipment.

CARE OF DENTURES

Encourage the sick person to wear dentures if he or she has them. They will improve the patient's ability to chew food, and will also improve speech and facial appearance.

Collect together
• Toothbrush
• Solution of dentifrice for dentures in a bowl
• A cup or bowl of water
• Tissues or disposable wipes
• Towel
• Plastic bag for soiled tissues or wipes
• Mouthwash in a cup
• Bowl or dish to spit into

1 Remove the dentures if the sick person cannot do so. To remove a full denture, hold it with a disposable wipe or tissue and tilt it away from the gum. To remove a partial denture, lift the metal-clamp with a tissue wrapped around your fingertip.

2 Soak the dentures in dentifrice solution in a small bowl.

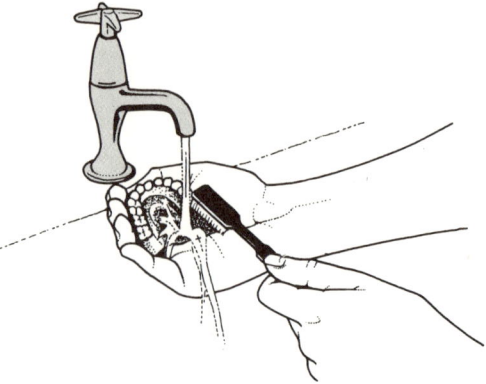

3 Take the dentures to the bathroom or wash-basin and brush each denture under running water, holding it in the palm of your hand.

4 Put the dentures in a cup or small bowl of clean water.

5 Take them back to the sick person.

6 Place a towel across her shoulders and help her to use a mouthwash.

7 Clean any of the patient's own teeth or ask her to do so if she can manage by herself.

8 Rinse the sick person's mouth well, wipe the gums with tissues and replace the dentures.

MOUTH CARE FOR SOMEONE WHO IS HELPLESS

Collect together
- Mouthwash in a small bowl
- Solution of sodium bicarbonate in a bowl
- Vaseline
- Denture container
- Toothbrush
- Toothpaste
- Metal teaspoon
- Towel
- Plastic bag
- Plastic disposable gloves, if you would prefer to use them
- Gauze swab or disposable wipes
- Tissues

Preparation

1 Wash your hands and put the equipment on the bedside table.

2 Explain the procedure to the sick person.

3 Wrap the towel under the patient's chin and round her shoulders to protect her clothing.

Cleaning

4 Put on the plastic disposable gloves, if used.

5 If the sick person wears dentures remove them and put them in the container.

6 Wrap a piece of gauze or a disposable wipe around the handle of a metal teaspoon and hold onto it with your index finger and thumb. Soak it in the sodium bicarbonate solution.

7 Gently clean the sick person's tongue from the back to the tip, using a new piece of gauze or wipe for each stroke.
▶ Take care to keep the spoon handle covered or you will damage the mouth.

8 Continue in this way until the tongue, the inside of the cheeks and mouth, and the gums have been cleaned.

9 Repeat the whole process using mouthwash solution, or the sick person may simply gargle with the mouthwash instead.

10 Clean any teeth.

11 Clean and rinse the dentures and replace them in her mouth.

12 Wipe and dry the sick person's lips and chin with tissues.

13 Cover the lips with a little vaseline to stop them becoming cracked and dry.

Finally

Clear away and clean all equipment; make the sick person comfortable; and wash your hands.

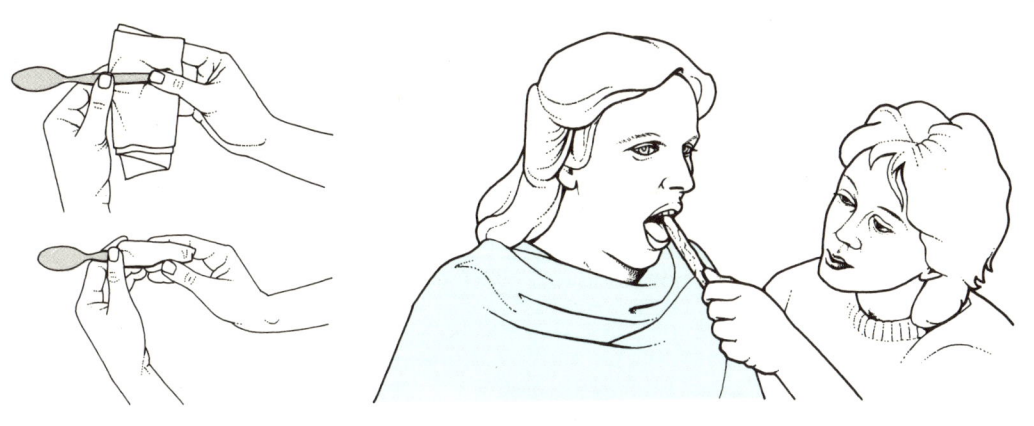

Care of the nose

Noses need very little attention in adults. If the nose becomes dry, it may later become sore so apply a little oily cream with a disposable wipe or gauze swab. Children's noses may need cleaning with damp wicks of cotton-wool.

Care of the eyes

Any discharge from the eyes should be mopped away with a damp wipe or cotton-wool ball, dipped in boiled, cooled water. Always wipe from the inner aspect of the eye (next to the nose) outward and use a fresh ball of cotton-wool for each stroke.

Elimination

Passing urine or faeces are two basic functions of the body. If the sick person is unable to get out of bed, or is not allowed out of bed by the doctor, this may cause a great deal of worry and stress.

For someone confined to bed, a bedpan and urinal can be used. Bedpans are made in metal or plastic. A woman may use a bedpan for passing both urine and faeces, while a man uses a bedpan for passing faeces and passes urine into a urinal, made of glass or plastic.

When you are asked to bring a bedpan or urinal, act promptly. Ensure privacy by closing the bedroom door and drawing the curtains, if necessary. Warm the bedpan or urinal by running the seat or spout under warm water; dry well.

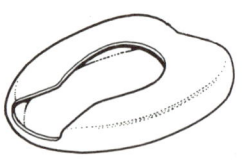

Bedpan

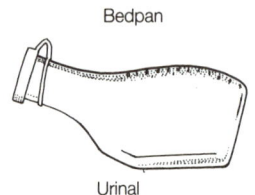

Urinal

Giving a bedpan

☐ Dust a little talcum powder onto the seat of the bedpan to stop the sick person sticking to it.

☐ You will need newspaper to place the used bedpan on and a disposable cover, such as a piece of paper or kitchen roll, for the bedpan after use. You will also need toilet tissue and a bell.

☐ It is most comfortable to sit up on a bedpan, supported by pillows.

☐ It is very important to lift the sick person clear when inserting or removing the bedpan, or you may damage the skin over the lower part of the back and buttocks.

☐ Unless the sick person is helpless, put the toilet paper and bell within reach and leave the room until he or she rings for you. Stay with a confused or helpless patient and wipe him or her clean, having removed the pan and rolled the sick person onto his or her side.

☐ Remove the bedpan in the same way as you put it in position, put it on a chair on some newspaper and cover it with a disposable cover.

☐ As you help the sick person off the bedpan, hold the pan by its side and not by the front or the back: this makes it less likely that your hands will be contaminated by the contents.

☐ You may find that the task of emptying a bedpan which has been used for a bowel movement rather unpleasant. The smell can be greatly reduced by leaving a stick air-freshener in the room, which makes the task more pleasant for you and less embarrassing for the sick person.

☐ Finally make the invalid comfortable.

Helping someone onto a bedpan
If the person is unable to sit up, ask her to lie on her back, bend her knees and press down against the mattress with the soles of her feet. Help lift her hips by putting one hand under the base of her spine, while you slide the pan into place with the other hand.

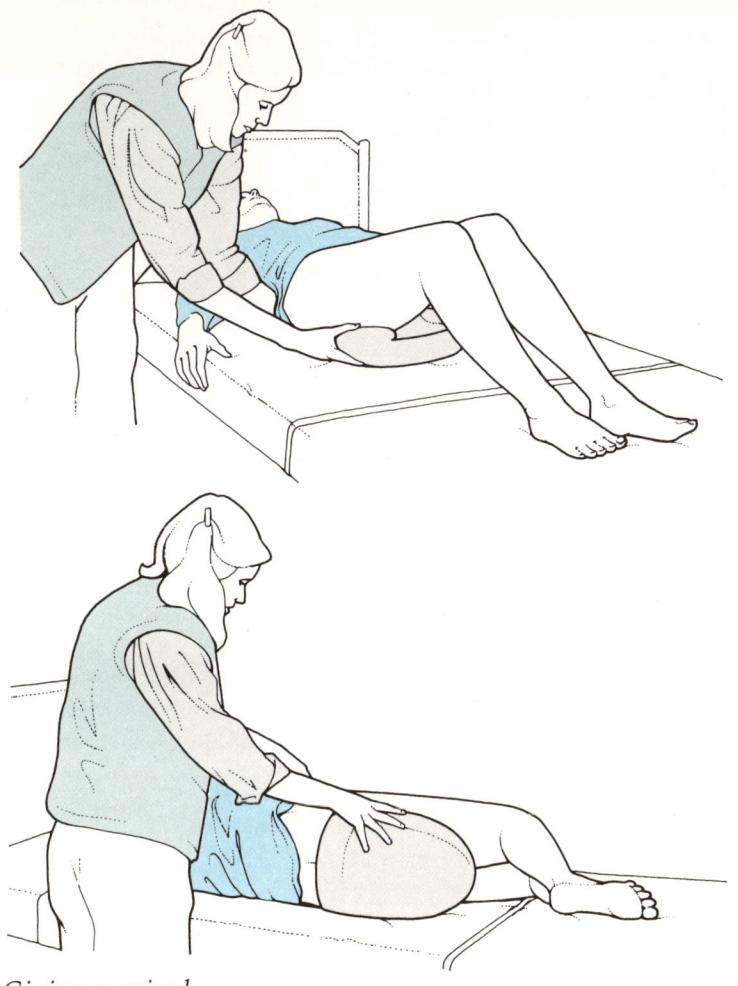

If the person is helpless, roll her onto her side and hold the bedpan against her buttocks; roll her onto her back so that the pan is in place. Make sure she is comfortable.

Giving a urinal

☐ Hold the urinal by the bottom so that the sick person can hold the bottle by the neck.

☐ Place the bottle between his legs making sure that it will not tip up and spill.

☐ When he has finished, cover the urinal with disposable paper and remove.

Cleaning a bedpan or urinal

☐ Empty the bedpan or urinal, unless the invalid's urine output is being measured or saved (see pages 92-94).

☐ Clean with a long-handled brush and soap and water. The brush should be soaked in a disinfectant solution after use, rinsed and dried.

☐ Rinse with cold water and dry thoroughly.

☐ Wash your hands and give the sick person a bowl of water, soap and towel to do the same.

Commodes or sanichairs

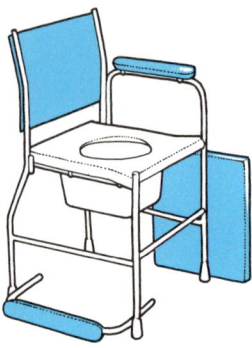

Commode

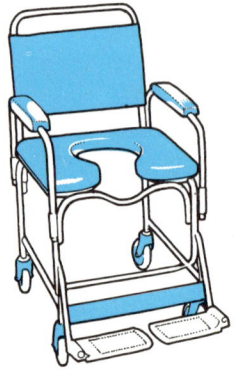

Sanichair

If possible, the sick person will probably prefer to get out of bed and use a commode – a chair fitted with a removable bedpan. A sanichair is another alternative: this is a chair that can be wheeled to the lavatory and used over the pan, or used at the bedside with a bedpan that slots in under the seat. Both a commode and a sanichair allow the sick person to be in a more natural position for defaecating.

Using a commode or sanichair

☐ Place the commode or sanichair beside the bed and remove the seat cover.

☐ Collect some toilet tissue and a bell, and put them within reach.

☐ Help the patient move from the bed to the chair (see pages 42-43).

☐ Leave the person in privacy if his or her condition permits. If necessary, wipe the person clean.

☐ Help the sick person back to bed, then remove the container or bedpan. Empty and clean.

Difficulty in passing urine or faeces

The sick person may be inhibited by worry that someone will walk into the toilet or the bedroom. However, it is not a good idea to lock the door: if he or she feels unwell or faints you will not be able to help. So make a cardboard sign saying 'engaged' or 'do not enter', which you can hang on the door to ensure privacy.

Worry about soiling the sheets may be a problem when using a bedpan. Use a commode or sanichair, or place a drawsheet or incontinence pad under the bedpan.

A man using a urinal may find it impossible to pass urine lying in bed so, if his condition permits, let him sit with his legs over the side of the bed with his feet resting on a stool. Or, again if his condition permits, he may be able to stand by his bed while he passes urine. Stay with him if he is unsteady on his feet. One way to stimulate the passing of urine is to turn on a nearby water tap or to pour water from one glass to another.

Sitting on a bedpan to pass faeces is particularly difficult as the normal position is sitting or squatting. So using a commode or sanichair, if the sick person's condition permits, is much easier.

Improvising bedpans, commodes and urinals

If you cannot buy, borrow or rent any of these items, you can improvise; improvisation can also be useful while you wait for equipment to arrive. Do make sure that improvised items are strong enough to take the invalid's weight and that the contents will not spill out when you are carrying them away for disposal. The equipment must also be comfortable for the invalid to use.

An improvised urinal

Any large glass jar can be used providing it will hold 1½ litres (2.7 pt) of fluid. An improvised urinal must be thrown away when the sick person has no further use for it.

MAKING A BEDPAN

Use a strong washing-up bowl about 28 cm by 28 cm (11 in by 11 in) and about 10 cm (4 in) deep. Insert this into a strong cardboard box of about the same size, and cut out a hole in the middle of the box. Make sure that you can remove the bedpan from the box without spilling the contents. Replace the box as soon as it becomes soiled, and throw it away when it is no longer needed.

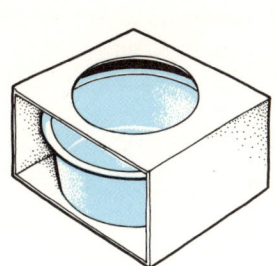

MAKING A COMMODE

Cut a hole, about 25 to 30 cm (10 to 12 in) in diameter, in the seat of a straight-backed wooden chair. Smooth the cut edges with sandpaper. If you like, you can pad the seat around the hole with material and cover with plastic or polythene to enable you to keep the seat clean with a disinfectant solution. Place a bucket directly under the hole. To make the commode look more like a chair, tack some material around the bottom of the chair.

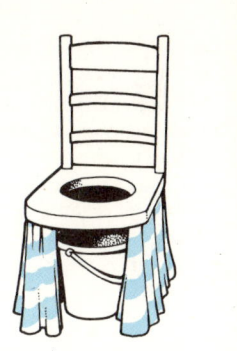

Incontinence

Someone who is conscious and aware of being incontinent, and is unable to prevent this, feels humiliated and anxious. Incontinence may be permanent due to injury, disease, infection or ageing. On the other hand, it may be a temporary condition following a fit, or due to fear or forgetfulness. The patient may be unable to control his or her bladder or bowels, or both. A sick person will need to know that he or she is loved and accepted despite this problem and will be helped to regain control over his or her bladder or bowels.

The bed and linen

The bed should have a firm mattress and be at the right height for the caregiver (see page 18). Protect the bed with some plastic sheeting and cover the sheeting with a drawsheet (see page 27). Change the bed linen as often as necessary to keep the bed dry and clean.

Incontinence pads, placed under the sick person's buttocks, reduce the amount of washing to be done. An incontinence pad consists of several layers of absorbent disposable material, with a moisture-proof backing. This plastic backing should never be put next to the sick person, as it makes the skin sweat and creates soreness. The pads must be changed as soon as they become wet or soiled.

A substitute can be made at home from layers of newspaper or padding covered with a piece of material, put on top of a piece of plastic sheeting; the whole bundle is then put inside a pillowcase. After use, dispose of the newspaper or padding and wash the plastic and the pillowcase. There are other incontinence aids, including plastic-backed, absorbent pants: your local chemist can advise you on what is available.

If you are looking after an incontinent person, ask him or her to wear tops only rather than long nightdresses or pyjama trousers, to save washing. Buy plenty of large plastic bags for soiled disposable materials. A deodorant stick or wick makes the room smell pleasanter and the sick person will feel less embarrassed. Offer a commode, bedpan or urinal every couple of hours and you may prevent soiling of the bed. If the sick person soils the bed in between, make a note of how often and when he or she requires toileting and offer it at those times.

CHANGING AN INCONTINENCE PAD AND DRAWSHEET

Collect together
- A clean drawsheet
- Clean incontinence pad
- Disposable plastic gloves
- Bowl of hand-hot water
- Soap
- Paper towelling, tissues or wipes
- Barrier cream, if prescribed
- Large plastic bag
- Basket for dirty linen
- A chair

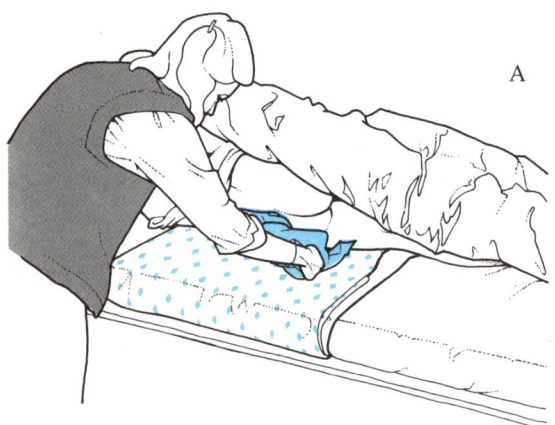

A

Preparation

1 Explain to the sick person what you are going to do.

2 Close the windows and ensure privacy.

3 Place the clean drawsheet and incontinence pad on a chair at the foot of the bed.

4 Place the large plastic bag and dirty linen basket at the bedside.

5 Fill the bowl with hand-hot water and put it on the bedside table along with the tissues or wipes, gloves and barrier cream (if used).

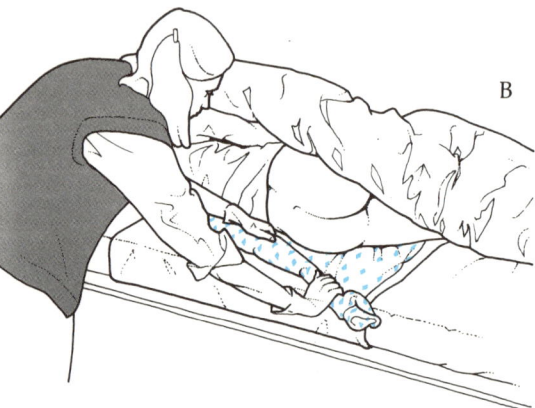

B

6 If the sick person is sitting upright, remove the backrest and some of the pillows, leaving her comfortable. If the patient is breathless, leave her sitting upright.

7 Fold the bedclothes to one side.

8 Put on your disposable gloves.

9 Turn the person onto one side (see page 36). Check that she is still covered by the bedclothes on one side, and is not in danger of falling out of bed.

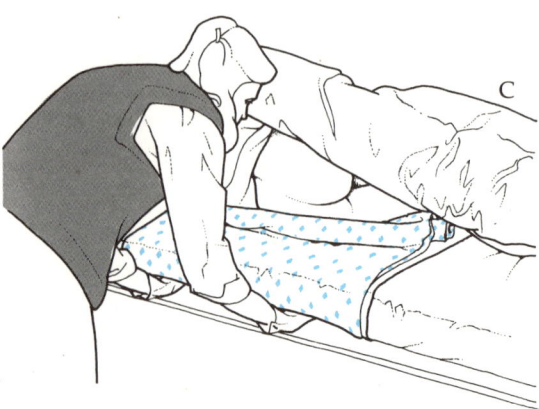

C

Cleaning up

10 Fold the incontinence pad over the contents and remove (A). Discard into a large plastic bag.

11 Untuck the soiled drawsheet and roll it up toward the sick person (B).

12 Clean the soiled area with disposable tissues or wipes soaked in soap and hand-hot water. Rinse and dry thoroughly. Clean gently from the front toward the anus. Do not rub. Rinse and pat dry, using each wipe only once.

13 Apply a barrier cream, if necessary. These waterproof creams are used to prevent the skin breaking down.

Remaking the bed

14 Straighten the bottom sheet and plastic sheeting. Pull the sheet tight, making sure that there are no wrinkles. This helps to prevent pressure sores (see page 78).

15 Taking the clean drawsheet, lay it on top of the plastic sheeting. Roll one half up against the sick person's back and tuck the other end in under the mattress (C).

16 Roll up one half of the clean incontinence pad and place the roll up against the sick person's buttocks, on top of the rolled-up drawsheet. Lay the rest of the pad over the drawsheet (D).

17 Roll the sick person toward you over the rolled-up linen.

18 Wash the buttocks on the other side.

19 Pull through the soiled drawsheet (E) and put it in the dirty linen basket. Discard the plastic gloves into the large plastic bag.

20 Straighten the bottom sheet and plastic sheeting, pull tight and tuck in under the mattress. Pull through the clean drawsheet and incontinence pad (F). Tuck in the drawsheet.

21 Make sure the incontinence pad is in the right position. It should be flat under the sick person's buttocks.

22 Roll the sick person to the centre of the bed, onto her back.

Finally

Rearrange pillows and make sure the sick person is comfortable; replace the top covers; clear away and clean all equipment; wash your hands; and re-open any windows that you closed.

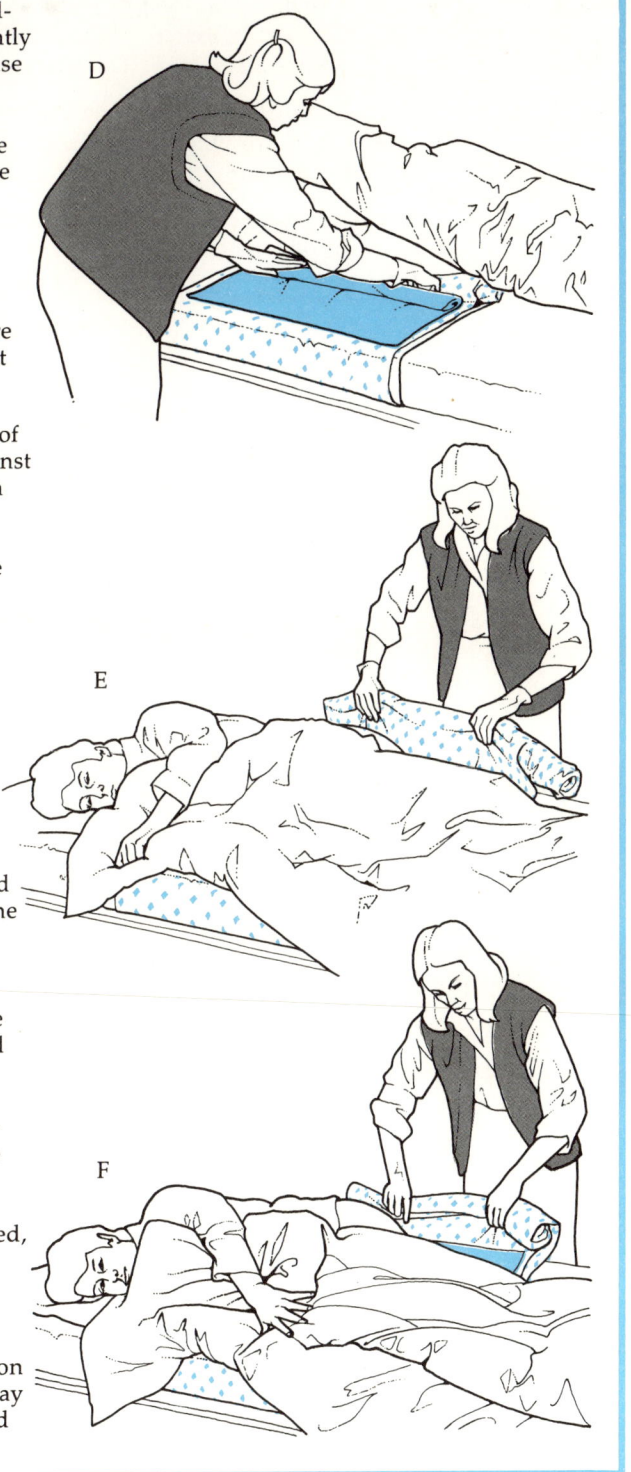

Catheters

Some patients may need a urinary catheter. This is a soft plastic tube, which is passed into the bladder by a nurse or doctor. A small inflatable balloon holds it in the bladder. The catheter is attached to a sterile disposable plastic tube, which in turn is attached to a drainage bag.

☐ The catheter should be taped to the sick person's inner thigh with Skinfix or Elastoplast; make sure that he or she can move without pulling on the catheter.

☐ The plastic tubing and drainage bag should be hung either on the bed or on a special stand.

☐ The tubing must not be kinked or obstructed, for example by being tucked in with the bedclothes under the mattress.

☐ While the catheter is in the bladder you can reassure the sick person that urine will only pass through the catheter, without any conscious effort on the part of the patient. The urine simply drains into the bag.

☐ The urine bag holds about 1.5 litres (2.7 pt) and will need emptying at least once a day. At the bottom of the urine bag there is an outlet valve or a tap for this purpose.

☐ Leg drainage bags are often used for active people who need to wear a urinary catheter permanently. They can be taped to a leg or pinned to the inside of a trouser leg or skirt. They need to be replaced by a larger urine bag during the night.

Make sure that the catheter is taped securely to the thigh, and that the tube can bend freely without kinking.

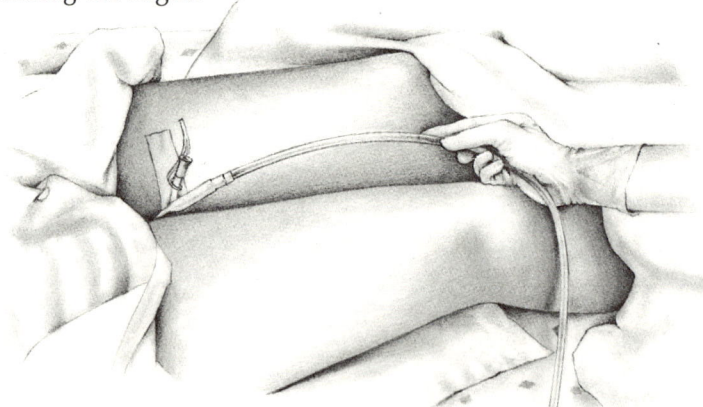

Infection

The main problem that besets people who have catheters on a long-term basis is infection. If the sick person gets a urinary tract infection he or she may complain of pain and discomfort in the lower abdomen and have a raised temperature. If the urine is infected it will smell fishy and may look hazy or cloudy, in which case inform your doctor, who may ask for a specimen of urine.

To prevent infection:
○ Make sure the catheter is kept clean
○ Be very careful when emptying and changing the urine bag
○ Make sure that the sick person drinks plenty of fluids, unless the doctor has restricted fluids for some medical reasons

TO EMPTY A URINE BAG

Collect together
- A clean, disinfected jug
- A wipe and a little antiseptic solution in a small saucer or bowl
- Disposable gloves
- Plastic bag

Preparation

1 Wash your hands and put on the disposable gloves.

2 Put the plastic bag on a table or chair near the urine bag to be emptied.

3 Put the wipe into the antiseptic solution and leave it to soak for a few seconds.

Emptying the bag

4 Place the clean, disinfected jug under the valve or tap at the base of the urine bag.

5 Leaving the urine bag on its stand or attached to the bedside, press the valve or turn the tap at the base of the bag. Keep the opening under the valve or tap well away from the sides of the jug to prevent the opening from becoming contaminated. Infection can track back up from here to the bladder and cause a urinary tract infection.

6 Allow the urine to flow into the jug.

7 Release the valve or turn off the tap.

8 Clean the valve or tap with the wipe soaked in antiseptic solution and discard into the plastic bag. This helps to prevent infection.
▶ Squeeze out any excess fluid before wiping.

9 Cover the jug and dispose of the contents, observing and recording the amount if necessary (see pages 92-94).

10 Discard your gloves into the plastic bag.

Finally

Rinse the empty jug under running water, and clean it with disinfectant solution; then wash your hands.

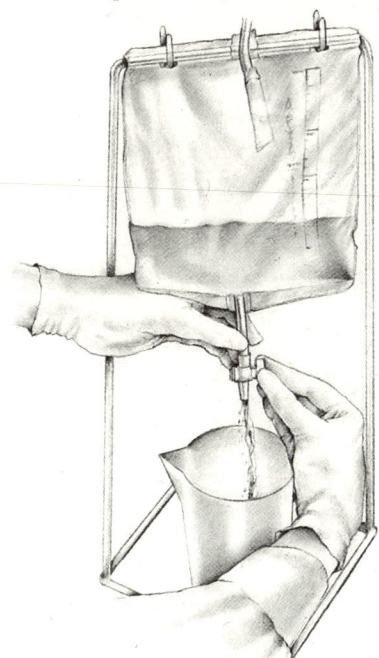

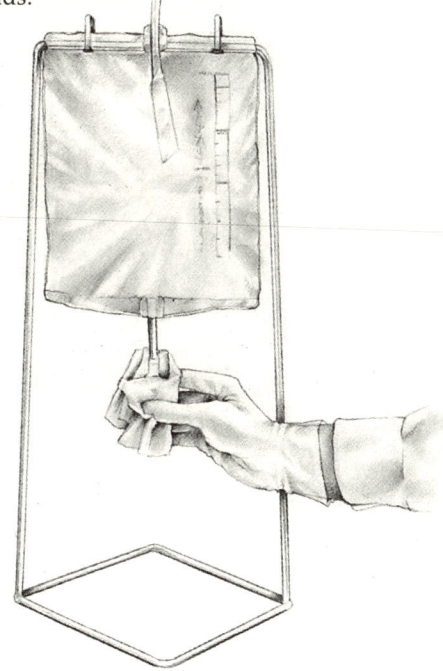

CHANGING A URINE BAG

The urine bag will need to be changed weekly or more often if the bag is leaking or if it becomes encrusted with organic deposits.

Collect together
- A new urinary drainage bag
- Two plastic or metal gate clips
- A pair of disposable gloves
- Plastic bag for disposable rubbish
- Skinfix or Elastoplast
- A pair of clean scissors

Preparation

1 Wash your hands.

2 Fold back the top covers from the foot of the bed until the catheter is visible and remove the Skinfix or Elastoplast.

3 Put on the disposable gloves.

4 Cut open the bag containing the new drainage bag and check that the tap or valve is closed. Leave the new urine bag in its outer bag – this will keep it sterile.

5 Put one plastic or metal clip on the catheter. Place the other on the urine drainage bag tube. This will prevent the urine from running out when you disconnect the catheter from the drainage bag.

6 Hold the catheter in one hand and disconnect it from the drainage tube, taking care not to touch the open end of the catheter. Discard the old urinary drainage system into the plastic bag.

7 Still holding the catheter in one hand, take the new drainage system, open it and join it to the catheter, without touching the end of the catheter or the new drainage system (see below). Make sure that the equipment does not touch anything unsterile.

8 Take the gate clips off the catheter. Attach the drainage bag to a stand or to the bed. Make sure that the catheter is not twisted or kinked. Reapply Skinfix or Elastoplast to the thigh.

Finally

Replace the top bedcovers; clear away and clean all equipment; make the sick person comfortable; and wash your hands.

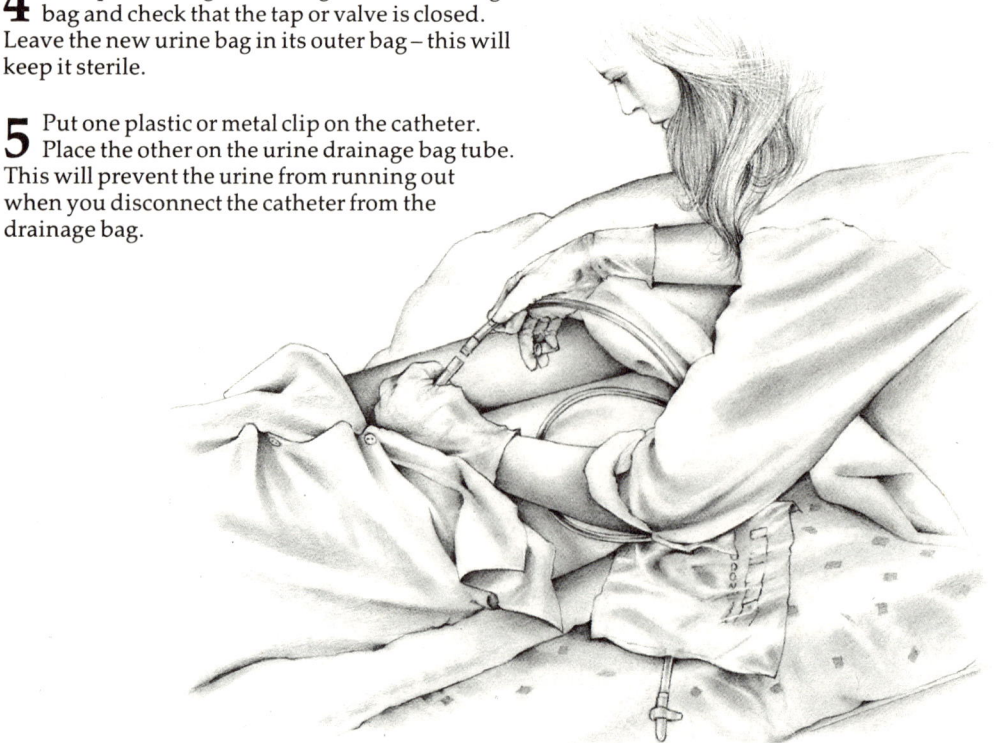

CATHETER CARE

If the sick person is allowed to have a bath, the catheter can safely be soaked in water. Drop the tubing over the side of the bath and either attach the bag to the side or put it on its stand beside the bath. Replace the Skinfix or Elastoplast afterwards.

Cleaning the catheter

If the sick person is unable to get into a bath, use the following technique twice a day to remove crusts and secretions, to prevent infection and to make him or her more comfortable.

Collect together
- A bowl filled with hand-hot water
- Soap
- Disposable gloves
- A plastic bag for used wipes
- Skinfix or Elastoplast
- New incontinence pad
- Disposable wipes

Preparation

1 Wash your hands.

2 Fold back the bedclothes from the foot of the bed until the catheter is visible.

3 Put an incontinence pad under the sick person's buttocks.

4 Put on the disposable gloves.

Cleaning

5 With a soap-and-water-soaked disposable wipe or swab, with one downward stroke, wash the side of the vulva in a female and the penis in a male, then discard the wipe into the plastic bag. Make sure that you use each wipe once only in a downward direction.

6 Then repeat the procedure down the other side and down the centre until the whole area has been covered. This action ensures that you are washing away from the catheter.

7 Repeat the whole procedure with plain water and then with dry wipes.

8 Then clean the catheter. Take a soap-and-water-soaked wipe and, with a downward stroke from top to bottom, clean down one side of the catheter. Make sure you do not pull on the catheter.

9 Repeat down the other side and down the centre, using a new wipe each time.

10 Repeat with plain water and dry wipes.

11 Take off your disposable gloves and discard them into the plastic bag.

12 Renew the Skinfix or Elastoplast on the sick person's thigh.

13 Remove and discard the incontinence pad.

Finally

Replace the bedclothes and make the sick person comfortable; clear away and clean the equipment; wash your hands; and open any windows that you closed.

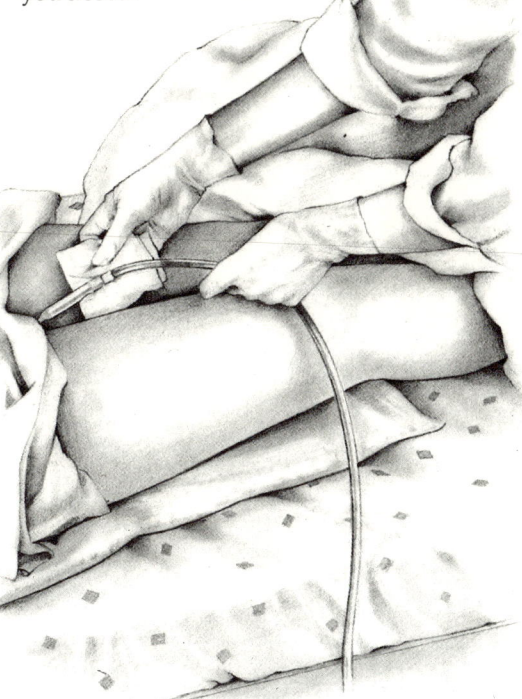

Pressure sores

The weight of the body presses down on certain areas as the sick person lies in bed or sits in a chair. If the pressure is not relieved by the sick person changing position, the blood supply to the affected parts is reduced and the tissue cells die, the skin breaks down and pressure sores develop. First the skin becomes red, then there will be a small break in the skin which, if left untreated, will break down further. A deeper ulcer will form and, as these sores usually develop over an area where the bones are near the surface, the bone may become visible. It is important to prevent this by giving regular pressure-area care.

Avoiding pressure sores

The weight of the bedclothes can aggravate pressure sores, so use a bedcradle to keep the covers off the invalid's heels, toes and knees (see page 56). Make sure that you do not irritate the skin by leaving wrinkles or crumbs in the bed, or by dragging on the skin when lifting the sick person on or off a bedpan. Most important, encourage the sick person to move about as much as possible.

Pressure areas
Pressure sores are likely to develop in certain areas, if the sick person lies in any position for too long. Pressure areas for particular positions are indicated here by the shaded areas.

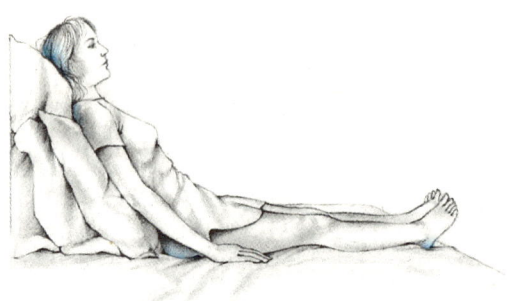

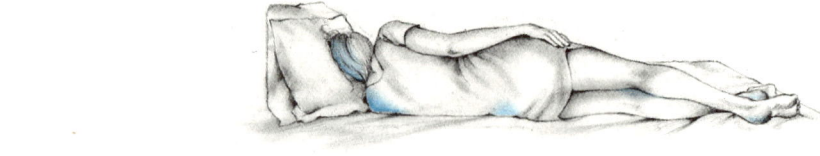

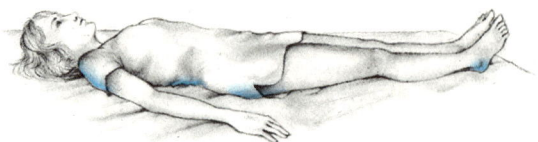

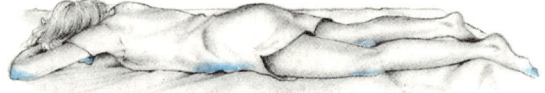

EXERCISES FOR THE SICK PERSON IN BED

Someone who is confined to bed for some time may have difficulties caused by poor circulation and lack of exercise. He or she may also find walking and standing difficult when allowed up. The following exercises help to prevent these problems. They also have the significant advantage of making the sick person feel he or she is doing something to feel better.

Relearning to walk

When a sick person first gets up, start by suggesting that he or she walks very short distances, and increase these gradually as the convalescent becomes stronger. Agree on a realistic distance that you can both work toward, so that the sick person feels that progress is being made and does not become discouraged.

Breathing

This simple exercise helps to prevent respiratory complications and can be done in bed. Ask the sick person to breathe in to the count of four, and then out to the count of four; he or she should breathe gently through the nose. He or she should keep breathing in this rhythm for several minutes, and repeat the exercise three or four times a day.

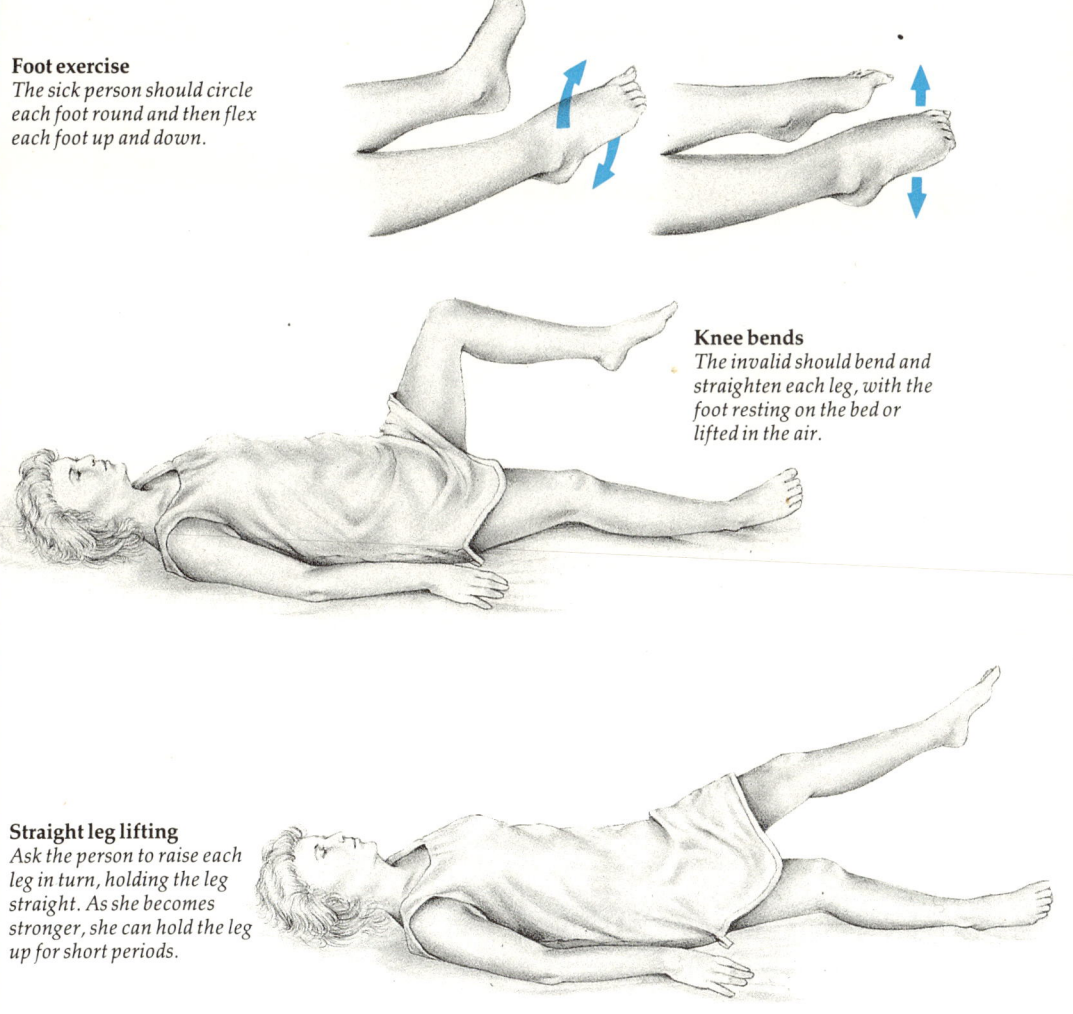

Foot exercise
The sick person should circle each foot round and then flex each foot up and down.

Knee bends
The invalid should bend and straighten each leg, with the foot resting on the bed or lifted in the air.

Straight leg lifting
Ask the person to raise each leg in turn, holding the leg straight. As she becomes stronger, she can hold the leg up for short periods.

If you are caring for someone helpless, you should change their position every 2 to 4 hours, or more frequently if the skin becomes red and sore. Turn the sick person in the following sequence – from right side to back to left side to front, and back onto the right side. If the invalid is breathless, keep him or her in an upright position and move from right side to back to left side to back and then back onto the right side again (see pages 35-37).

Keeping the skin clean and dry also helps to prevent pressure sores. Wash the sick person once a day, or more frequently if needed – if he or she is incontinent, for example. But avoid rubbing the skin and be sparing with soap: over-use of soap removes the natural oils in the skin that keep it supple. A silicone or barrier cream may be prescribed to protect the skin. If, despite these measures, pressure sores do develop, tell your doctor.

Sheepskins

Sheepskins are used to help prevent pressure sores developing, as the natural oils produced by the sheepskin keep the skin in good condition; however, they do not relieve the pressure. Make sure the skin is in contact with the wool – the sick person should wear no clothes below the waist. Ask your chemist or pharmacist where you can buy them.

To make a sheepskin for a sick person to sit on, cut a piece of sheepskin into an oblong 50 cm by 70 cm (20 in by 27 in). To make a boot for the heel cut a shape 20 cm by 20 cm (8 in by 8 in) and attach a Velcro tape to either side. Alternatively, you can use a large sheet of foam rubber with holes cut in the rubber at the pressure points. This will keep the pressure points off the bed and help prevent pressure sores. A child's rubber swimming ring may also be useful and can be placed in a pillowcase.

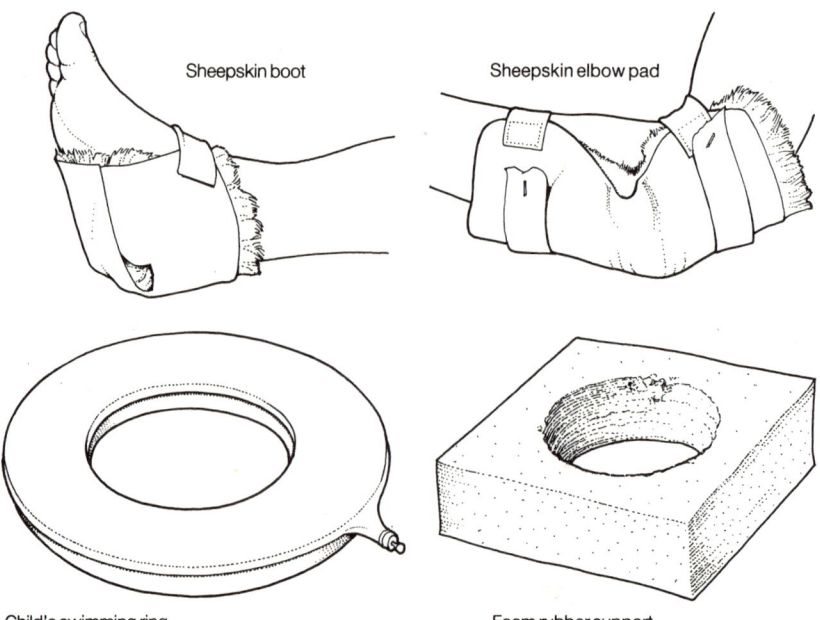

Sheepskin boot

Sheepskin elbow pad

Child's swimming ring

Foam rubber support

Rest and sleep

The amount of sleep required varies from person to person. The older you are, the less sleep you seem to need. Sleep is a time of mental and physical relaxation and the body needs this time in order to function properly. Someone who is suffering from lack of sleep may find it difficult to cope with everyday problems that he or she normally takes in his or her stride and judgement may become impaired. So it is important for both you and your patient to get adequate rest and sleep.

Settling a sick person down for the night

☐ Offer a bedpan, urinal, commode, sanichair or help to the toilet. Help with washing of hands and face.

☐ Help the sick person to clean his or her teeth and mouth (see page 66).

☐ Straighten the bedclothes and change any soiled linen.

☐ If the sick person is helpless, change his or her position in bed, making sure that he or she will be comfortable enough to sleep. Adjust the pillows and put an extra blanket on the bed, if required.

☐ A breathless sick person may be more comfortable sleeping in an armchair with blankets and pillows for warmth and comfort. A stool covered with a pillow will provide foot support.

☐ Changing a dressing may relieve pain and discomfort.

☐ Make sure that the bedside light, water, a glass and tissues are within reach. Also ensure that the sick person can reach a bell or can call for help during the night. Do not leave any drugs on the invalid's bedside table – it is easy to take an overdose by accident. It is especially important not to leave sleeping pills or pain pills on the table.

☐ Leave a window slightly open; make sure that the room is not too hot.

☐ Some people find that reading for a while helps them to get to sleep. Draw the curtains and put out the light when the invalid is drowsy.

Insomnia

There are some practical reasons why a sick person may be having trouble sleeping but if you have followed the list above these should not be a problem. More often than not all it takes to get the sick person to sleep is to give him or her a hot drink and sit and talk for a while. If this does not work, talk to the doctor. Too many broken nights sleep will soon leave you, the caregiver, exhausted and unable to care for the sick person efficiently. So sometimes it may be necessary for your doctor to prescribe a night sedation for the sick person so that you can get some sleep, too.

If the sick person does need you during the night it may be better for you to have a bed in the same room rather than sitting in a chair beside the bed. You may find there are nearby voluntary organizations or nursing agencies who arrange night nursing, perhaps for two or three nights a week. Ask your doctor if there is such a scheme in your area. If you do get someone to stay with the sick person at night make sure that you take full advantage of the help and that you have an early night.

Observing Your Patient

Part of your task as a caregiver is to monitor the sick person's condition and to alert your doctor to any changes that may be important. You are the person who is able to observe the invalid most closely and consistently, and much of the doctor's assessment of an illness may depend on what you and the sick person tell him. Mastering basic observation skills, such as taking a sick person's temperature and recording his or her pulse and respiration rate, will help you to assess the importance of any changes. If the doctor asks you to carry out more complex procedures at home, such as recording fluid balance, taking blood pressure or specimens, you must ask him to explain exactly what he wants you to do and, if possible, to give you a demonstration. Practise the procedure on a friend and only once you feel confident that you are doing it correctly, should you carry it out on the sick person.

Encourage the sick person to talk to you about how he or she feels; take note of what he or she says and if you are at all worried about any of the symptoms described, tell the doctor about them. Try to be open and honest with the sick person but, at the same time, avoid letting him or her see if you are worried by any change in his or her symptoms.

Signs to watch out for

Any sudden change in the sick person's condition which indicates a turn for the worse should be reported to the doctor. The following are a few of the signs and symptoms which you should report.

☐ Skin changes: pallor or a yellowish tinge to the skin or the whites of the eyes; sunken or dull eyes; blueness of the lips, fingertips or toes.

☐ Skin over a joint that feels hot when compared to the rest of the body; redness or swelling over a joint.

☐ Persistent redness over pressure areas.

☐ Skin that is unusually hot or cold to the touch.

☐ Frequent licking of the lips.

☐ A dry and unproductive cough which becomes loose and produces mucus; or a cough which produces blood-stained mucus.

☐ Noisy breathing; or difficulty in breathing when lying flat.

☐ Any obvious signs that the patient is in pain.

Observation skills

When you are taking a child's temperature, always explain what you are doing and why.

As caregiver, you will probably have to take the temperature of the person you are caring for; whether you need to use any of the other skills described below depends on the nature of the sick person's illness. In general, it is a good idea to become familiar with all the basic nursing procedures so that if you need them, you are clear about what to do and confident that you can do it correctly.

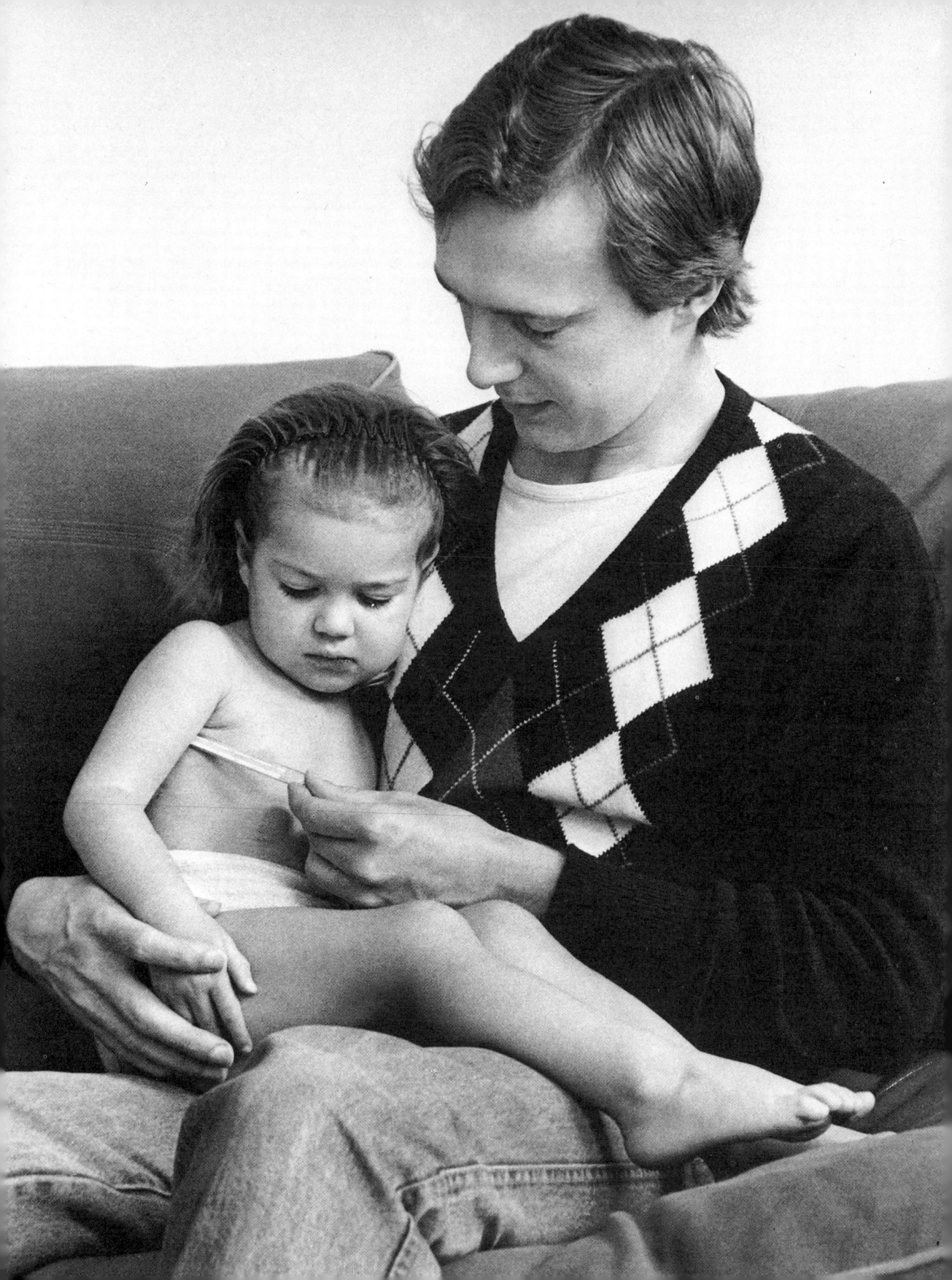

Temperature, pulse and respiration rates

In normal health, there is only slight variation in our temperature, pulse and respiration rates. When someone becomes ill, however, these rates may alter, and recording them at regular intervals throughout an illness is an effective way of monitoring a patient's progress. An infection, for instance, produces a raised temperature and a raised pulse rate. As the temperature and pulse rate return to normal, you can see a general improvement in the patient's condition.

Taking a temperature

A measurement of temperature can be taken under the tongue, under the arm, in the groin or in the rectum. There is a slight variation in the average temperature recorded at these different sites. The normal method of testing is under the tongue, for which the average rate is 36.9°c (98.4°F). Under the arm or in the groin, the average temperature is 36°c (97°F): these sites are used for people who are disturbed or confused or having difficulty breathing and also for young children, epileptics or anyone who is unconscious. The rectal method has an average temperature recording of 37°c (98.5°F) and is used for children under 2 years or for anyone who is unconscious. Fever strips are a useful method of reading a child's temperature, although they do not give as accurate a reading as a mercury thermometer. They are impregnated strips which, when pressed to the forehead, change colour to indicate a rise in temperature.

The thermometer

A clinical thermometer has a mercury rise with a scale, usually running from 35°c (95°F) to 42°c (107.6°F) or above. A small arrow or red line on the scale indicates what the average mouth temperature should be. A bulb at one end of the thermometer contains the mercury, which rises up as the thermometer is warmed. A kink between the bulb and the stem prevents the mercury falling back into the bulb once it has risen. To get the mercury back into the bulb, the thermometer must be shaken with a sharp flick of the wrist.

Mercury thermometer

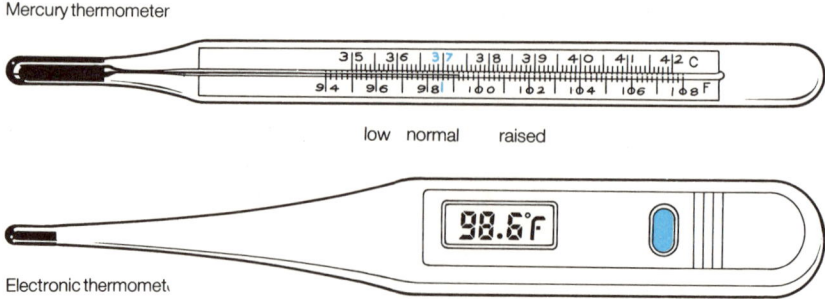

low   normal   raised

Electronic thermometer

An alternative to the clinical mercury thermometer is a battery-operated electronic one. A push-button switches it on and off. The temperature recorded in the tip is electronically converted to a digit, displayed in Fahrenheit or Celsius. There is much less danger of breaking these, but take care when cleaning to prevent water penetrating the body of the thermometer.

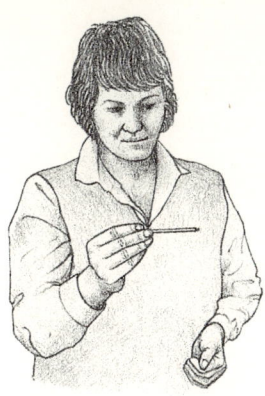

In a good light, slowly turn the thermometer round until you can see a silver band of mercury magnified against the frosted background.

Reading a thermometer

Hold the end of the thermometer furthest away from the bulb in your right hand. The point at which the column of mercury ends indicates the temperature level and the degree lines are clearly numbered along the scale so that you can read the temperature up to a tenth of a degree.

Once a temperature has been taken, the mercury will stay in position until shaken or until another higher temperature is taken. So, if you are unable to read the thermometer, you can safely wipe it dry and leave it for someone else to read.

Disinfecting a thermometer

A thermometer should be disinfected at the end of an illness, or after use if more than one person is using it. The thermometer should be washed (see below), then left to soak in alcohol (90% ethyl or isopropyl) or disinfectant. Ask your local chemist for advice on the best solution to use and leave the thermometer to soak for as long as indicated on the bottle. After soaking, rinse in cold water and dry.

TAKING A TEMPERATURE BY MOUTH

Collect together
- Clean clinical thermometer
- Tissues or wipes
- Plastic bag for disposal of wipes
- Chart or notebook and pen to record the reading
- Watch with a second-hand

Preparation

1 Wash and dry your hands.

2 Make sure the sick person is sitting or lying down and that he has not smoked or drunk anything hot or cold for at least 5 minutes.

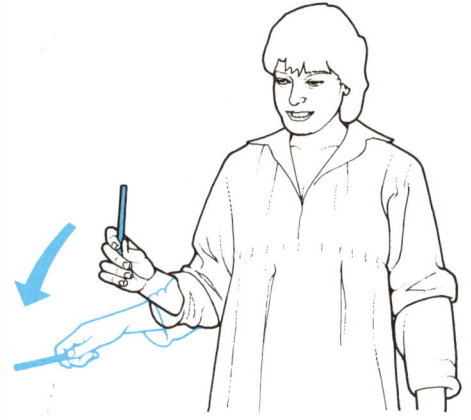

3 Shake the mercury down below the lowest reading on the thermometer, taking care not to accidentally knock it against anything hard.

Taking the temperature

4 Place the thermometer under the sick person's tongue. Ask him to keep his lips closed, not to talk and to take care not to bite the thermometer.

5 Leave it in position for at least 2 minutes or as long as stated on the side of the thermometer.

6 Remove the thermometer and wipe with a tissue. Discard wipe in plastic bag.

7 Read and record the temperature on a chart or in a notebook (see page 90).

8 Shake the mercury down and wash the thermometer in a bowl of cold water and washing-up liquid. Rinse in cold water and dry with a wipe. *Never* use hot water as this will push the mercury up too high and break the thermometer.

Finally

Dispose of the bag containing used wipes or tissues. Wash and dry your hands and make sure the sick person is comfortable.

Taking a temperature under the arm or in the groin

Use the same equipment and follow the same procedure for taking a temperature by mouth but, in addition, carry out the following measures.

☐ Wipe under the arm or in the groin beforehand to make sure the skin is dry, as the thermometer may slip on a wet surface.

☐ Make sure there are no clothes in the way of the thermometer.

☐ Keep the sick person's elbow by his or her side when taking a temperature under the arm – you can do this by holding the patient's forearm against his or her chest.

Taking a rectal temperature

This involves using a specially designed rectal thermometer and lubricating jelly. Otherwise, use the same equipment and follow the same procedure as for taking a temperature by mouth, apart from carrying out the following additional steps.

☐ Explain to the sick person what you are going to do beforehand.

☐ Before inserting the thermometer, lubricate the bulb of the thermometer with lubricant.

☐ Insert the thermometer 2.5 cm (1 in) into the back passage or rectum and hold in position for 1 to 2 minutes or as stated on the side of the thermometer.

☐ When you have finished taking the temperature, wipe the sick person's anus with a wipe or tissue.

The pulse

Each time the heart beats, blood is pumped through the arteries, causing a wave of momentary expansion which can be felt in the arteries near the surface of the body and where an artery passes over a bone. This expansion of the artery, or pulse, can be felt by gently pressing the artery against the bone with your finger. The most common sites for taking a pulse are at the wrist below the thumb, at the temple and at the angle of the jaw.

The pulse rate is the number of times per minute that the heart beat can be felt. A normal pulse rate for an adult is 60 to 80 beats per minute. For a baby, the normal pulse rate is 120 to 140 beats per minute; by 12 years of age, the rate has fallen to 80 beats per minute. Activity may double the pulse rate, but on resting the pulse should quickly return to normal. The rate may also be increased by fever, emotional states such as fear and anger, and extremes of hot and cold. It may be decreased by resting, as a result of a head injury or as a side-effect of certain drugs.

The rhythm of the pulse is normally regular and the beats evenly spaced; the volume of the pulse refers to the strength of each beat.

Any change in the rate, rhythm or volume of the pulse may mean that there has been a change in the sick person's condition. If on retaking the pulse a few minutes later there is still a significant change, call the doctor and ask his advice about what to do next.

Respiration

Breathing is the mechanism by which oxygen is taken into the lungs and the waste product, carbon dioxide, is exhaled. As air is breathed in, the chest expands in width and height and the diaphragm flattens, allowing air to be sucked into the lungs. From there it is carried round the body by the red blood cells in the arteries and supplied to all the cells in the body which require oxygen. The cells rid themselves of carbon dioxide, which is carried back to the lungs along the veins. This is then exhaled as the rib muscles and diaphragm relax and the air is forced out.

The respiration rate is the number of times per minute that the chest rises and falls. The normal respiration rate in an adult is 16 to 20 breaths a minute, and in a baby 32 to 50 breaths a minute. The rate may be increased by activity, fever, emotional stress and extremes of temperature; it may be decreased by rest, as a result of a head injury, some diseases or as a side-effect of certain drugs.

While recording a sick person's respiration rate, make a note of whether he or she is having difficulty breathing. The following are all signs of abnormal breathing and should be reported to the doctor with a note of how and when they started:

○ Noisy, wheezy or bubbly breathing
○ Unusually shallow or deep breathing
○ Excessive sighing and yawning
○ Difficulty in breathing when lying down
○ Waking up in the night unable to breathe
○ Wheezing, with difficulty breathing out – a sign of asthma

TAKING A PULSE AND COUNTING THE NUMBER OF RESPIRATIONS

Collect together:
• Chart or notebook and pen to record the reading
• Watch with a second-hand

1 Make sure the sick person is at rest, either lying or sitting down, and that her wrist and elbow are slightly bent with her forearm against her chest.

2 Place your first three fingers along the line of the artery in her wrist. Never use your thumb

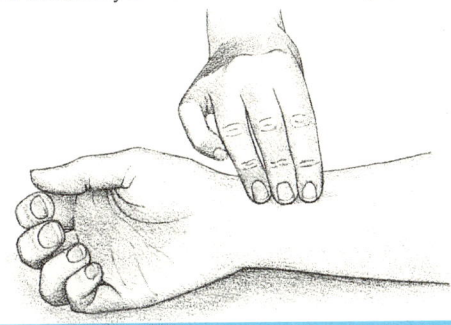

to feel a pulse, as you will be feeling the pulse in your own thumb.

3 Count the beats of the pulse for 1 minute, using a watch with a second-hand.

4 Make a note of the rate, whether the rhythm is regular and the volume is weak or strong.

5 Record the pulse on a chart or in a notebook (see page 90).

6 When you have finished taking the sick person's pulse, leave your fingers on her wrist and raise your eyes so that you can see the chest wall rising and falling. The sick person will not be aware that you are counting her respiration rate as she will think you are still counting her pulse rate. This is important, as once she becomes aware of you counting her every breath, her breathing may alter.

7 Record the respiratory rate.

Blood pressure

An increase in blood pressure, known as the 'systolic pressure', occurs every time the heart beats and blood is pumped into the arteries. The pressure then falls until the next beat. This lowered pressure is known as the 'diastolic pressure'. These pressures can be measured by using a sphygmomanometer or blood pressure measuring scale. The normal levels for systolic pressure are 110 to 140 millimetres of mercury, and for diastolic pressure, 70 to 90 millimetres of mercury. This is expressed on paper with the systolic figure over the diastolic in the following way – 120/80. Levels are affected by emotion, posture, age and disease. Arteries become less elastic with age and blood pressure tends to rise.

TAKING BLOOD PRESSURE

Collect together
- Stethoscope
- Sphygmomanometer
- Chart or notebook for recording the reading

Preparation

1 Wash and dry your hands.

2 Make sure the sick person is lying or sitting down unless the doctor has specifically asked you to record his blood pressure while he is standing up.

3 Roll up the clothing on his upper arm – if it is going to restrict his arm in any way when rolled up, remove it altogether.

4 Place the sphygmomanometer on a table or chair beside the sick person, at the same level as his arm. Position it so that you can see the measuring scale clearly.

Recording blood pressure

5 Place the arm band around his arm with the tubes to the front and tuck in the end (A), or close with the Velcro or clips provided.

6 Connect the manometer to the arm band (B).

7 Feel for the pulse in his wrist and, with the other hand, close the valve in the rubber bulb and pump up the arm band until you can no longer feel the pulse (C). Note of the level of the sphygmomanometer – this will give you an idea of systolic blood pressure and, therefore, an idea of how high to inflate the arm band when you take

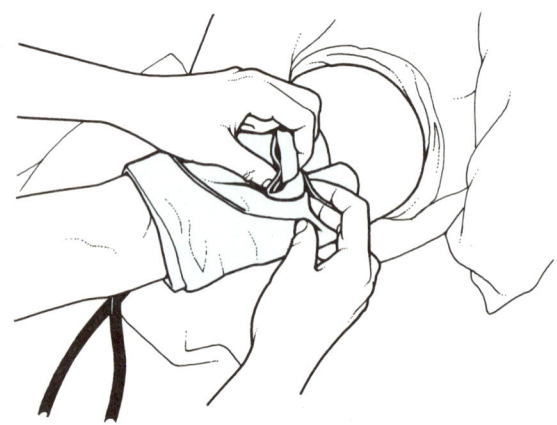

A

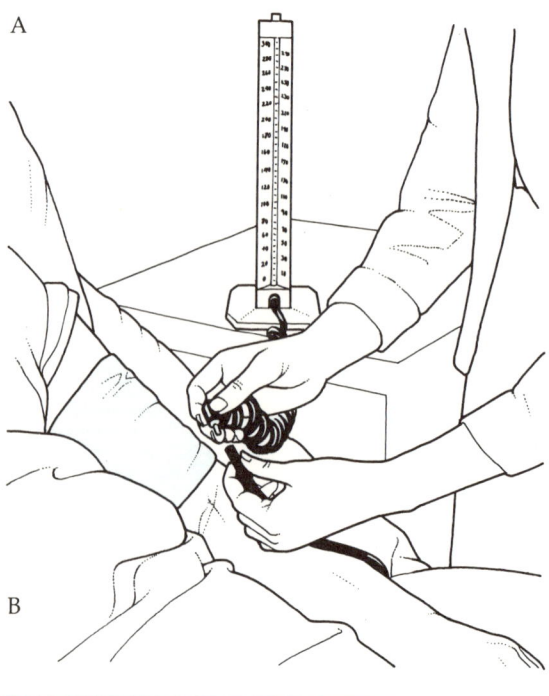

B

If the doctor does ask you to record the sick person's blood pressure, make sure you know what the average levels should be in his or her case and whether the doctor wants to be told if the recordings are abnormally high or low. If the reading is abnormal, try not to show any anxiety. Reassure the patient that you are taking his or her blood pressure in order to monitor his or her progress. Check it again in 10 minutes and if it is still abnormal, call the doctor and ask him what you should do next. Before taking the sick person's blood pressure, check with the doctor as to how much he has told the patient about his or her blood pressure and how much he or she is likely to understand.

the actual reading. Inflating the arm band unnecessarily highly can cause great discomfort.

8 Deflate the arm band and feel for the pulse in the crook of the arm.

9 Place the hearing pieces of the stethoscope in your ears and the other end over the artery in the crook of the sick person's arm (D).

10 Close the valve and inflate the arm band until the reading is just above the systolic pressure you have already noted. You should no longer be able to hear the beat through the stethoscope.

11 Loosen the valve and deflate the cuff slowly. As you do so, you will hear a faint tapping sound which is the systolic pressure – make a note of the level at which the tapping started. As the mercury falls, it is quite normal for the tapping to change to a knocking sound.

12 The sound will then change to a muffled murmur which is the diastolic pressure – make a note of the level at which the murmuring started. In the USA, a complete disappearance of sound is taken as the diastolic pressure – a difference of 5 to 10 mm mercury.

13 Record the readings on a chart or in a notebook (see page 90).

14 Remove the cuff and empty it of air by flattening it with your hand. Fold it up and put it away.

Finally

Replace any clothing and make sure the sick person is comfortable.

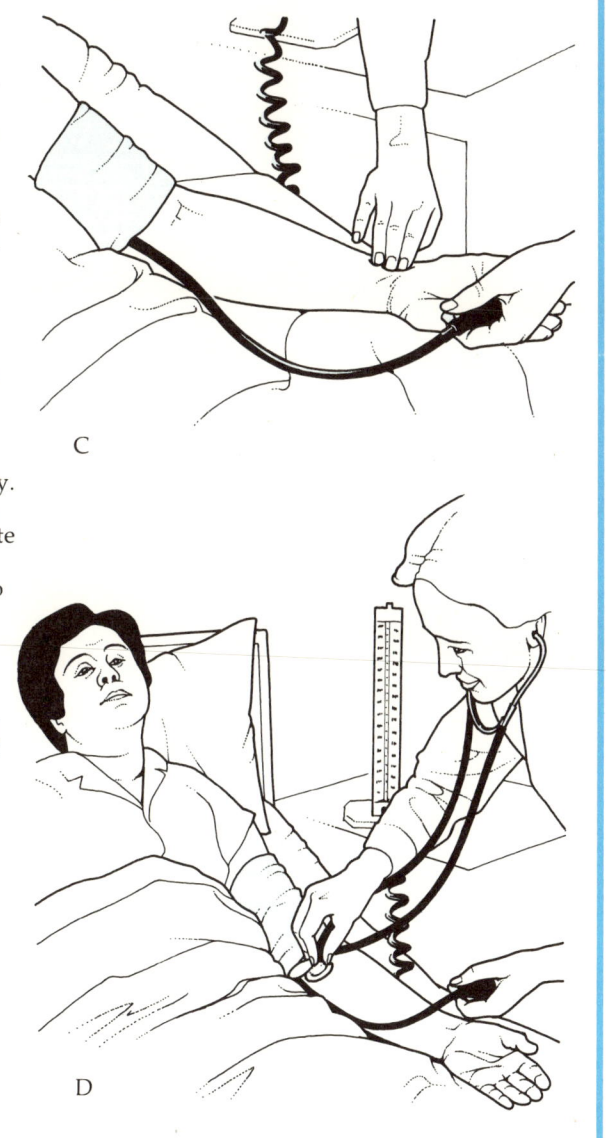

C

D

Recording temperature, pulse and respiration rates and blood pressure level

At the beginning of an illness, the patient's temperature, pulse, respiration and blood pressure need to be checked frequently and at regular intervals as they will then act as reliable indicators of any change in his or her condition. They should be marked clearly on a piece of graph paper or in a notebook along with the date and time taken so that the doctor is quickly able to see how the patient has progressed since his last visit. If you change the method by which the temperature is taken, make a note of the change.

Keep the chart or notebook in a safe place near the patient's bedside so that it is easily accessible.

	DAY	TIME	TEMPERATURE IN CENTIGRADE	PULSE	RESPIRATION	BLOOD PRESSURE
						120/80
4 hourly	MAY 1	6 AM	36.8	78	18	130/86
	"	10 AM	37	82	20	126/80
	"	2 PM	37.8	86	22	122/84
	"	6 PM	38	90	24	120/80
	"	10 PM	37.8	70	22	128/86
	"	2 AM	37.4	62	19	130/90
6 hourly	MAY 2	6 AM	37	50	17	130/90
	"	12 NOON	37.2	70	20	130/86
	"	6 PM	37.5	76	20	130/90
	"	12 M'NIGHT	38	100	20	120/90
Twice daily	MAY 3	10 AM	37	80	20	126/90
	"	10 PM	36.8	80	20	140/95
	MAY 4	10 AM	36.5	90	19	140/100
	"	10 PM	36.2	76	20	140/90
Daily	MAY 5	10 AM	36.5	80	18	126/96
	MAY 6	10 AM	37	73	20	120/83
	MAY 7	10 AM	36.8	70	20	110/70
	MAY 8	10 AM	40	90	24	

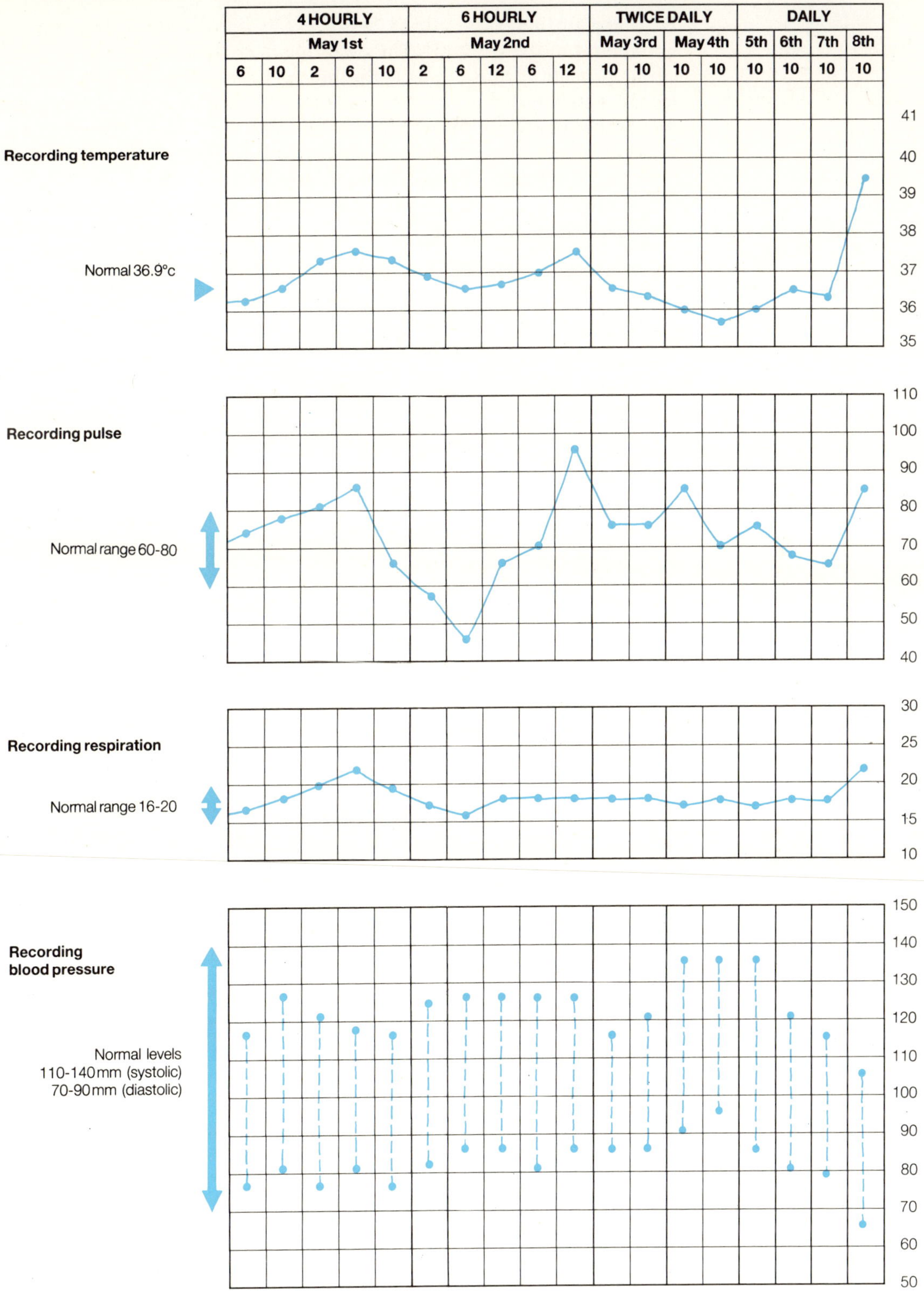
4 HOURLY
6 HOURLY
TWICE DAILY
DAILY
May 1st
May 2nd
May 3rd
May 4th
5th
6th
7th
8th
6 10 2 6 10 2 6 12 6 12 10 10 10 10 10 10 10 10
Recording temperature
Normal 36.9°c
41 40 39 38 37 36 35
Recording pulse
Normal range 60-80
110 100 90 80 70 60 50 40
Recording respiration
Normal range 16-20
30 25 20 15 10
Recording blood pressure
Normal levels
110-140 mm (systolic)
70-90 mm (diastolic)
150 140 130 120 110 100 90 80 70 60 50

Recording fluid balance

With certain illnesses, it may be necessary to record the sick person's intake and output of fluid. This is rarely necessary for someone who is being nursed at home, but if the doctor does ask you to keep such a record, you should take careful note of the patient's intake and output. In some cases of kidney disease it is essential to keep such a record, but the sick person will usually be quite capable of doing so without your help. If you do not have two jugs marked in millilitres or fluid ounces, try to buy them. You can, however, work out the capacity of an ordinary jug and mark it on the inside.

☐ Measure any fluids offered to the patient carefully in a jug and make a note of how much the sick person drinks and the time of day at which it is drunk.

☐ Make a note of all urine passed by measuring it in a jug. If you throw it away by a mistake or if the sick person is incontinent or passes urine while in the toilet, make a note of the fact and tell the doctor, otherwise the chart becomes inaccurate and misleading.

☐ If the sick person vomits, this should also be measured and recorded.

☐ If the sick person has diarrhoea, you should record the time it was passed. Check with your doctor beforehand if it is really necessary to measure the exact amount.

☐ If the patient is sweating, make a note of the fact.

☐ At the end of a 24-hour period, add up the total intake and output. Keep the chart or notebook to show to the doctor, and start a fresh one for the next 24 hours.

As long as you record everything that is taken in and everything that is passed out in fluid form, it does not matter which system of recording you decide to adopt.

Taking and observing specimens of sputum

Sputum is a substance which is coughed up from the respiratory tract and which consists mainly of mucus. If a sick person is producing sputum, make sure he or she has a disposable pot or container with a lid into which he or she can spit. The pot should be kept near to the patient, plus a box of tissues and a bag to put the used tissues in. Throw away the pot frequently and replace it or, alternatively, burn the pot along with any used tissues.

If you are asked to save a specimen of sputum for the doctor, first give the sick person a mouthwash and then ask him or her to cough and spit a small amount into a container. If the doctor asks for a description of the sputum and the sick person is unable to tell the doctor, then you must describe it to him as it may be of importance in deciding the type of treatment to be given. The doctor may need to know the following details about the sputum produced:
○ The amount, colour and smell
○ Whether it is watery or sticky
○ Whether it contains any blood
○ Whether it is frothy

Whether you are recording fluid intake or output in millilitres or fluid ounces, the structure of the chart remains the same.

DATE: TUESDAY 4 MAY					
TIME	INTAKE IN MLS		OUTPUT IN MLS		NOTES
	Type	Amount	Type	Amount	
8	Tea	150	Urine	500	
9	Water	50			
10	Coffee	150	Urine		Incontinence
11					
12	Lemonade	150			
13			Urine	200	
14	Coffee	150			
15	Water	80			
16			Urine	300	
17	Tea	150			
18	Water	100			
19					
20	Coffee	150			
21					
22	Chocolate	200			
23					
24					
1					
2					
3			Vomit	100	Blood stained
4					
5					
6			Urine	100	
7					
	TOTAL INTAKE 1,300		TOTAL OUTPUT 1,200		

Taking and observing specimens of vomit

When the muscles of the stomach wall are irritated, the contents of the stomach are ejected as vomit. There is no need to measure the actual amount vomited unless the doctor specifically asks you to do so. If the vomit contains something other than undigested food, it is probably a good idea to cover the bowl containing the vomit and let the doctor look at it himself. It will probably be a help to the doctor if you can make the following observations.

☐ Find out from the sick person whether he or she felt any nausea or pain prior to vomiting and whether or not the pain was relieved by vomiting.

☐ Find out from the sick person when he or she last ate.

☐ Note whether the vomit was projectile (forcefully ejected).

☐ Take a note of whether the vomit contained partially digested food; whether it resembled a clear watery fluid or a yellow or green sticky fluid; whether or not it contained streaks of blood, or particles resembling ground coffee, which might be an indication of slow bleeding from the stomach, as in the case of a gastric ulcer.

☐ If the vomit smelt foul like faeces, make a note of the fact.

Taking and observing specimens of urine

The amount of urine passed on average is 500 ml (0.85 pt) less than the total amount of fluid taken in. For example, if a sick person drinks 2 litres (2.6 pt) of fluid, approximately 1½ litres (3.5 pt) of urine will be passed, but if the weather is hot and he or she is sweating a lot or if his or her bowel actions are loose and watery, the urine output will be less.

The doctor may ask for the sick person's urine to be tested with a reagent strip, which you can buy at your local chemist. Instructions for their use are clearly printed on the bottle and an explanatory leaflet is enclosed in the package. These strips of paper are impregnated with substances which react with the substances in urine.

The container for the urine sample must be deep enough for the test area of the strip to be inserted. Dip the strip into a fresh urine sample, draw the strip out against the container to remove any excess urine and compare the test area with the colour chart on the side of the reagent strip bottle.

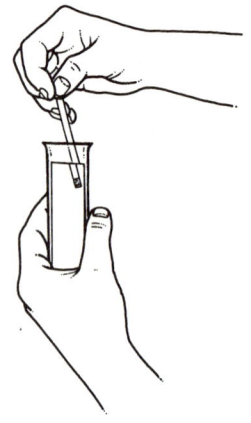

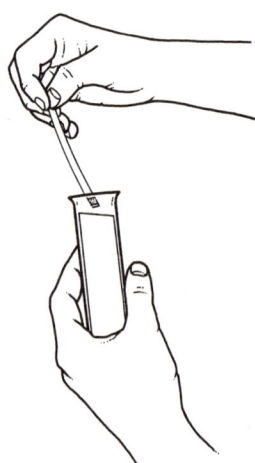

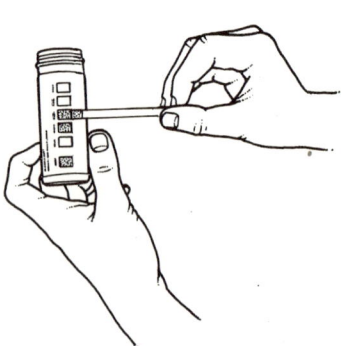

A sample of urine for testing must be a fresh sample passed into a clean bedpan, urine bottle or jug, and then poured into a clean, transparent container for testing. The doctor may ask the sick person to produce a midstream sample of urine, which means that the sample must be uncontaminated by the area around the urethra. The genital area should therefore be cleaned with soap and water before the urine is passed. The sick person should start to pass urine and then stop in midstream and pass some urine into a sterile container such as a sterile jug, and then pass the rest of the urine into the toilet or bedpan. The urine sample should then be transferred from the sterile container into the specimen bottle provided.

It may help the doctor if you can describe the sick person's urine to him. You should make a note of any of the following signs.

☐ Urine which is darker or paler than usual – an indication that it is more concentrated or more dilute than would normally be the case.

☐ Red-coloured urine – an indication that there may be blood present; smoky-coloured urine – an indication that there may be a small quantity of blood present.

☐ Dark orange or brown urine – an indication that bile may be present, as found in people suffering from jaundice.

☐ Cloudy urine – an indication that blood, pus or excess mucus are present.

☐ Hazy urine which smells fishy; this is usually a sign of infection.

If urine is left to stand, any blood, pus or mucus present will show up in the deposit which forms at the bottom of the specimen.

Taking and observing specimens of faeces

Most healthy people open their bowels once or twice a day and the faeces or stools passed are soft, dark brown and with a characteristic smell. They are mainly made up of undigested and indigestible food, mucous membrane, mucus, bacteria and water.

Any abnormal stool passed by a sick person should be reported to the doctor. To obtain a specimen from the sick person, ask him or her to urinate first so that the specimen is not contaminated by urine. Ask the sick person to pass the stool in a bedpan or commode. When he or she has finished, take the bedpan or commode into the bathroom and remove a small sample of the stool with a wooden spatula. Place the sample in a clean jar with a screwtop or in the specimen jar provided, and make a note of the time it was taken.

The doctor may ask you to describe the sick person's faeces to him. The following list will give you an indication of what the doctor may be looking out for.

☐ Hard stools – an indication of constipation.

☐ Frequent, loose stools – an indication of diarrhoea. Very watery stools are an indication of severe diarrhoea.

☐ Bright red blood in the stool – an indication of bleeding from the rectum.

☐ Dark tarry and sticky stools – an indication of a condition known as melaena where blood has undergone changes in the digestive tract.

☐ Black stools – an indication that the sick person may be taking iron.

☐ Green stools – in children, an indication of undigested food.

☐ Pale, bulky, greasy, offensive stools – an indication that the sick person may be suffering from liver or gall bladder problems.

Home Treatments

Treatments exist for most illnesses and conditions and many can be carried out successfully at home. If a treatment is prescribed by a doctor, it is up to you as caregiver to find out from the doctor exactly what has to be done. Do not hesitate to get back to him if you are unclear about something, and if you are still in doubt, you can always ask for a practical demonstration.

It will help your patient if you give an impression of confidence and faith in what you are doing. Do not expect instant results – a treatment may have to be repeated at regular intervals over a period before there are any visible signs of improvement. If it becomes obvious that it is having no effect or if there are signs of an adverse reaction, talk to the doctor before stopping the treatment.

Giving treatments

☐ Collect together all the equipment you are going to need beforehand and take it to the bedside or wherever you are treating the patient.

☐ Tell the sick person exactly what you are going to do and ensure that he or she has privacy, if required.

☐ Make sure the sick person is in the most comfortable and appropriate position.

☐ Wash and dry your hands before and after the treatment.

☐ Always read the label on the bottle or packet containing the treatment carefully and follow the instructions closely.

☐ Talk to the sick person during the treatment and explain what you are doing and what he or she can do to help.

☐ Watch the sick person's reaction to what you are doing: stop the treatment and consult your doctor if it is obviously making the patient unwell. Do not stop a prescribed course of medicine or drugs without talking to the doctor first about the problems and effects they are having; he may be able to prescribe an alternative.

☐ After the treatment, replace any clothes or bedclothes that you have removed and make sure the sick person is comfortable.

☐ Clear away, clean or dispose of any used equipment.

Baths

When giving medicines, always stay with the sick person to make sure that she takes the correct dose and does not choke.

Baths with an additive are prescribed to treat skin conditions and are very soothing particularly if the sick person is suffering from itchy skin. Some of these additives may make the bath very slippery so take extra care when helping a sick person in or out of the bath: a non-slip mat on the bottom of the bath helps. Salt or saline (a solution of salt and water) baths are very soothing following an operation. Taken daily they help to

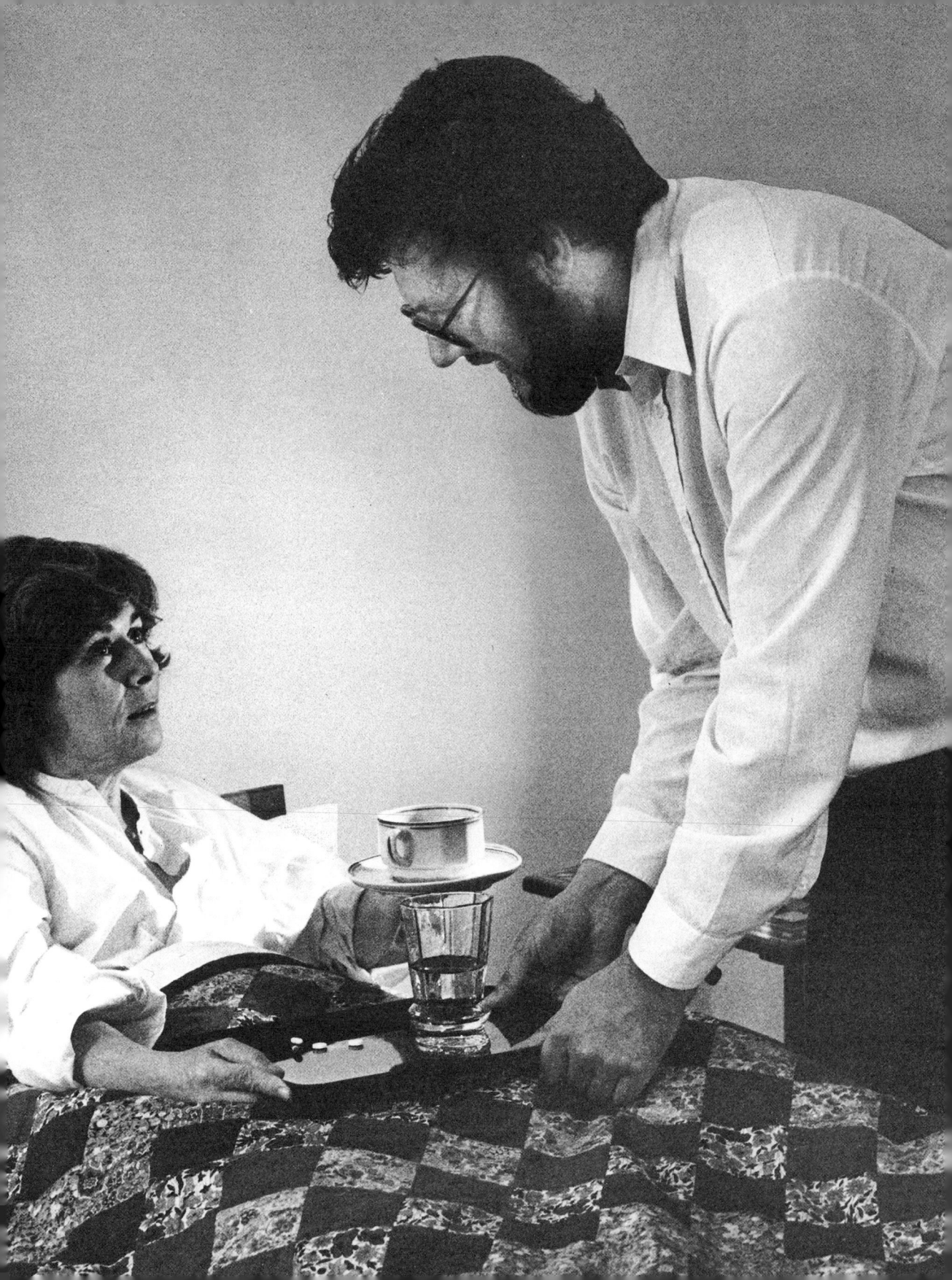

keep the wound clean and encourage healing. However, a sick person should only take these baths if advised to do so by the surgeon, doctor or other health professional.

Find out about the following details from your doctor.

☐ Exactly how long the sick person should stay in the bath in order for the additive to take effect.

☐ The correct temperature of the water and the exact amount of additive to be used.

☐ How often the patient should take this bath.

☐ How the patient's skin should react and when you can hope to see some improvement.

☐ What the signs of an adverse reaction are and what you should do if this occurs.

Shampoos

There are medicated shampoos on the market which help to clear dandruff. It is important to follow the manufacturer's and doctor's instructions precisely for effective results. Lice can also be treated effectively by shampooing the infected head with a specially formulated shampoo or a special lotion. These may be prescribed by the doctor, although some are available without prescription and may be obtained from the local chemist. A shampoo will usually have to be left on for a short time, and a lotion may have to be left on for as much as 12 hours. Treatment may have to be repeated again after a week. To prevent the spread of head lice, treat with shampoo as soon as possible and avoid contact with other people until treatment has taken effect.

Ear, nose and eye drops

Many drops are contained in plastic dropper bottles. Remove the cap and the upside-down bottle becomes a dropper. Do not contaminate the tip. Should contamination occur, clean twice with soap and water, rinsing after each wash, then drying. Some drops, however, come as a solution in a small bottle with a dropper – a glass tube with a rubber bulb on the end, which screws into the top of the bottle. When using such a dropper for the first time, fill it and raise it just above the level of the solution in the bottle to see how much pressure is required to produce a drop. Eye drops must be instilled with great care and very gently and should not be allowed to fall directly onto the cornea. Do not allow the dropper to touch the sick person's eye, skin or eyelashes. If the glass tube does get contaminated in this way do not return it to the bottle or reuse it. Rinse it out with boiling water and allow it to cool without touching anything. Do not reuse or replace it in the bottle until it has cooled. Always check how many drops should be given and in which ear, eye or nostril.

Eye ointments

The ointment usually comes in a small tube with an applicator at the end. To apply the ointment, pull down the lower lid and squeeze a thin layer of ointment along the inside of the lower lid.

INSTILLING EAR, NOSE AND EYE DROPS

Instilling ear drops
Ask the sick person to lie on her side with the affected ear uppermost. Hold the top of the affected ear and pull up and back as you instill the drops. This will straighten the ear canal and ensure that the drops have maximum effect. Ask the sick person to stay in this position for a few minutes. Massage the affected ear gently, just in front of the opening, to ensure that the drops have penetrated successfully.

Instilling nose drops
Ask the sick person to blow her nose gently and then to sit down with her head tipped back. Tilt the sick person's head slightly to one side when instilling the drops and hold the opposite nostril closed. Ask her to breathe in and out of her mouth and, as she does so, instil two or three drops (as prescribed) into each nostril. Ask her to keep her head tilted back for a few minutes following instillation of the drops.

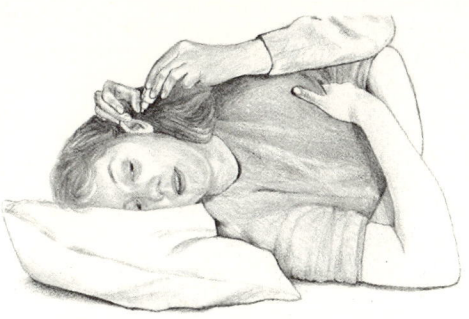

Instilling eye drops
Ask the sick person to sit or lie down and to look up. Place your index finger on her cheek just below the eye and gently draw down the lower lid away from the eye. Hold the dropper in your other hand about 5 cm (2 in) above the eye and allow one drop to fall into the lower part of the eye. Repeat as many times as required. Wipe her eyelashes with a disposable tissue or piece of gauze.

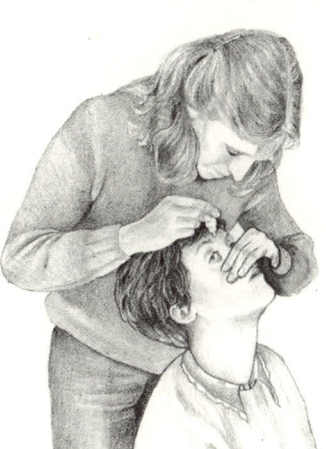

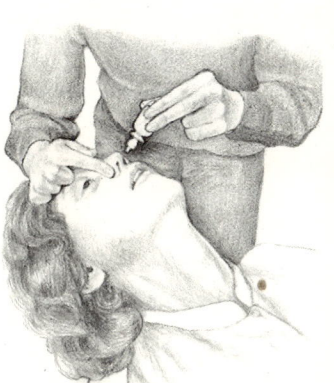

Heat treatment

Heat treatment has a soothing effect on the body: it helps to reduce muscle tension, relieves pain and encourages healing. There are various types of heat treatment in use but whichever you use, try to ensure that it cannot burn the patient or yourself. Stay with a sick person while he or she is having heat treatment.

A hot compress is a very effective way of applying heat to the body. A hot-water bottle on top of the compress keeps the compress hot for longer. A hot-water bottle can be used on its own to apply heat but take care to wrap the bottle in a pillowcase or small blanket if it does not already have a case. Heat can also be applied by using an electric blanket or pad, but make sure the appliance is safe and in good repair; do not use it anywhere near water.

Ultraviolet and heat lamps

If the doctor prescribes the use of a heat lamp or an ultraviolet or sunlamp, find out from him which part of the sick person's body should be exposed to the lamp and for how long and how far away the lamp should be. Write down the instructions and follow them carefully.

Make sure that you follow the manufacturer's instructions carefully too. A sick person receiving this type of heat treatment should always wear goggles to protect the eyes.

If the area being treated becomes red, painful or even blistered and swollen, this is a sign that the sick person's body is suffering from over-exposure to the lamp.

Cold compresses

A cold compress can be used to stop bleeding, reduce bruising and swelling and to relieve pain, as the cold causes the blood vessels to constrict. An ice bag has the same effect as a cold compress but remains cold for much longer and does not have to be changed so frequently. An alternative to making an ice bag is to buy a sealed ice bag from a department store. It will stay cold longer and is just as effective.

HOT AND COLD COMPRESSES

To make a compress, use a towel or a piece of lint folded double. For a hot compress, soak in water which is hot but not painful to touch, wring out and apply to the affected area. Replace when it becomes cool. For a cold compress, soak in ice-cold water, wring out and apply to the affected area. Replace as it becomes less cold.

To make an ice bag, fill a plastic or waterproof bag full of ice cubes or crushed ice. Remove any excess air and seal the bag. Wrap it in a cloth, so that any condensation which forms on the outside will not drip onto the sick person. Place the ice bag over the injury. Replace when necessary.

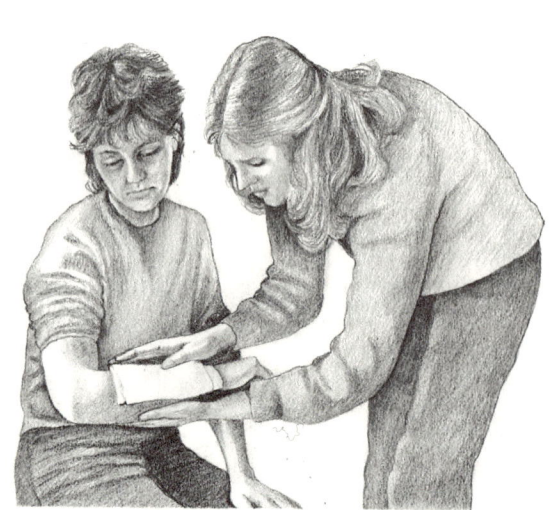

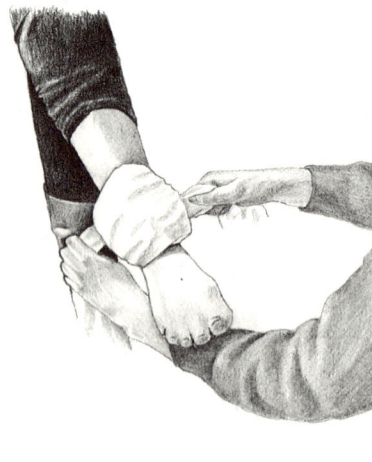

TEPID SPONGING

If a sick person's temperature reaches 40°C (104°F), sponging with tepid water is an effective way of bringing the fever down. Always check with your doctor before trying tepid sponging.

▶ This procedure should *never* be carried out on a baby under the age of 1 year without medical supervision or with cold water, as the child may go into shock.

Collect together
- Luke-warm water in a bowl
- One or two sponges or flannels
- A bath towel

1 Undress the sick person, lie her on a towel and fold back the bedclothes.

2 Check and record the sick person's temperature.

3 Soak the sponge in the tepid water and wring out some of the excess fluid; it should still be very wet.

4 Start at the sick person's head, and with long smooth strokes, sponge the entire body, gradually working downward. Try to let the sponge soak back up some of the water.

5 Do not allow the invalid to become chilled.

6 Check her temperature again during the sponging and stop when you have reduced the temperature by 1°C or 2°F. To continue may make her condition worse.

7 When you have finished sponging, pat her body dry with a towel and dress her in cool light clothes.

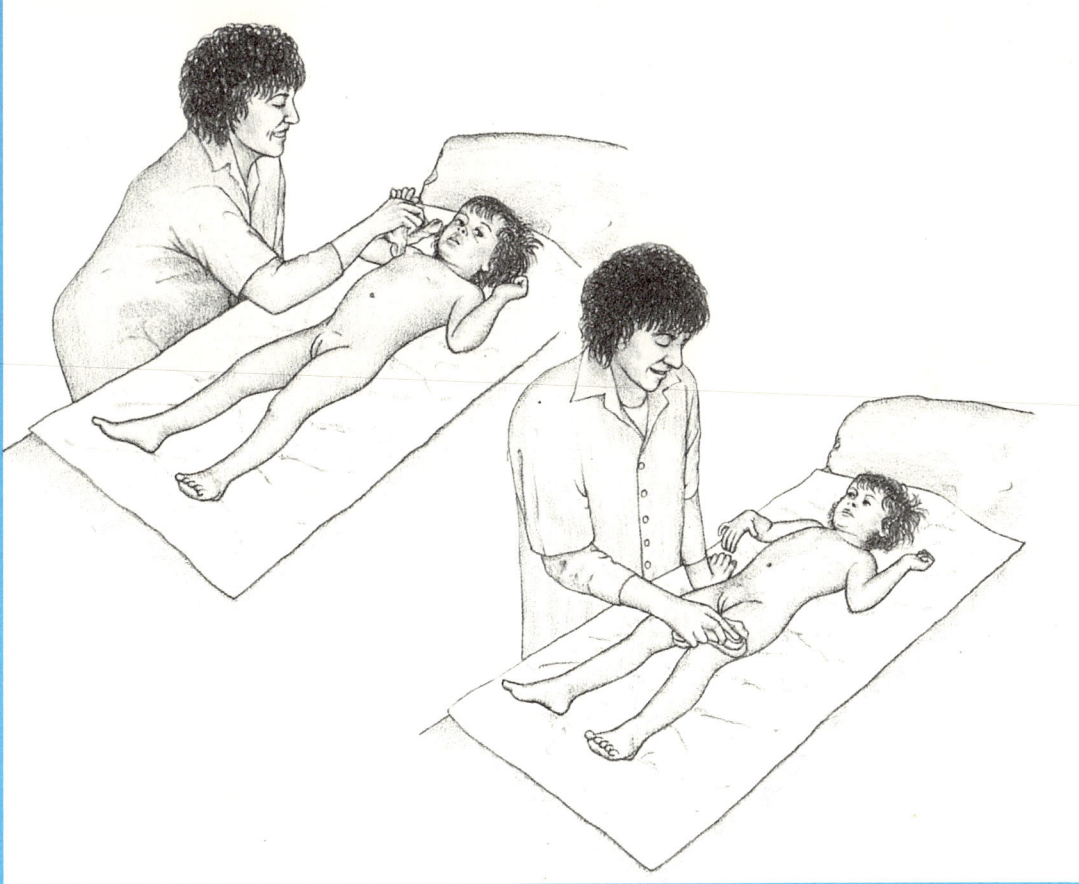

INHALATIONS

Inhalations are used to relieve a heavy cold, to clear a blocked sinus and to loosen a tight chest. Plain hot water is very effective but various substances, such as pine or eucalyptus oil or menthol crystals, can be added for increased effect. If menthol crystals are used, the instructions on the packet should be read carefully and care taken not to use more than the recommended dose.

Collect together
- Bowl
- Nearly boiling water, made up with 150 ml (5 oz) cold water and 450 ml (15 oz) boiling water
- Added inhalant, for example pine oil, eucalyptus or menthol crystals
- Towel
- Pot to spit into and tissues

Preparation

1 Explain to the sick person what you are going to do and tell her what she can do to help. Make sure she is warm and in a comfortable sitting position.

2 Wash and dry your hands.

3 Collect the above equipment and place it on a firm table or bedtable.

Inhaling

4 Place the bowl of water with added inhalant on the table in front of the patient.

5 Ask her to bend her head over the bowl and to breathe in through her mouth and out through her nose. She should continue inhaling like this for 15 minutes.

6 Make sure that there is a pot for her to spit into and tissues within her reach.

7 It is not necessary to place a towel over the sick person's head. By putting her head over the bowl, enough steam will be inhaled. If she does prefer to use a towel, there is no reason to stop her.

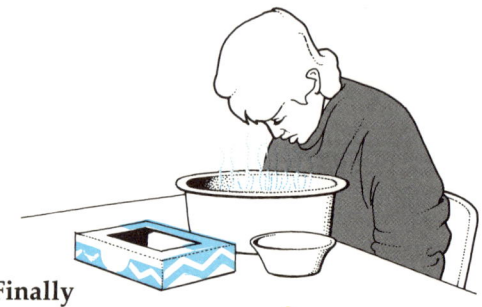

Finally

Dry her face with a towel and make sure she is comfortable. Clear away and clean all equipment and wash and dry your hands.

Pressurized aerosols

These are used for treating asthma and contain drugs which help to relieve the spasm which occurs in the airways (see page 168). The pressurized aerosol, if used correctly, can prevent or at least cut short an asthmatic attack. The sick person will need to be taught how to use the aerosol by a doctor or health professional. He or she should observe the following basic rules.

☐ The user should breathe out fully before placing his or her lips around the opening.

☐ He or she should release the metered dose at the start of a deep breath in through the mouth, then hold the breath for a short time to allow the drug to be absorbed.

☐ The dosage should be restricted to two puffs, inhaled one at a time – the second 5 minutes after the first, or as instructed by the doctor.

☐ Relief usually lasts about 3 to 4 hours. The dose should not be repeated more frequently than at 4-hourly intervals. If the inhaler has no effect, seek medical advice immediately.

Oxygen

All the cells in the body need oxygen. This is brought to them by the haemoglobin in the red blood cells which carries oxygen from the lungs to the body tissues. Haemoglobin is made up of protein and iron and combined with oxygen is called oxyhaemoglobin. This is a bright red substance and gives the skin its normal colour. Once the tissues have taken up the oxygen from the haemoglobin, it becomes reduced and darker in colour.

Too little oxygen and too much carbon dioxide make a person breathless and his or her skin takes on a bluish colour, especially at the tip of the nose and ears, lips, fingers and toes. This lack of oxygen can damage the tissues, especially those in the brain. The doctor may well prescribe oxygen therapy to correct this. Those who require oxygen may be suffering from a respiratory disease such as chronic bronchitis, from emphysema or from heart disease.

Oxygen is supplied in cylinders. A special attachment fitted to the top of the cylinder contains an indicator to tell you how much oxygen is in the cylinder; there is also a control device, so that you can give the oxygen at the correct rate, and a tap, with a special spanner or key for turning it, which should always be kept beside the cylinder. A length of tubing with an oxygen mask on the end of it is attached to the cylinder. Small portable cylinders are also available.

Safety points

The presence of concentrated oxygen in a confined space increases the risk of fire breaking out, so it is very important to take note of the following cautionary points.

☐ Do not smoke in the same room as the oxygen cylinder.

☐ Keep a fire extinguisher nearby.

☐ Cylinders should not be used near an open fire or gas flame, nor should they be used near lamps, radiators or other heating devices.

☐ Do not use electric appliances such as electric blankets, heating pads or razors anywhere near an oxygen cylinder.

☐ Nylon carpets can be a hazard as they produce static electricity and sparks. Bedclothes and nightclothes made of nylon also produce static electricity and are therefore a potential danger.

☐ Do not use oil or grease around the oxygen connectors which join the various pieces of equipment.

☐ Oxygen cylinders must be secured in a position where they will not be knocked or tripped over.

☐ Always store any spare oxygen cylinders in a cool area, preferably outside the person's home.

☐ Ask your doctor, chemist or pharmacist for advice on how many cylinders should be stored at any one time and where is the best place to store them.

☐ Explain the risks to any visitors and do not allow them to smoke.

Some systems of giving oxygen

If you have not given oxygen before, you can manage successfully if you follow the doctor's instructions closely. He will tell you which mask to use, at what rate and for what length of time. Do be sure that you ask the doctor if you are worried or uncertain about any part of the treatment. You can help to make the whole procedure a less frightening experience for the patient by observing the following points.

☐ Make sure the mask fits correctly and is comfortable.

☐ Explain to the sick person exactly what you want him or her to do.

☐ When the sick person first uses oxygen, stay with him or her for a while to provide reassurance and to observe any reactions. If the sick person is frightened stay there until he or she is calmer. Reassure the patient that the oxygen will help him or her to breathe more easily.

☐ Encourage the patient to breath fairly slowly and deeply.

☐ Change the mask and tubing frequently – preferably daily if you have enough supplies or as often as recommended by the doctor.

☐ Oxygen therapy leaves the sick person with a very dry mouth, so give plenty of fluids, if allowed, or frequent oral hygiene (see page 65).

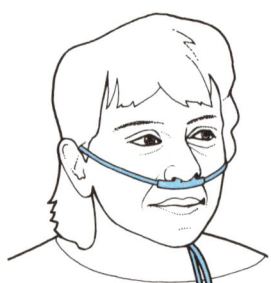

Nasal cannula

Nasal cannula

Most sick people prefer to have oxygen given this way as there is no need for a mask over the face and it is much more comfortable. A tube about 2cm (1in) long is inserted into the nose; it should be lubricated with water-soluble jelly beforehand. The flow of oxygen is usually set at about 4 to 6 litres per minute, or as prescribed by the doctor.

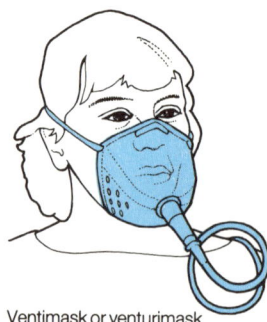

Ventimask or venturimask

Ventimask or venturimask

This method of giving oxygen is used for people suffering from chronic lung disease (see page 169). The masks give precise, controlled low oxygen concentrations and come in 24, 28, 32, 35, 40 and 50 per cent oxygen settings – this ensures that the percentage of oxygen to air given is correct. The oxygen flow rate is printed on the side of each mask. The side of the mask is perforated and the excess gas and carbon dioxide breathed out by the sick person escape through these perforations.

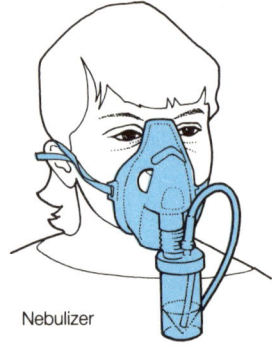

Nebulizer

Plastic face mask

This is a method of giving oxygen at a high concentration to someone with heart failure or suffering from low blood pressure. These masks are normally used only in hospital and a sick person at home is unlikely to use one.

Sometimes the oxygen may need to be moistened when high concentrations are being used. If your doctor suggests this, you will need to attach a humidifier to the cylinder head attachment. The humidifier contains water and the oxygen is moistened as it flows through the water to the sick person. Drugs may be prescribed to be given with the oxygen. The drug is measured and placed in a special container which replaces the humidifier, called a nebulizer. The oxygen then flows through the nebulizer, picking up the prescribed drug on its way.

Suppositories

Rectal suppositories are conical in shape and are made of substances that will melt when inserted into the rectum. They can contain drugs. In the treatment of migraine, for example, the drug is slowly absorbed through the rectum as the suppository dissolves.

They can also be used to produce a bowel action. Those most commonly in use stimulate the rectum and soften the contents by lubricating them. Unless the sick person is extremely constipated, they will take effect in about 15 minutes. Glycerine suppositories contain a small amount of glycerine and on melting provide good lubrication. A bowel action usually follows in about 30 minutes.

HOW TO GIVE A SUPPOSITORY

Collect together
- One or two suppositories, as prescribed
- A disposable glove or a finger stall
- A small bowl of warm water
- A gauze swab or square
- Paper or plastic bag in which to dispose of used materials
- Bedpan or commode and toilet paper

Preparation

1 Have a bedpan or commode and toilet paper near the bed.

2 Wash your hands.

3 Explain to the sick person what you are about to do.

4 Ask him to lie on one side with his knees drawn up toward his abdomen. Keep him covered with a blanket or sheet to avoid embarrassment and to give him warmth.

5 Put your glove or finger stall on. A finger stall should go on your index finger.

Inserting the suppository

6 Take the suppository out of its wrapping.

7 Dip the pointed end of the suppository into warm water.

8 Pass the suppository through the anus and up into the rectum, about the length of the index finger.

9 Remove your finger and wipe the sick person's anus with a gauze swab.

10 Discard the used swab and glove or finger stall into a bag.

11 Ask the sick person to retain the suppository for as long as he can, if possible for 15 minutes. Then help him to the toilet or onto the commode or bedpan.

12 Check to see what sort of bowel action he has had and note whether or not the suppository has been effective.

Finally

Make sure he is comfortable. Clear away the equipment and wash and dry your hands.

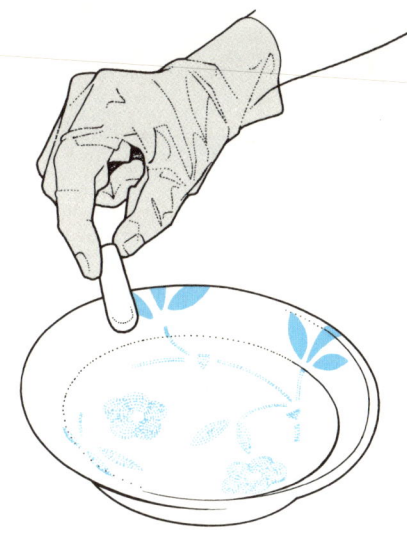

Enemas

An enema is the introduction of fluid into the bowel. It is used to empty the bowel and to give water and drugs. In the home the enema is most commonly used to empty a constipated bowel when suppositories have failed to work. A disposable enema is easy to use in the home and can be administered by the patient. It consists of a small plastic bag with a nozzle attached, containing about 150 ml (5 oz) of fluid.

Enemas should never be given unless advised by the doctor. The patient should first be encouraged to eat a diet containing substantial amounts of fibre and fluid and to take regular exercise. If the patient remains constipated, a mild laxative can be given and, if necessary, a suppository. Only when all of these methods have failed, is the doctor likely to recommend that an enema is given.

TO GIVE A DISPOSABLE ENEMA

Collect together
- A disposable enema pack placed in warm water about 40°c (104°F) – this should warm the enema to about 38°c (100°F]
- Disposable gloves
- Swab or square of gauze
- Lubricating jelly
- Plastic bag for disposal of rubbish
- Bedpan or commode and toilet tissue

Preparation

1 Place a bedpan or commode and toilet tissue beside the bed.

2 Wash and dry your hands and put on disposable gloves.

3 Explain to the sick person what you are about to do and ask her to turn onto her side as for giving a suppository.

Giving the enema

4 Remove the cap on the end of the enema nozzle and lubricate the end with a little lubricating jelly on a gauze square.

5 Dispose of the used gauze swab into the rubbish bag.

6 Insert the nozzle up into the rectum through the anus, and roll up the plastic bag so that the contents are expelled into the rectum.

7 Remove the nozzle and wipe the anus; put the empty enema bag into a rubbish bag.

8 Leave the sick person in a comfortable position and ask her to retain the enema for a few minutes at least, until the bowel is stimulated.

9 Help her onto the commode, bedpan or toilet, and observe the resulting bowel action.

Finally

Help the sick person back to bed or into a chair and ensure that she is comfortable. Clear away the equipment and wash and dry your hands.

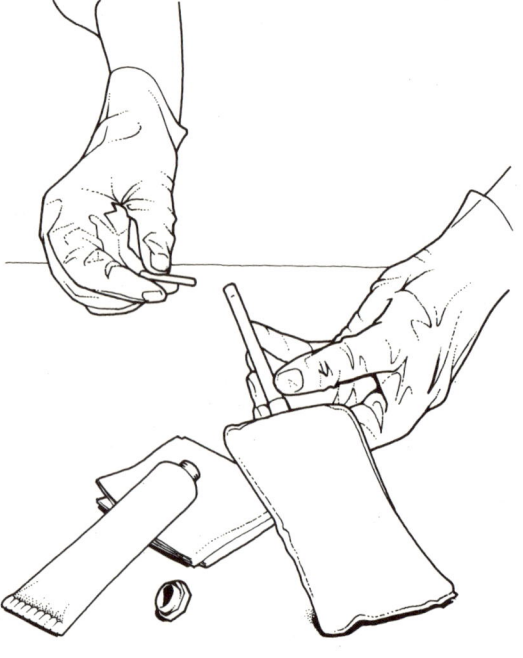

Administering medicines at home

Medicines or drugs are substances which are given to sick people as treatment for a disorder or to relieve symptoms of disease. They can be given by mouth in various forms. Alternatively, they can be injected, applied to the skin or can be given as pessaries.

General points

☐ Medicines prescribed for one individual should never be given to someone else who appears to be suffering from a similar complaint.

☐ A doctor will prescribe a certain amount of a medicine (the dose), to be given a certain number of times a day for a prescribed length of time. These instructions should be strictly adhered to or the sick person may get too little or too much of the drug and this will affect his or her response to the treatment.

☐ Always finish a course of treatment that has been prescribed, even if the sick person seems to be recovering.

☐ Never increase a dose if you feel a drug is not having the required effect. Talk to the doctor about it and discuss the problem.

☐ When a sick person has finished a course of prescribed medicine, throw away any left-over drugs.

☐ Always check for use-by-dates on over-the-counter medicines and throw away any which are over the recommended date. Medicines stored for long periods lose their potency or become dangerous.

☐ Ask your chemist for advice on correct disposal of medicines. Do not just throw them into the dustbin. If you cannot get advice, flush them down the toilet.

☐ If you know the sick person is allergic to a drug, make sure that the doctor is aware of this. Make sure that the doctor knows what other medicines the sick person is taking as some medicines may change their action when combined with others.

☐ If you are responsible for someone taking his or her medicine, you should ask the doctor about possible side-effects. Some people are allergic to certain medicines and may suffer symptoms such as nausea and vomiting, dizziness, diarrhoea, skin rashes, itching, extreme restlessness, headaches and confusion. There may be swelling of the ankles and legs or a sudden change in behaviour. If any of these signs or symptoms occur, consult the doctor.

☐ All medicines should be stored in a locked cupboard out of reach of children. Some medicines are attractively coloured and children may mistake them for sweets.

☐ Always read the label and check that you are giving the right dose at the right time to the right person.

☐ Never leave a bottle of tablets beside a sick person's bed, especially night sedation. It is so easy to wake in the night, forget that you have already taken your sleeping pills and take some more.

Oral medicines

Liquid form

Liquid medicines should be measured into a medicine glass, into a plastic measure or onto a teaspoon. Protect the label with the palm of your hand when you are pouring the liquid to prevent any of it dripping onto the label and making it messy and difficult to read. Hold the medicine glass at eye level so you can see exactly how much you are pouring in. Some mixtures are in suspension and will need to be shaken well. If the medicine tastes unpleasant, follow it with some fruit or a favourite drink.

Tablets or capsules, or other forms

Tip the tablet or capsule onto a spoon or into a medicine glass without touching it. Ask the sick person to place the tablet or capsule on the back of his or her tongue and to swallow it with a mouthful of water. Some tablets are designed to be put under the tongue until dissolved. Capsules should be swallowed whole and not broken open or chewed. Large tablets can be broken in half or crushed between two spoons and mixed with jam or jelly. Some tablets are designed to be dissolved in water. Check how much water should be added beforehand.

Powders can be stirred into water or put on the tongue and swallowed with a drink. Check with the doctor which method is appropriate.

Pastilles are drugs in a flavoured gelatine base and should be sucked.

Lozenges are drugs in a compressed form. They are usually flavoured and designed to be sucked.

Linctuses are syrupy liquids, containing drugs, and should be given undiluted for the best effect. They have the disadvantage of causing dental decay due to their high sugar content, so regular oral hygiene is especially important.

ANTIBIOTICS

Antibiotics are used to treat infections. There are many different kinds on the market and each one is used to treat a specific infection.

Special points

- Antibiotics are not necessarily given for all infections
- They should always be prescribed by a doctor
- Always give an antibiotic at the time stated and in the correct dose or they may not be as effective against the infection
- Always complete the entire course of antibiotics or the drug may not have the required effect and the infection may return. Even if the sick person feels better after a few doses of the antibiotic, he or she must still complete the course

- Check with the doctor that none of the drugs already being taken by the sick person will conflict in their activity with the antibiotic
- If the sick person is allergic to penicillin or any other antibiotic, make sure the doctor is aware of the fact

Some common side effects

- Skin rashes and raised temperature
- Diarrhoea. If the patient is female and taking an oral contraceptive, the effectiveness of the contraceptive may be impaired as long as the diarrhoea continues. It is therefore necessary to use some other form of contraceptive for the rest of the cycle
- Thrush in the mouth or vagina. Thrush is a fungal infection which produces white patches on the tongue, gums and even the throat

Medicines for the skin

The following are medicines for external use only and should not be taken by mouth.

Lotions are solutions which, when applied to the skin, have a cooling effect as they evaporate. They may come in the form of a suspension – an insoluble substance suspended in liquid. Use a piece of gauze to dab it onto the skin: do not use your fingers.

Creams are thin ointments which can be directly applied to affected areas. Use a piece of gauze to apply the cream to the skin.

Antibiotic powders can be put directly onto infected areas.

Pastes are thick, porous and absorbent and should be applied by using a gauze swab or a wooden spatula.

Liniments are drugs in an oily base and should be applied with a gauze swab or square.

Ointments are greasy and heavy and should be applied using a gauze swab or square.

By injection

The injection most usually given at home is insulin, used commonly in the treatment of diabetes (see page 180). Even quite young children can learn to inject insulin.

Anyone needing an injection will be given a demonstration by his or her doctor or another health professional.

By vagina

Pessaries are drugs in a fatty base which are similar in shape but smaller than suppositories. They are inserted as high into the vagina as possible. The best time to insert them is before going to bed to sleep – this allows the drug prolonged contact with the upper part of the vagina, during which time it can be absorbed.

FAMILY MEDICINE CABINET

The cabinet should be kept locked and well out of reach of children. A typical family medicine cabinet may contain:

- Paracetamol for adults and children – for relief of fever or pain

  Aspirin is no longer given to children, as it may cause Reyes syndrome. It should never be taken by anyone with a tendency to bleed, a history of gastric problems or taking anticoagulants. If in doubt, ask your doctor or chemist for advice.

- Kaolin mixture – for diarrhoea. This should not be given to babies or toddlers
- An antacid such as aluminium hydroxide – for minor stomach aches and pains

- A cough mixture, such as linctus simplex, for painful dry coughs, although a warm drink with honey also works well
- Vapour rub – to make steam inhalations or rub on chests for dry coughs and sore throats
- Antiseptic cream – for septic spots and sores
- Aqueous cream – for minor rashes
- Calamine lotion – for dabbing on rashes, bites and stings
- A few packets of sterile gauze swabs
- Plasters of various sizes and shapes
- Packet of paper tissues
- Packet of cotton-wool
- Thermometer
- Eyebath
- A pair of tweezers
- 5 ml dosage spoon
- A measuring glass
- A pair of hand scissors

Diet and Nutrition

Eating a well-balanced, healthy diet is important for everyone's physical and mental well-being. A convalescent needs a wholesome, nutritious diet to regain strength and to build up resistance to further disease. A sick person may well suffer from a temporary loss of appetite, and as caregiver, it is as well to allow yourself to be guided to a certain extent by your patient's likes and dislikes – a loss of appetite may be a clear indication that the body is not yet ready for food. When the sick person starts to feel hungry again, offer food which you know he or she will like and try to make meals as attractive and varied as possible. At the same time, take care not to forget your own needs and those of the rest of the family and try to adapt meals so that they are suitable for everyone. Rich sauces, strong seasonings and flavourings can be added once the invalid's portion has been removed. Certain foods may aggravate the sick person's condition and should be avoided; the sick person's doctor may refer him or her to a qualified dietitian who will advise on any such restrictions (see the chapter on **Medical and Surgical Problems**).

For a chronically sick person confined to bed, meals should be light and contain sufficient fibre to prevent constipation resulting from inactivity (see page 171). Small, appetizing meals given at regular intervals can help to break up and brighten an otherwise uneventful day.

Basic nutritional requirements

Our bodies need food for energy and warmth, and for growth, repair and replacement of body tissues. Children in particular need a varied, nutritious diet to maintain their growth rate. Nutritional requirements vary according to age, activity and state of health, but in general a healthy diet should contain reasonable amounts of protein, fibre, minerals and vitamins but not too much fat or sugar. Health professionals are now recognizing the fundamental role that a healthy diet has to play in the prevention of many illnesses.

Basic recommendations for a healthy diet include cutting down on refined carbohydrates such as sugar, limiting intake of fat and salt and increasing intake of whole grains, cereals, fresh vegetables and fruit. Addictive stimulants such as caffeine (found in tea, coffee and cola drinks) and alcohol should be taken only in limited quantities, if at all. Processed foods containing preservatives, colouring and flavouring should be avoided whenever possible, as some of these additives are suspected of aggravating allergies and other health problems. There is an increasing range of additive-free convenience foods, which are useful.

To function normally, the body requires a minimal amount of dietary fat, but most people in developed countries eat far more than they need, increasing their vulnerability to heart disease and other complaints. Salt, if taken in excess, can aggravate a tendency to high blood pressure and is best used sparingly by adults and not at all by babies and young children. Wholefoods, fresh vegetables and fruit all have a high vitamin,

Mealtimes with the sick person can become enjoyable social occasions for the whole family: even if you do not eat at the same time, you may like to sit and talk as the invalid eats.

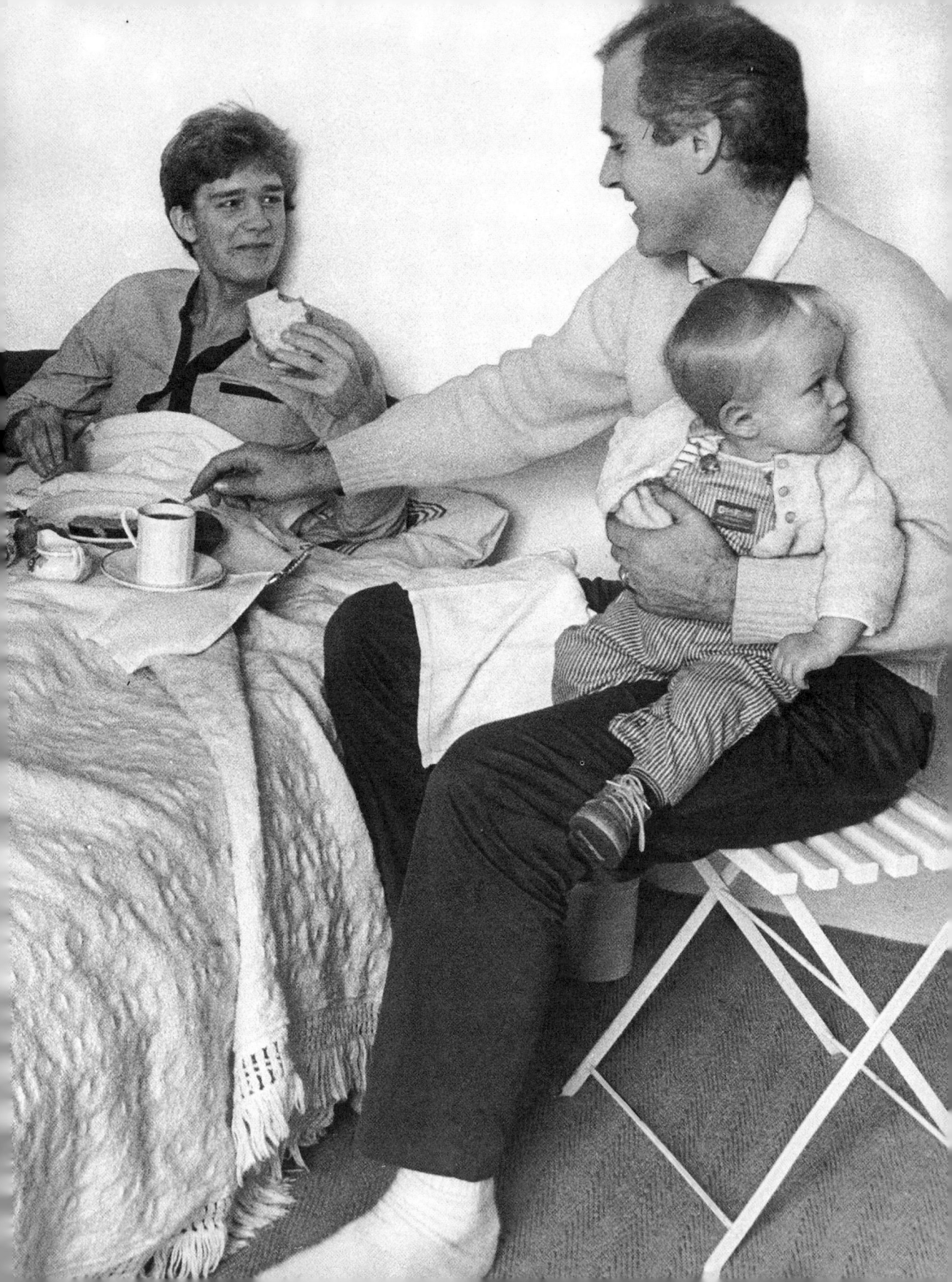

mineral and fibre content and should be eaten whenever possible instead of refined and processed foods. Dietary fibre is now considered to have an important role to play in the prevention of cancer of the intestine and heart disease. You can increase your intake of dietary fibre by eating wholemeal bread and pasta, brown rice, pulses and beans, muesli, bran and plenty of fruit and vegetables. A healthy diet should

NUTRIENT	REQUIRED FOR	SOURCES	DEFICIENCY MAY LEAD TO
Carbohydrate: sugar, starch and cellulose, or fibre	Energy	All foods made with flour, cereals and bread, fruit and vegetables, nuts and pulses	Malnutrition
Protein	Strong bones, growth and repair of muscle tissue	Animal protein: meat, poultry, fish, eggs, milk and cheese. Vegetable protein: peas, baked beans, lentils, nuts, cereals and root vegetables	Poor growth and malnutrition
Fat	Energy	Butter, milk, cheese, oils from fish and vegetable sources and meat	Loss of fat-soluble vitamins (A, D, E, K)
Water	Essential for the life of all body cells and involved in nearly all bodily functions	Nearly all food contains water, especially fruit and vegetables	Dehydration
Calcium	Healthy development of bones and teeth, blood clotting and normal nerve and muscle function	Yoghurt and milk, cheese, bread, tinned fish, and green leafy vegetables	Twitching muscles and cramps. Osteomalacia (softening of the bones). Rickets in children where bone growth is delayed
Iron	Prevention of anaemia (vitamin C aids absorption)	Red meat, liver, eggs, cereals, pulses, green vegetables and wholemeal bread	Iron deficiency anaemia – symptoms include fatigue, headaches, poor concentration and lowered resistance to infection. Those at risk include menstruating women, alcoholics and those suffering from bleeding piles and ulcers
Salt	Maintenance of the water balance in the body and to regulate muscle and nerve activity	Many types of food	Cramps

also contain a sufficient quantity of water – the average adult requires 3 litres (5 pt) daily, of which 1.5 litres (2.5 pt) should be taken as drinks. Mineral water, fruit juices and herb teas are excellent drinks, containing no refined sugar, fat or additives.

The chart below tells you which foods contain which nutrients, and how deficiencies affect the body.

NUTRIENT	REQUIRED FOR	SOURCES	DEFICIENCY MAY LEAD TO
Vitamin A	Growth and resistance to infection	Fats, fish-liver oils, dairy products, carrots, tomatoes and dark green leafy vegetables	Night blindness. Infections of the mucous membranes of the nose, throat and gastrointestinal tract
Vitamin B complex	Healthy development, maintenance of nerve cells and red blood corpuscles	All types of vitamin B are found in wholemeal bread, oats, kidney, liver and dairy products. This vitamin is water-soluble and can be destroyed in cooking	Cracks and dermatitis around the mouth, nose. lips and eyes. Anaemia. In extreme cases, beri-beri and pellagra
Vitamin C	Wound healing, growth and development of bones	Breast and formula milk. Orange and blackcurrant juice. Most fruit and vegetables, although cooking can destroy this water-soluble vitamin	Poor resistance to infection and poor healing. Swollen, bleeding gums. Pains in limbs and joints, generalized anaemia. Prolonged deficiency leads to scurvy
Vitamin D	Regulates calcium absorption	Herrings, sardines, eggs and dairy products. The body manufactures vitamin D when exposed to sunlight, although dark-skinned people living in cold climates manufacture less Vitamin D than light-skinned people	Rickets and stunted growth in young children. Osteomalacia (softening of the bones) in adults
Vitamin E	Its function is not fully understood	Wheatgerm, wheatgerm oils, soya beans, nuts, seeds, green leafy vegetables, eggs, fish and meat	
Vitamin K	Normal blood clotting	Leafy green vegetables, cereals, milk, eggs and polyunsaturated fats	Tendency to bleed

Coping with loss of appetite

If the person you are caring for is suffering from a temporary loss of appetite, the sort of diet most likely to appeal is what is known as a light diet – easily digestible, containing plenty of nourishment and very little bulk. It should also contain enough fibre to prevent the sick person becoming constipated. The following list gives a selection of foods which can be included in the diet and those which are difficult to digest and therefore best avoided.

Foods to include

- Lean meat, fish, poultry and eggs
- Savoury dishes made with milk, milk puddings and cheese
- Beef and vegetable extracts served as clear soups, or chicken soup with brown rice
- Wholemeal bread, scones and crispbreads
- Vegetables, unsweetened fruit juices and fruit such as honeydew melon, grapes, puréed dried apricots, sultanas, prunes, baked eating apples and poached pears
- Vegetable juices served hot or cold with dry toast or crispbread

Foods to avoid

- Any foods which the sick person dislikes
- Boiled cabbage, sprouts, turnips, cucumber and unripe melon
- Fried and fatty foods, including pork, ham, gammon and other fatty meats
- Overcooked meats
- Raw onions
- Smoked and highly spiced or highly seasoned foods
- Any other food that adversely affects the sick person

Useful hints

☐ Encourage the sick person to eat simply cooked food, either grilled, baked, steamed or boiled. Do not spend hours slaving over a hot stove making elaborate, rich food as it will probably not be eaten.

☐ Always try to select a menu which you know will please.

☐ Always grill food rather than frying it. Someone confined to bed and unable to take exercise will have difficulty digesting greasy foods and the extra calories can lead to weight gain.

☐ Serve up small portions of attractive-looking food, taking care with presentation and using garnishing for added colour and interest. Never use chipped or cracked plates or glasses and make sure that any cutlery or linen you use is clean.

☐ Make sure the sick person has been to the toilet, washed his or her hands and is comfortable, before taking in a meal.

☐ Encourage the sick person to take time over and enjoy meals. If he or she enjoys eating with you, bring in your own meal on a tray.

☐ If a sick person really does not want to eat, buy a fortified milk drink from the chemist. Available in sweet or savoury form, these drinks are useful as a temporary source of nutrients but should be given in moderation, as their bland taste can blunt the sick person's appetite for other foods. Other fluids must be taken in addition to prevent dehydration.

Helping a sick person to eat

Some sick people will have difficulty feeding themselves. Someone recovering from a stroke, for instance, will probably need to be fed by you to begin with. The following suggestions may help you to make the meal a more pleasant experience.

□ Make sure the sick person is sitting in a comfortable, upright position.

□ Sit down on a chair next to the bed and place a napkin across his or her shoulders.

□ Using a dessert spoon or fork, gently but firmly put a small amount of food into the sick person's mouth.

□ Allow time to chew and swallow before offering the next mouthful. Do not feed the sick person so slowly that he or she becomes bored and loses interest, nor so fast that you risk choking him or her.

□ Make sure that the food stays hot by covering dishes or using a hotplate if you have one.

□ Offer a drink at least once during a meal.

□ Make sure that you know what to do if an invalid does choke on food (see page 201).

It is important for the sick person's dignity and self-respect that he or she is able to eat independently again as soon as possible. If the patient has difficulty holding a knife or fork, make use of some of the ideas for modified cutlery shown below.

Manufactured eating aids

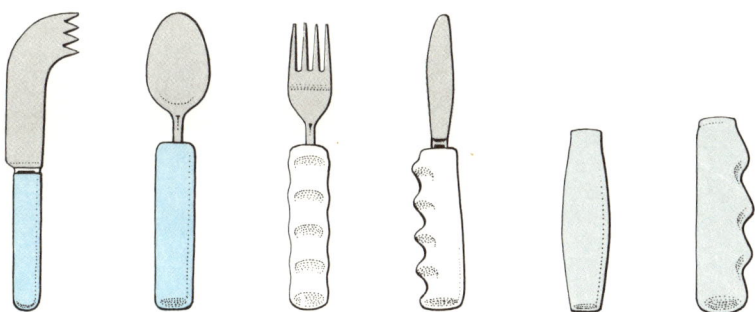

Improvised eating aids

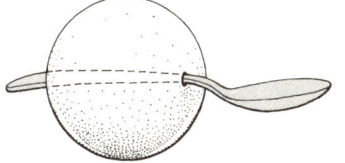

Using a spoon pushed through the centre of a rubber ball

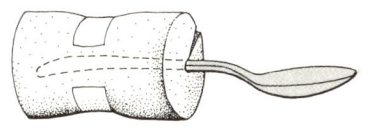

Using a spoon with foam rubber taped around the handle

Feeding sick children

Sick children often have no desire to eat. There is no need to be alarmed if this is the case, as a sick child will come to no harm without food for a few days, as long as he or she continues to drink plenty of fluids.

Useful hints

☐ Encourage a sick child to drink by offering a refreshing drink in a brightly coloured cup, with perhaps a curly straw for added attraction. Well-diluted, unsweetened fruit juice, mixed vegetable juice or a hot fruit drink are all acceptable drinks for a sick child. Bottled or filtered water often has a better taste than tap water.

☐ Offer something to drink at least every 2 hours and more frequently if the child requests it.

A SAMPLE DAY'S MENU FOR A SICK CHILD

Breakfast
Unsweetened apple juice
Porridge or muesli and milk
Fresh fruit

Midday meal
Scrambled egg and wholemeal toast
with grilled tomato,
lightly cooked mushrooms,
carrots and peas
Orange juice jelly
Blended banana and yoghurt drink

Evening meal
Home-made chicken broth with
ABC pasta and wholemeal bread
Fresh fruit and yoghurt
Warm malted milk

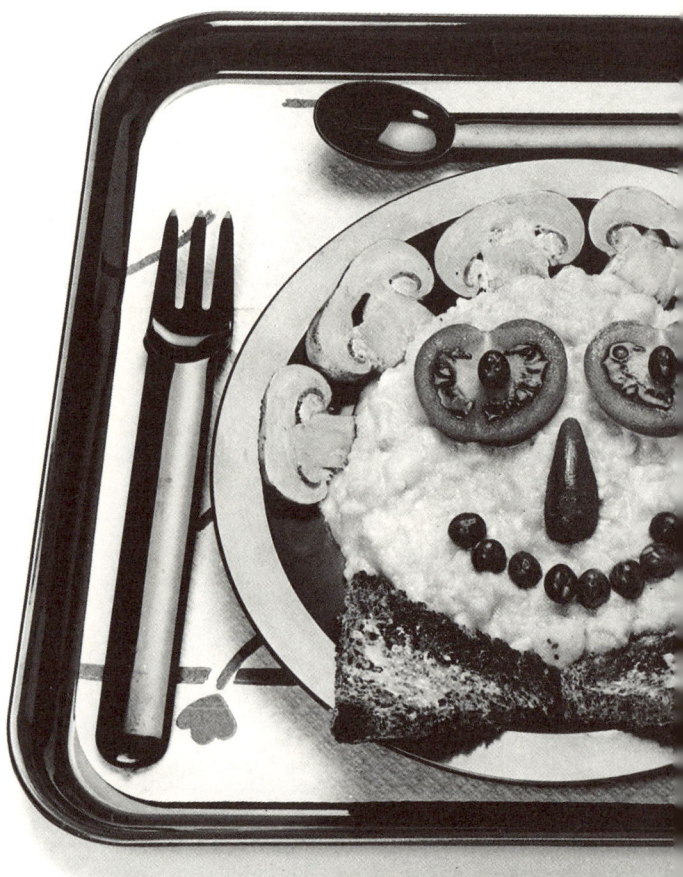

□ Avoid giving a sick child fizzy drinks as the sugar content is likely to increase any feeling of nausea.

□ Avoid giving drinks which contain artificial colours, flavouring or preservatives. The orange colouring tartrazine has been linked by some doctors with behavioural problems in children.

□ Let the child's own appetite act as a guide to the sort of food you offer him or her to eat, unless a special diet has been prescribed by the doctor. A sick child may want to eat only jelly or ice cream, or may prefer just a dry biscuit or toast.

□ Once appetite has been regained, offer a well-balanced diet to help rebuild the child's strength and stamina.

Blend together one banana (peeled and cut into pieces) and one cup of yoghurt, with honey to taste

Stir 3 teaspoonfuls of agar agar or 1½ teaspoonfuls of gelatine into ½ pint (0.25 litres) of orange juice and turn into a mould to set

Use mushrooms, tomatoes, carrots and peas for the hair, nose, eyes and mouth

Feeding the elderly An elderly person's diet may be inadequate for a variety of reasons. Loss of the sensation of taste, badly fitting dentures or a sore mouth may lead to a poor appetite. Alternatively, an elderly person may be unable to afford to eat properly, have difficulty in getting to the shops or problems with preparing food – in any of these cases a doctor will be able to advise on what help is available. If the person you are caring for is elderly, encourage him or her to eat a well-balanced, nourishing diet and help the person identify and prepare such a diet.

Useful hints

☐ Protein in the form of meat, eggs, cheese or lentils should be an important element in the diet. Encourage two helpings of these protein-rich foods a day, plus 0.6 litre (1 pt) of milk to be taken in drinks, puddings or soups.

☐ Give a serving of any or a combination of the following at least once a day: lightly cooked, fresh, leafy green vegetables; root vegetables such as carrots, swedes or potatoes; tomatoes or fresh fruit.

☐ Foods that contain fibre help to prevent constipation and other

**A SAMPLE DAY'S MENU
FOR AN ELDERLY PERSON**

Breakfast
Fresh orange juice
Porridge or other high-fibre cereal
with milk
Wholemeal toast with butter or margarine
and preserve
Tea or coffee

Midday meal
Macaroni cheese with lightly
cooked carrots and broccoli
Yoghurt and baked pears
Tea or coffee

Evening meal
Grilled fish, baked potato and
spinach
Cheese and biscuits or fresh fruit
Warm malted milk

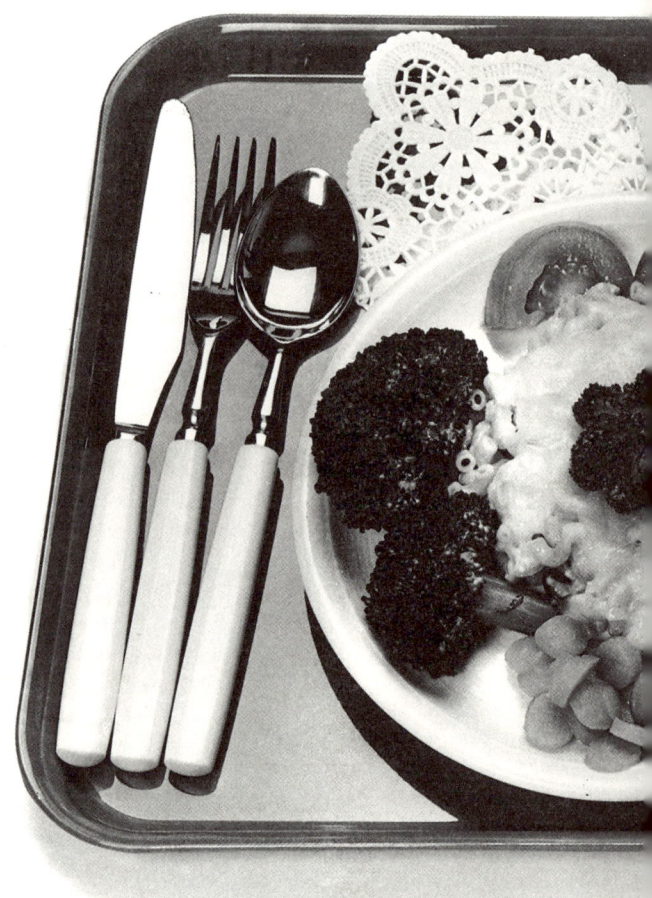

digestive disorders. Bran is most effective when served with milk or cooked with soup, stew or porridge. It should never be given dry as it will swell in the stomach and cause discomfort.

☐ Preserves, cakes, pastry, fried foods, buttered potatoes and sugar all provide energy but should only be given in moderation or the sick person may become overweight and will find it harder to keep fit and mobile.

☐ Give plenty of fluids in the form of juices, soup, milk, plain water and moderate amounts of weak tea and coffee. The use of strong tea and coffee should be discouraged as the high caffeine content can lead to disturbed sleep, heart palpitations and indigestion.

☐ If he or she is used to drinking alcohol occasionally, allow this to continue in moderation if the doctor permits it. *Never* give alcohol to an elderly person if he or she is suffering from extreme cold (see page 136).

☐ Encourage an elderly person to eat small meals frequently and at least one good meal a day containing a sufficient quantity of protein, vegetables and whole grain cereal.

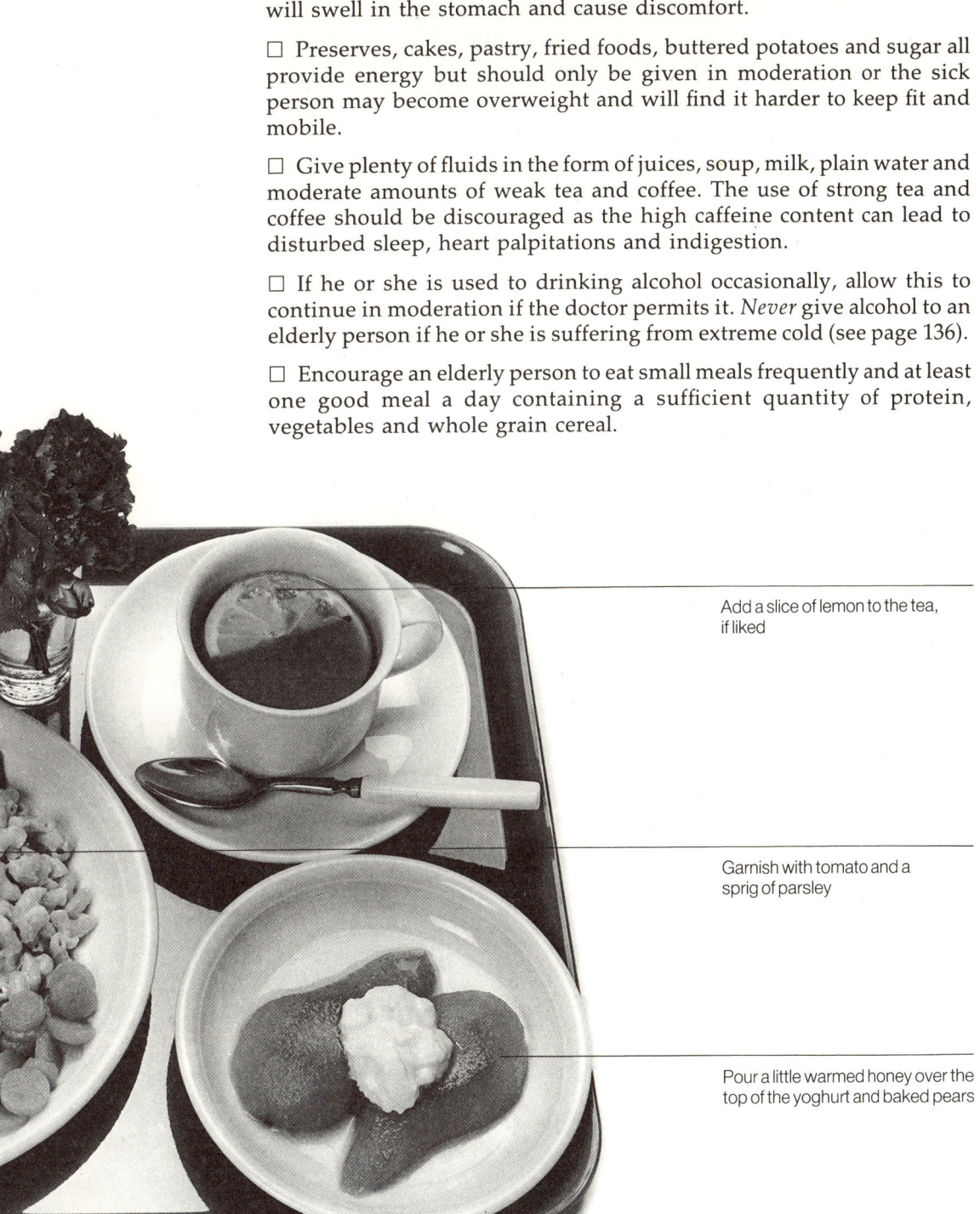

Add a slice of lemon to the tea, if liked

Garnish with tomato and a sprig of parsley

Pour a little warmed honey over the top of the yoghurt and baked pears

Special diets

The person you are caring for may require a special diet for a variety of reasons: simply to gain or lose weight or as part of the treatment for a condition in which it is essential that certain foods are excluded from the diet, or eaten only in moderation. If this is the case, the doctor will prescribe a special diet and refer the sick person to a dietitian who will give detailed instructions on how to manage the diet (see the chapter on **Medical and Surgical Problems**). The following list outlines some of the more common diets recommended.

To regain weight

A sick person who has lost a great deal of weight because of an illness needs a short breaking-in period when the extra calories and protein needed are given in a concentrated, easily digestible, liquid form. Fortified milk feeds can be bought from the chemist and are supplemented with a wide range of nutrients. Glucose is a useful way of increasing energy intake as it is less sweet than sugar and can be added to food in larger amounts; other substitutes containing concentrated amounts of calories are available on prescription and have an advantage over glucose in that they are less likely to cause diarrhoea.

After this breaking-in period, the sick person can continue with a normal diet and should be encouraged to eat high calorie foods until the necessary weight has been regained. Nutritious foods with a high calorie content include cheese, milk, nuts, seeds, dried fruits and homebaked, whole grain pastries.

To reduce weight

A sick person may be overweight from eating too many sugary foods or drinking too much alcohol and, by cutting down on these, will automatically lose weight. However, if this is not the case, the sick person will need to eat a low-calorie diet – low in fat and refined carbohydrates and preferably high in fibre. Buying a calorie chart will enable you to choose foods of low calorific value but you must make sure that the diet you have chosen can be realistically adhered to and that it supplies all the essential nutrients. Crash diets are often unbalanced and lacking in essential nutrients and can have adverse effects on the sick person's metabolism over a long period. The sick person should aim to lose around 1 kg (2 lb) per week.

Whether the sick person is trying to lose or regain weight, record his or her weight at the beginning of each week.

Chronic diarrhoea

If the person you are caring for is suffering from chronic diarrhoea, tell the doctor immediately so that a cause can be established. He may prescribe a special diet and will probably advise the sick person to avoid highly seasoned foods and perhaps milk products.

Constipation

A sick person suffering from constipation should check with the doctor on appropriate dietary measures. However, it is generally a good idea to include a substantial amount of roughage in the daily diet. Encourage an increased intake of wholemeal bread, whole grain cereal foods and plenty of fruit and vegetables. Prunes, figs, oranges and rhubarb all have a laxative effect. Adding cooked or moistened bran to food and drinking plenty of water will also help.

Raised temperature

A sick person with a raised temperature is likely to sweat a great deal and should therefore drink plenty of fluid, even if he or she does not feel like eating anything. Offer a choice of nourishing drinks at least every 2 hours. Offer fruit drinks frequently, with added glucose if necessary. Make sure that plenty of water, slightly chilled, is readily available.

If the sick person is becoming dehydrated owing to a lack of fluid, his or her skin will feel dry. Pinch a little of the skin on the back of the sick person's hand and, if well-hydrated, the skin will quickly fall back into place; if the sick person is becoming dehydrated, the skin will have lost some of its elasticity and will remain pinched together longer. However, dry skin in an elderly person is not a reliable indication of dehydration as skin automatically loses moisture and elasticity with age.

After surgery

If the sick person has not been put on a special diet by the doctor prior to the operation, diet should be monitored so that he or she is neither overweight nor underweight. After the operation, the sick person will need carbohydrate and fat for energy and protein, vitamins and trace elements, such as zinc, to repair and replace affected tissues; and all the other components of a well-balanced diet, including sufficient fluids. If he or she is not eating solid foods, any fluids given should supply the required nutrients in the form of liquidized or puréed foods, fortified meat broths, milk drinks and real fruit and vegetable juices.

When the appetite is so poor that sufficient of these nutrients are not taken, specially formulated drinks are available as a high calorie supplement or replacement for the day's meals. The aim should always be to return the sick person to a normal diet as soon as possible.

SAMPLE MENUS FOR SPECIAL DIETS

**SAMPLE MAIN MEAL
FOR REGAINING WEIGHT**
Pineapple juice
Scrambled egg, creamed fish or chicken
or cheese and onion flan with vegetables
and mashed potato
Homemade wholemeal apple pie

**SAMPLE BREAKFAST
FOR CONSTIPATION**
Fruit juice
High-fibre cereal with bran and milk
Wholemeal toast with butter or margarine
and preserve
Fresh fruit

**SAMPLE MAIN MEAL
FOR REDUCING WEIGHT**
50 to 80 g (2 to 3 oz) of grilled meat or fish
Lightly cooked carrots and one potato
Fruit – fresh or stewed without sugar
A hot drink with skimmed milk

**SAMPLE MAIN MEAL
FOR A RAISED TEMPERATURE**
Strained chicken soup
Grilled fillet of plaice, grilled tomatoes and
a small helping of creamed potato
Fruit dessert or fresh fruit

**SAMPLE BREAKFAST
FOR CHRONIC DIARRHOEA**
Fruit juice or water
Soft scrambled egg
White toast with margarine and preserve

**SAMPLE MAIN MEAL
FOR AFTER SURGERY**
Orange juice or vegetable soup
Grilled fish, savoury mince, roast meat or
braised liver with vegetables
Rice pudding with fruit or a fruit dessert
Milk or water

Special Needs

Whoever you are caring for, you have to be aware of that person's individual needs and preferences. However, some groups have particular needs in common – this chapter discusses the special needs of children and babies, of the elderly, of the handicapped or disabled, and of invalids who are terminally ill. Nursing someone in any of these categories has particular difficulties and requires particular skills; it is also often especially emotionally demanding. Support groups can be very helpful in providing a place to share problems and to learn from others in the same situation as yourself. The chapter on **Medical and Surgical Problems** gives you more detailed information about the nursing needed for each particular health problem.

SICK BABIES AND CHILDREN

One of the main problems about caring for a young child, especially a baby, who is sick is that it may be very difficult to find out what is wrong or how the child is feeling. It can also be difficult to explain to a child what is likely to be involved in a treatment for an illness, or to persuade a young one to accept whatever medicine, treatment or restrictions are necessary.

Calling the doctor

It can be particularly hard to know whether to call the doctor if you have a young child who seems a little below par – who is perhaps unusually fretful, or who has passed an abnormal-looking stool, for example. Waiting for a few hours to see how the situation develops often helps to clarify your choice. If the child is pale, listless, has no interest in favourite foods or does not want to play, you can be fairly sure that something is wrong. Remember that parents are usually the best judge of how sick their child is: after all, you know what he or she is like when well. On the whole, if the child looks and seems well, it is unlikely that there is anything seriously wrong. However, some symptoms do call for medical attention, either immediately or within the course of a day or two; how urgent they are depends on the age of the child. Whatever the situation, if you are worried, you should feel free to call your doctor to discuss the problem.

When a baby should see a doctor

Contact your doctor urgently if your baby has any of the following signs or symptoms. If you are unable to get in touch with your doctor, take your baby, wrapped up in a blanket or shawl, by car or taxi to the nearest hospital with an accident and emergency department. Failing this, call an ambulance:

Warmth and closeness with others can do a great deal to contradict the sense of isolation that sick or disabled people may feel.

○ Refusing to feed at all, combined with crying, weakness or unusual quietness and indifference to anything going on

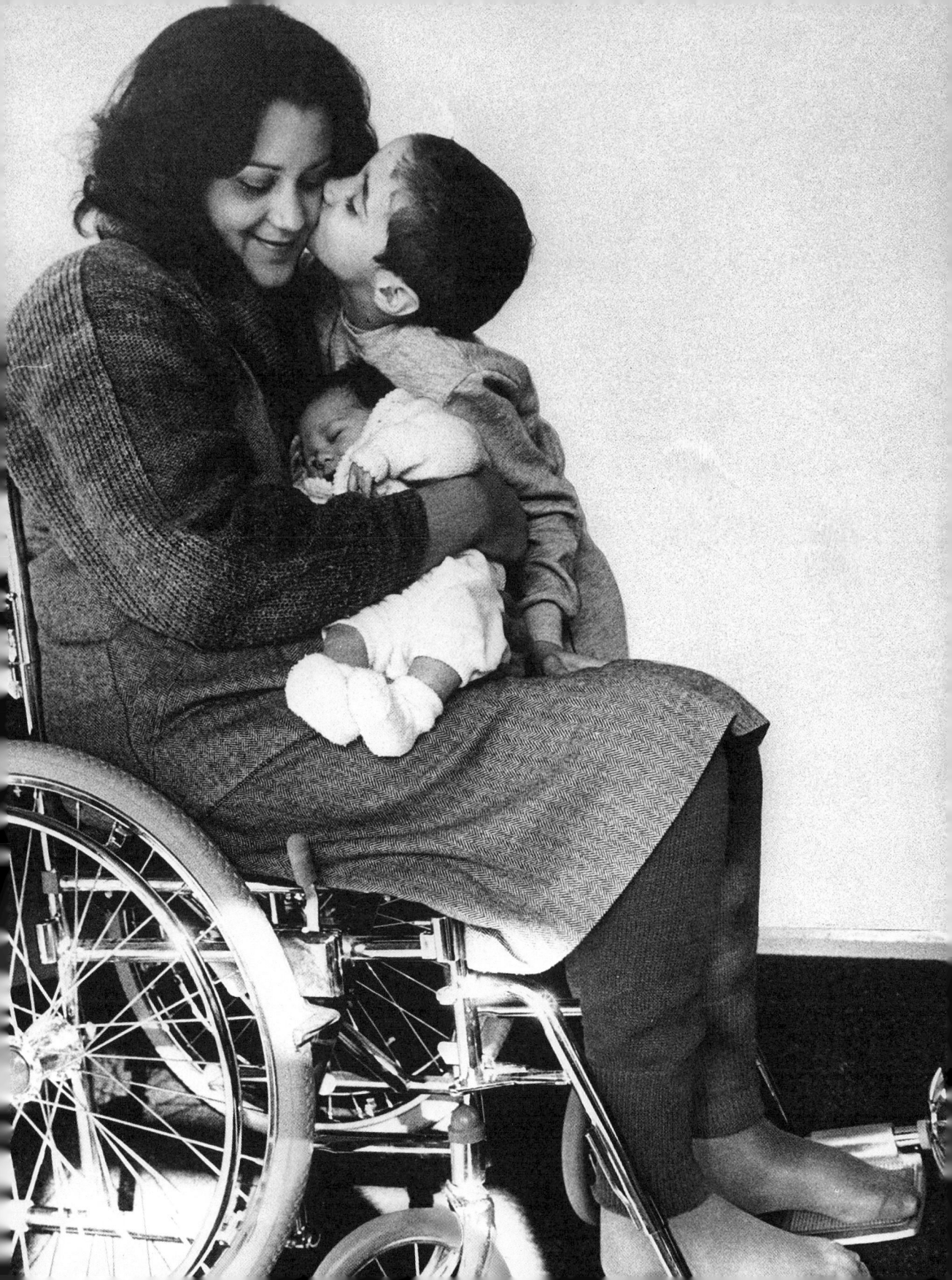

○ Fits or convulsions
○ Severe and persistent pain. It can be difficult to assess when a baby is in pain but you should be suspicious if the baby cries persistently and cannot be comforted by feeding, nappy-changing or plenty of cuddling and attention, and also gives some indication of pain – drawing up the knees in the case of abdominal pain or pulling at an ear or lying constantly on one side in the case of earache
○ Severe and frequent diarrhoea and vomiting, lasting for more than 2 hours especially in young babies
○ Breathlessness or a blue tinge to the skin
○ A serious injury, such as a scald or burn, bleeding that cannot be stopped, an injury to the head or suspected poisoning

When a child should see a doctor

The commonest causes of illness in children are the infectious diseases of childhood, such as chickenpox and measles; common coughs, colds and sore throats; and stomach upsets.

A child who is about to develop an infectious disease or another illness may become quiet and lacking in energy. He or she may refuse to eat, have a raised temperature, a runny nose and be irritable. Often the child is unusually clingy and wants more attention and cuddles than normal. Some children revert to behaviour that they had grown out of: they may wet the bed, for example. As the disease develops, more definite symptoms appear, such as a rash or raised temperature. You should call the doctor if your child has any of the following problems or symptoms:
○ Persistent or recurring earache
○ Frequent vomiting (several times per hour over a period of 2 hours or longer
○ Frequent diarrhoea (several watery stools per hour, persisting for more than 2 hours)
○ Diarrhoea and vomiting with a raised temperature and pains in the stomach
○ Difficulty in breathing
○ A temperature over 39.5°c (103°F)
○ A fit or convulsion
○ A serious injury

Childhood infectious diseases

If immunization is available against a particular infectious disease, this is usually the best course of action. Some diseases can bring with them unpleasant complications in adulthood, and so it is better if a child can get over German measles, chickenpox and mumps at an early stage.

Other diseases, such as whooping cough and measles, are unpleasant at any age, and possibly dangerous. There are inoculations available against both diseases, but if your child has not been immunized, you should avoid any contact with anyone who has either disease. If your child has had one of the childhood infectious diseases, you should not allow him or her to return to school, or to mix with others in crowded places such as shops or cinemas, until recovery is complete. Although

Disease	When a child is no longer infectious
Measles	4 to 5 days after the child's temperature is normal
Mumps	Until after all the swelling has gone down
Chickenpox	When the scabs have all dried up
German measles	A week after the rash first appears
Whooping cough	About 3 weeks after the coughing spasms start

you may feel that your child is on the way to recovery, if he or she is not past the infectious phase of the illness, there is still a chance that the infection may be passed on to an adult or another child. Remember also to restrict visitors to those who have had the infection.

You may find that when your child first goes to school or playgroup, he or she catches a series of colds and minor infections. This can be worrying but remember that children gradually build up their own resistance and grow out of this vulnerability to minor illnesses. A good, well-balanced diet (see page 110), plenty of fresh air and a sensible routine help to keep a child healthy.

Consulting the doctor

Before the doctor sees the child make a note of anything special that you want to ask or tell him. Keep anything that you need to show him, like vomit or a soiled nappy.

Once the doctor has seen the child and given advice, ask him if there are any special problems to watch out for, and if they do occur whether he wants to be informed. Make sure that you know what sort of care is required for the child; whether any medicines are to be given and how to administer them; and if there are any special treatments to be given and how to give them. If you do not understand what the doctor says, ask again. You may find it helpful to write down what he says, or to have the doctor write down any instructions for you.

Medicines given by mouth

These should be given by you in a matter-of-fact fashion. Once a child sees that you are likely to let him or her get away without taking the medicine, then you may have a battle on your hands. There is no need to be harsh or unkind, just firm. While it is not usually a good idea to bribe a child, you may like to reward a child for taking medicine with a favourite drink or treat of some sort and plenty of praise.

Do not be tempted to give a second dose within the safe period of time written on the packet or bottle, even if you feel that the original dose had no effect on the child. If your child vomits and you are worried about whether or not you should repeat the dose, call your doctor and ask for his advice.

Different types of medicine

Most medicines for young children are now available in syrup form, which children usually find easier to take than tablets or capsules. There are often several different forms of a particular drug, so if your child dislikes the form that has been prescribed, ask your doctor if there is an alternative.

If tablets have to be taken, you may like to offer them crushed between the back of a teaspoon and a bowl of another, and mixed into a small amount of jam or, if a tablet is difficult to crush, soak it in a drop or two of water for an hour or so before crushing it. Check with your doctor or chemist that this will not affect the medication.

Never put a crushed tablet into water, or any other drink or food, as only part of the dose may be taken. The exception is soluble tablets, which are designed to be dissolved in water. If your child is prescribed capsules, you should offer them with a drink – never try to open them.

Always read the instructions on a bottle or packet of medicine very carefully and be sure you know how much has to be given and when.

If a child refuses medicine

Most children take medicine without much fuss. If, however, a child refuses to take medicine or spits it out when you put it in his or her mouth, and you and the doctor are convinced that the drug is necessary, there is a way that you can make the child take it. This method is only suitable, and usually only necessary, for children up to the age of 5 or 6 years old.

Enlist the help of another adult. Put a large towel, sheet or blanket around the child's shoulders to keep his or her arms well tucked in. Ask your helper to hold the child firmly but kindly in this position. Have a glass of the child's favourite drink ready as a reward as soon as the medicine has gone down. Gently spoon the medicine into the child's mouth, a little at a time. If he or she spits it out, ask your helper to hold the child's mouth open while you spoon the medicine to the back of the mouth so that it goes straight down the throat. Never forcibly hold a child's nose and pour medicine in any form down the throat as the child may choke.

It is important not to lose your temper while doing this, but however gentle you are, your child will need some comforting after this: try to give reassurance and to restore the child's pride.

If the child opens her mouth to protest, you have only to hold it open while the other person spoons in the medicine. If you have to open her mouth, press gently down on her chin with your thumb or thumb and index finger.

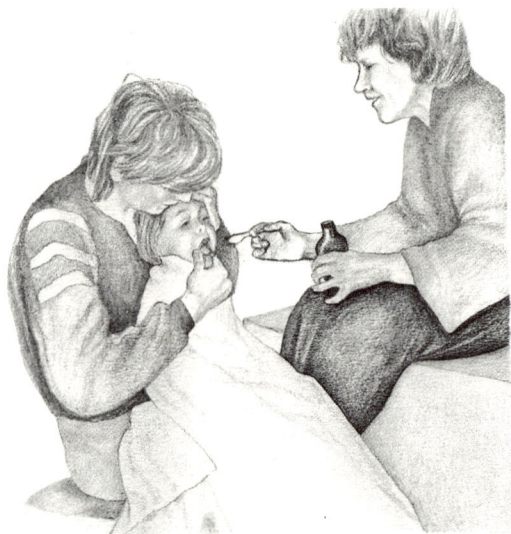

Rest in bed

Unless the doctor has specified bed-rest, there is no need to confine a child to bed or to insist that nightclothes are worn. Very few children actually enjoy being in bed, but when feeling unwell some may go to bed quite happily, while others may prefer to be curled up on your knee, or to sit in an armchair or on the sofa, wrapped up in a blanket.

As a caregiver, particularly if you are a busy mother with other young children to look after, you will probably find it much more convenient to have the sick child downstairs in the family room. It means there is less running up and down stairs, and there is ready-made entertainment around in the form of other members of the family, which gives you time to do all the really necessary chores around the house. If you are busy in the kitchen, there is no reason why you should not make your child comfortable on a pile of cushions on the floor.

If your child is confined to bed

☐ Make sure that the child's hands are washed after using the toilet. It is sometimes better to use a pot in the child's room. Not only does this mean that he or she does not have to walk or be carried to the toilet, but it is easier to see exactly what type of stool is being passed and a specimen can be saved if one is required.

☐ Gently washing the child's face and brushing his or her hair makes the invalid feel fresh and comfortable.

☐ Regular teeth-cleaning and use of mouthwashes help keep the mouth fresh, especially if there is any vomiting or soreness in the mouth.

☐ Change the bedclothes when soiled and make the bed at least once a day. In between times, tidy and smooth the sheets when necessary.

☐ Nightclothes should be light and comfortable; a change of clothes before settling for the night often helps the child to sleep better.

Entertainment

Keeping a child happy and occupied while he or she is unwell can present problems. Most children love to be read to, especially curled up next to an adult, although they may prefer the comfort and reassurance of familiar stories and even those intended for a much younger age group. It is a good idea to have a box hidden away with some small surprises – perhaps a new or unread book, a jigsaw puzzle, a packet of crayons or a colouring book. However, a child who is feeling really unwell will probably be happy just to watch television or doze. He or she may want your company, but there is no need to suggest games.

These are some simple ideas for entertaining a sick child; you will probably be able to invent many more:
○ Hand puppets
○ Simple cutting out – provide old magazines, old birthday and Christmas cards, blunt scissors
○ Jigsaws
○ Colouring books
○ Sewing cards
○ Scraps of material to make dolls' clothes
○ Simple card games

A tray makes a good base for puzzles or cutting out, and a bedtable (see page 18) is also useful. If a child is ill for a long time, it is quite possible to arrange painting, modelling and other messy activities in bed. Use an old sheet to cover the bed, and lots of newspaper on the floor to cut down on the cleaning up.

Sleep

Be guided by the child's own desire for sleep, but try to stick to normal sleeping times as much as possible without being rigid. If the child is sleeping more during the day, he or she may need less sleep at night. Once the child is up and about again, his or her normal pattern will become re-established.

Food and drink

The chapter on **Diet and Nutrition** gives detailed advice on feeding a sick child. Remember that it is particularly important to give a child plenty of fluids at regular intervals, especially if he or she is feverish. This is because children and babies easily become dehydrated.

Your attitude to your child's illness

Your attitude as caregiver toward the sick child is very important. Try to achieve a balance between being loving and caring and being over-protective and fussy. Your company and attention is what the child needs most, but if you appear unnecessarily anxious or make life far more pleasant than normal you may create problems for yourself.

A child who is normally dry at night may wet the bed when ill, and a child who normally washes and cleans teeth independently may suddenly want you to do it. There is no need to worry – your child will soon return to independence when he or she is feeling better.

To make time to give the extra attention and cuddling that a sick child is likely to want, you will probably need to drop all but the essential chores that need to be done. When a small child is ill you may find that you get more sleep if you sleep in the same room until he or she is over the worst.

Vomiting

Some children become very frightened when vomiting, so if your child does vomit, hold his or her forehead with your hand and give reassurance that everything will be all right. Once it is all over, it is soon forgotten. If being with a child who is vomiting makes you feel sick then, keeping the child close to you, turn your head to one side to avoid the smell and very quietly breathe in and out through your mouth slowly and deeply, concentrating on your breathing – it really does help.

Practical tips

☐ Cover the pillows with plastic sheeting, stuck down with adhesive tape. Then replace the pillowcases. If the child vomits over the pillow, you only have to wash the case and replace the plastic.

☐ Do *not* give pillows, with or without plastic covers, to children under a year old. A baby who may vomit should be propped on one side with a thick, rolled-up towel behind his or her back to prevent rolling. If the baby lies on his or her back, there is a danger of choking or suffocation on vomit.

☐ Keep a bowl covered with a cloth beside the child, so that he or she does not have to dash to the bathroom.

☐ Use paper tissues instead of cloths or handkerchiefs for clearing up. This reduces both the washing and the spread of germs.

Raised temperature or fever

A fever is usually defined as a temperature above 38°c (100.4°F), taken orally, and is one of the body's responses to infection. Children tend to run high temperatures as a result of quite minor illnesses. If you suspect that a child has a raised temperature, feel his or her forehead with the back of your hand, then feel your own forehead. If the child's forehead feels hotter than yours, he or she probably has a raised temperature, so check it with a thermometer or a fever strip (see page 84).

To bring down a fever

☐ Call the doctor and discuss any treatment.

☐ Give paracetamol in either syrup or tablet form according to the child's age. Be careful to give only the amount prescribed on the packet or bottle.

☐ Remove blankets and any warm bedclothes: one sheet is probably enough. Do not be tempted to wrap up a child in blankets.

☐ Dress the child in cotton loose-fitting nightclothes or a cotton T-shirt and pants.

☐ If the child's temperature reaches 40°c (104°F), sponging with warm water is an effective way of bringing the fever down (see page 101). Always check with your doctor before trying tepid sponging.

☐ Give plenty of fluids.

☐ Keep the child in a warm room at a constant temperature, with some ventilation but not a draught.

☐ An electric fan may help. Do *not* use the fan while sponging the child – it is highly dangerous to have electrical equipment in use anywhere near water.

Convulsions or fits

Children between the ages of 1 and 4 years old are sometimes prone to fits or convulsions when they have a high fever. These fits are very rarely dangerous but can be frightening. The following are signs of a fit:
○ There is twitching of the muscles in the face, arms and legs
○ Sometimes the eyes turn upward or squint
○ There may be froth around the mouth
○ Sometimes the child holds his or her breath

What to do

☐ Try to keep calm and reassure the child, who may be very frightened.

☐ Protect the child from hurting him- or herself but do not restrain the child in any way. The floor is probably the safest place as there is nowhere to fall.

☐ Loosen any constricting clothing around the chest and neck. If possible, take off outer clothing to help reduce the fever.

☐ Following the fit the child may become unconscious for a short while. Put the child into the recovery position (see page 198).

☐ Call the doctor and inform him about the fit. Ask if you should tepid sponge your child to bring the fever down. If you cannot get in touch with a doctor and the child's temperature is still high, you should tepid sponge in any case to reduce the risk of another fit (see page 101).

Rashes

If a child has an itchy rash, it can be very difficult to prevent scratching. Discuss any treatment with the doctor. Give the child a warm bath with some bicarbonate of soda in the water, then pat him or her dry with a towel after the bath and apply some calamine lotion. This is refreshing and helps to reduce the irritation. Dress the child in cool, loose-fitting and preferably cotton clothes. Plenty of things to do, such as drawing, cutting out or doing puzzles, helps to keep a child's mind off the itching.

Coughs

Very small children may find coughing very distressing and frightening, and so may be happier in your arms. Whooping cough can be particularly distressing at night: a child may find it comforting and reassuring to move into the parents' room.

Long-term illness

Some diseases affecting children can last for months or years, in which case they may be known as 'chronic' disorders or diseases. Cystic fibrosis, diabetes mellitus, epilepsy, asthma and leukaemia are all examples of long-term illnesses. Sometimes the child may recover from the problem. Or he or she may outgrow the disease, as in the case of asthma. Or the disease may be controllable, allowing the child to live a normal active life, as in the case of diabetes.

Sometimes the outlook is not so good and the child's health deteriorates, perhaps leading to death. The section on **Care of the Dying** deals with this subject in greater detail.

Whatever type of long-term illness you are coping with, you have to adapt to the prospect. When you are first told about the illness, the most natural reaction is to ask why it has happened to you and what you have done to deserve this. Whatever the problem, it is in fact extremely unlikely that you could have done anything to prevent it. Talk to your doctor and ask his advice. Find out the address of a support group. Talk to someone who has been through the same experience, ask how they coped, what help they had and from where. There is no need to feel that you have to cope all on your own – no one expects you to do so.

Be honest about what is going to happen to the child. There is nothing worse than saying 'it will not hurt' or 'they are not going to do anything to you', when the reality is the opposite. It is far better to tell the child gently and simply what is about to happen. If a blood test is to be done, say so. Most children cope very well when they know the truth and will only learn to distrust you if you disguise the truth. If the child has to face treatment which is unpleasant and painful, try to plan a treat or something to anticipate to help focus his or her attention ahead.

A young child needs you to organize any treatment, medicines and other therapy that must be given, but an older child should be encouraged to take over. This usually works well until adolescence when the teenager may suddenly rebel, perhaps eating the wrong food, missing medications or failing to keep appointments. So, although it is sometimes difficult to be firm with a child you know is ill, continuing discipline is needed, combined with a great deal of love and understanding.

Other children

Children can be very cruel to each other and may be unkind to a child who seems different, making jokes about a special diet or about self-injections. The best defence that your child can have is a good understanding of the disease and a supportive family. Talk to your child's teacher, who can then be on the look-out for any difficulties.

Sometimes other children in the family become jealous of all the attention a sick child gets. Alternatively, a husband may become jealous of the amount of time that his wife is spending 'fussing' over the child, or vice versa. Each family has to work out its own happy medium as everyone in the family, especially other children, must be able to lead a full life. However, most brothers and sisters of a sick child are only too willing to help and care. A younger child will usually accept a sick brother or sister without question, as the younger child will not have known any other way of life.

It is the caregiver who may find it most difficult to cope with looking after both a sick child and a baby or toddler or other siblings. If you should find yourself facing this problem or any other family difficulty, talk to your doctor or another health professional, or get in touch with someone at the support group. You will be surprised to find how much it helps to talk over the problem with someone in the same situation.

Going into hospital

No one likes to think that their child is likely to be admitted to hospital but it is a good idea to introduce some discussion on the subject with every child, as you never know when your child may be hospitalized in an emergency. One of the best ways to introduce the idea is in play: 'doctors and nurses' is a common game, in any case. Dolls or children themselves can act out care and treatment, taking on different roles, and this sort of play increases a child's understanding of what happens in a hospital. Never use the doctor or hospital as a threat or the child may come to see treatment as a punishment.

There are plenty of children's books about going into hospital. So if you are a little unsure about what hospitals are all about, you can learn at the same time. These books show pictures of nurses in uniform, doctors in white coats, the beds in the ward area and children in the wards, and they can generally convey the atmosphere of a hospital.

If you know in advance that your child is going into hospital, the staff will probably show you both the children's ward and give you a guided tour. There is often a booklet about hospital life that gives information about what to bring for the child, including suitable toys to bring in, and about visiting hours, along with plenty more information.

The staff in children's wards are especially skilled in caring for children and will be very aware of the needs of the child's parents as well. As a general rule, parents are encouraged to stay with their child, especially if the admission is an emergency. Some children's wards have special units where parent and child can stay, with the parent taking over a large share of the day-to-day care. Priority is given to parents of children aged 6 months to 4 years, to the mentally handicapped of all ages, to breast-fed babies, to physically-handicapped children, to very sick children and those living a long way from home.

Settling in

To help your child settle into the ward, you may like to try the following ideas.

☐ Include a favourite toy or teddy, clearly labelled with the child's name, in the child's bag.

☐ If the child uses a dummy or comfort rag, even if you think he or she is a little too old to do so, make sure that it is in the bag. This is not the time to break this kind of habit.

☐ Make sure that the nursing staff know about any special names used for going to the toilet.

☐ They should also know about any allergies or strong food dislikes, and what the normal feeding routine is. If you are in the process of weaning, tell them exactly how far you have got and what solids are being taken.

☐ Make sure the staff are aware of any fears that the child has and whether nightmares or sleepwalking are a problem.

☐ Tell the staff whether the child normally sleeps in a cot or a bed. A child who is used to sleeping in a bed at home will not take kindly to being put in a cot just because he or she is in hospital.

☐ If the child is called by a nickname at home, make sure that the staff know, so that they can carry on using the same name.

☐ If you cannot stay in the hospital with your child, make sure that you visit regularly and frequently. Send lots of letters, cards and postcards. Encourage other friends and relatives to do the same.

☐ When you leave the child, say when you are coming back and make sure that you are back by then.

☐ Leaving a young child with something of yours, such as a soft T-shirt, can be a great comfort.

Going home

Before leaving the ward, find out what care is needed at home (see pages 152-153). Once the child is home from hospital, talk about what has happened, the hospital, the people there, the whole experience. A young child may find it easier to act the whole business out in play, or you can ask for a drawing.

CARE OF THE ELDERLY

The process of aging begins as soon as we are born, but the rate at which different people age varies greatly. The changes that occur as we get older may eventually lessen our independence. This may mean that a frail elderly person is no longer able to look after himself or herself and has to move in with a relative or into a nursing home. If, as is usually the case, a person is very attached to his or her own home and would much rather stay there, a better solution is to make life easier in that home so that he or she can remain independent for longer.

Another alternative is to find accommodation where someone is available to keep an eye on the elderly person. This may be a flat or apartment with a warden who is responsible for all the elderly living there, or a home for the elderly in which residents can have their own rooms while joining others for meals and social activities. The solution depends on how mobile and independent the person concerned is. Perhaps he or she simply finds the household chores difficult, in which case the answer may be to employ someone to come in a few times a week to help with these. Talk to your doctor and see what he can suggest; see also the Appendix: **Where to Find Help**.

Mobility

The longer elderly people can remain independent and manage everyday activities for themselves, the better. Going to the shops, meeting friends, or expeditions to the cinema, theatre or a social club all help to keep up an active interest in life.

An elderly person, even though otherwise mobile, may spend too long sitting in a chair. If possible, help him or her to get up and move around for a short period every hour. Sitting for long periods tends to cause stiff joints and increased difficulty in getting about.

Comfortable feet are essential for mobility. The elderly should wear well-fitting, low-heeled shoes and should pay regular visits to the chiropodist to make sure their toenails are kept in good condition – these tend to become thicker and more difficult to care for with age. If the feet have a tendency to swell, make sure that the elderly person uses a footstool when sitting down (see page 56).

Gardening

Gardening is an activity that many people enjoy, certainly getting great pleasure from the end result; it keeps the mind and body active, stimulates the appetite and creates a sense of independence and achievement. It is a good idea to think ahead and plan the garden with old age in mind. Flower beds may be raised to a height which makes them easier to tend. There are various kinds of kneelers for those who find stooping difficult and long-handled tools are also useful garden aids.

Practical tips

You may sometimes feel that it is simpler and quicker for you to do things for the elderly person, but it is much better for him or her if you help but do not take over. There are many practical aids that may help the elderly person to remain independent.

☐ Make it easier for the elderly person to dress without help by replacing zips and buttons with Velcro and giving front fastenings to clothes.

☐ Shoe horns, combs and brushes should have long handles and nail clippers are easier to manage than scissors.

☐ Put a stool by the bath to simplify getting in and out and put a non-slip mat in the bath to prevent slipping and falling (see page 63). Or you might consider the installation of a shower instead; a plastic chair placed under the shower may enable the elderly person to sit and wash unaided.

☐ Handrails next to the bath, shower and toilet are easily fitted.

☐ Raising the level of the toilet seat also helps the elderly to be more independent.

☐ A walking frame or stick will help anyone who is unsteady on their feet to get about (see pages 53 and 156).

☐ Make sure that the bed is the right height (see page 18): if it is too high, the elderly person has to drop onto his or her feet when getting out; if too low, the person has to heave him- or herself up when getting up. For advice on comfort in bed, see pages 18 to 20 and 54 to 56.

The elderly person's chair should have a seat that is not too low – about 45 to 65 cm (18 to 26 in) off the ground – and not too deep, so that getting up is easy. It should have a high back and strong arms for pushing on when standing up. If this is a problem, an ejection seat may help: these can be bought from a furniture shop, or you may see them advertised for sale in the newspaper.

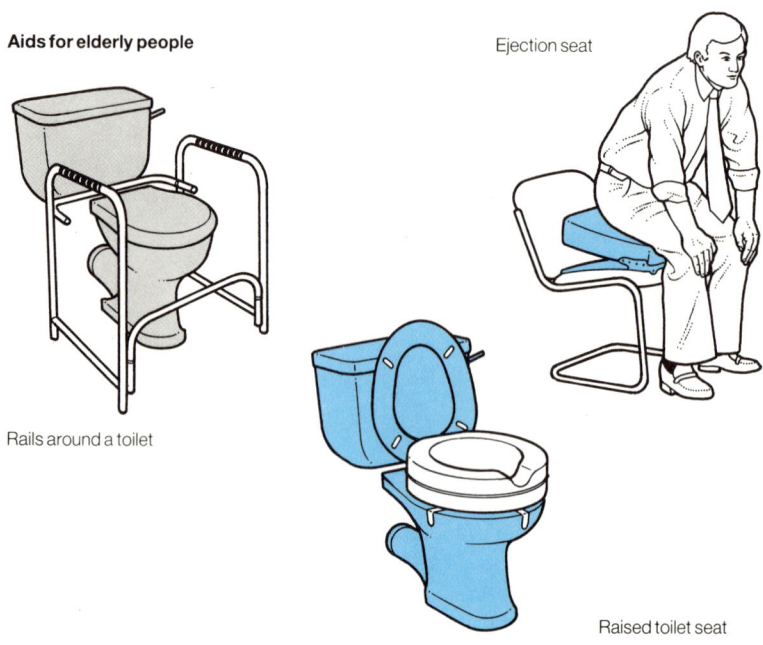

Aids for elderly people

Ejection seat

Rails around a toilet

Raised toilet seat

Home safety

Elderly people are particularly vulnerable to accidents. Falls are the most common problem and the elderly often hurt themselves quite badly as the result of what may seem a minor fall, as their bones are more brittle and therefore break more easily. Balance is also a problem and when the elderly start to fall they are often unable to right themselves. Once an older person has had a fall, he or she may be frightened that it will happen again and so may stay sitting in a chair or retire to bed. Reassurance is needed and of course you must do everything you can to ensure that he or she can move about safely and confidently.

☐ Make sure that there are no worn edges to carpets or light flexes to trip up the elderly person.

☐ Floors should not be too highly polished and slippery.

☐ Passages and stairways should be well lit; tidy away children's toys and other items left lying about.

☐ Light switches should be easy to find.

☐ Fires should have a guard and oil heaters should not be in a position where they can be knocked over.

☐ Gas taps and cookers should be regularly inspected for leaks; gas and oil stoves should only be used in rooms with adequate ventilation – an elderly person may become unconscious before realizing that anything is wrong.

☐ Store all medicines in a safe place and make sure that the elderly person can read the labels. Especially if he or she is taking sleeping tablets, keep the bottle in the cupboard and not at the bedside to prevent accidental overdose.

Another important aspect of safety is security – both in the home and outside. Sadly, today many old people are very vulnerable; they have grown up in a time when burglary, vandalism and attacks on the elderly were rare. Many do not appreciate the dangers and continue to leave doors unlocked and windows open, or to go shopping with a purse in an open basket in full view of any intending thief. Try to persuade any elderly friends or relatives to have secure door and window locks fitted and a chain put on the front door. The crime prevention officer at your local police station will advise.

Keeping warm

An older person's body is not as efficient at preserving normal body temperature as a younger person's. One of the dangers of cold weather for the elderly is that they may not realize that they are as cold as they actually are.

If the expense of heating the whole house is too great, or if heating in a bedroom is inadequate, it is probably better for the elderly person to live in one room that is warm, and to have his or her bed moved into that room during the cold weather.

Encourage the elderly person to wear layers of clothes, preferably woollen. Wearing a hat and gloves indoors is also a good idea: it may seem a little silly but it is worth looking odd to avoid suffering from cold.

At night, he or she should put on extra clothes including bedsocks and a woollen hat. If the bedroom is not used during the day, ensure that it is well heated before the elderly person goes to bed. Warm the bed with a hot-water bottle or an electric blanket, but remember that hot-water bottles must never be used at the same time as an electric blanket, and that electric blankets should be turned off before the person goes to bed. Ordinary electric underblankets should not be used if the person is incontinent or likely to spill drinks on them. Any sort of heating appliance should be serviced regularly to avoid accident.

Exclude draughts from windows, doors and floorboards. You can seal cracks with newspapers, and clingfilm applied to the inside of window frames acts as a type of double glazing. The chimneys of old unused fireplaces can be blocked with metal or brick or any other non-flammable material. Be careful not to block up any source of ventilation that is necessary.

If you know that someone elderly is on their own, take in a thermos of hot soup or tea, and encourage the person to eat well by bringing in the occasional meal or making a meal in that person's own home. Better still is an invitation to share a meal with you and your family. If possible, make regular visits to check that the elderly person is well, even if he or she thinks you are fussing.

Hypothermia

If an elderly person becomes chilled, he or she may develop hypothermia or a low temperature. Learn to recognize the signs and symptoms.

☐ The sick person may be slow, dazed or even unconscious.

☐ The skin may be pale or blue and very cold to the touch – not only the skin that is exposed but the skin that is covered with clothes. The skin may also look puffy.

☐ Pulse and breathing rates (see pages 86-87) are slower than normal. Sometimes it is very difficult to feel a pulse or hear a heartbeat, so do not rush to attempt resuscitation (see page 196). If the person is breathing, the heart is beating even if you cannot feel or hear it.

☐ Temperature may not register on an ordinary thermometer that goes down to 34°C (94°F) because it can be as low as 26°C (79°F) before the person dies. If he or she is drowsy, dazed or unconscious take the temperature under the arm, not in the mouth (see page 86).

Rewarming must be slow to avoid the danger of heart failure. If the body is heated too quickly by direct heat, the blood vessels in the skin dilate which in turn deprives the heart and other vital centres of blood. The same applies to giving alcohol. It is also important not to rub or massage cold hands or arms, feet or legs; nor should you try to get the patient to exercise.

☐ Put the patient to bed with plenty of loose covers, or wrap him or her in blankets or coats. Do not give a hot-water bottle or use an electric blanket.

☐ If the patient is conscious, give sips of warm, sweet drink. Do not give hot drinks or alcohol.

☐ Warm the room up to at least 27°c (80°F).

☐ Call for a doctor urgently or get the sick person to hospital.

Bowels

The elderly often experience problems with their bowels. They have a tendency to suffer from constipation because their bowel function slows down, and they are less mobile, take less exercise and perhaps find it difficult to get to the toilet.

It is not a good idea to give laxatives without first asking the doctor. Constipation can be relieved or prevented by a diet which includes plenty of fibre, as well as plenty of fluids – at least 2 to 3 litres (3 to 5 pt) per day – and by taking as much exercise as possible. Ensure that the elderly person is able to get to the toilet in good time, especially if he or she is confined to bed.

Constipation can sometimes cause incontinence. Faeces retained in the bowel become drier, harder and progressively more difficult to pass, as water is reabsorbed from them through the bowel wall. As more hardened stools accumulate in the bowel, they eventually become impacted. At this stage, the sufferer may develop what seems like diarrhoea but is in fact fluid leaking past the impacted stool. This may be difficult or impossible for the person to control and so lead to incontinence. If you think this might be what is wrong get the doctor's advice: you may need to give suppositories or an enema (see pages 105-106).

Constipation sometimes has the effect of making an elderly person mentally confused, so bear this in mind if his or her behaviour becomes a little strange or out of character.

Bladder

Many elderly people have difficulty controlling their bladder function. This may be because they are unable to get to the toilet in time, in which case you may be able to solve the problem simply by providing a commode or urine bottle (see pages 70-77) by the bed at night. It may be that the person is a little forgetful and just does not remember to go to the toilet. Reminders from you and help getting to the commode or along to the toilet at regular intervals may help. He or she will probably need to urinate every 2 to 4 hours. By making a note of when a person's individual need arises and reminding him or her at the appropriate times, you may avoid accidents.

It may be tempting to restrict fluids for someone who is incontinent but this is in fact likely to make the situation worse. If the elderly person does not take plenty of fluids, he or she risks becoming dehydrated or developing a urinary infection and is more likely to become constipated. However, it is sensible to avoid giving large amounts of fluid at night before the person goes to sleep.

Sometimes an elderly person may leak a small amount of urine when coughing, laughing or sneezing. This is called stress incontinence; in a woman it is often the result of childbearing and gets worse as she grows older. Try and get her to see the doctor about the problem. In men, an enlarged prostate (see page 178) often leads to dribbling.

Illness and the elderly

Many illnesses affecting the elderly are minor and can quite well be managed at home but it is always best to ask the doctor's advice. If the illness is severe enough to keep the patient in bed, you should definitely call the doctor. Long periods in bed may cause problems such as stiff joints, chest infections and problems in passing urine or opening the bowels. There is also a danger of pressure sores developing. The chapter on **Day-to-day Care** discusses caring for someone in bed.

Sometimes when an elderly person falls ill, he or she becomes mentally confused. This may only be temporary, but it does mean that the doctor may have difficulty finding out about the events leading up to the present illness. You may be able to help by telling the doctor about the patient's past medical history, or any signs and symptoms that have developed recently, for example:

○ passing of blood in the stools or urine (see pages 94-95)
○ chest pain
○ loss of appetite
○ loss of weight
○ headaches
○ weakness in arms or legs

Hearing problems

Often the hearing of an elderly person is not as sharp as it used to be. By speaking loudly, without actually shouting, you can make yourself more easily heard. Speak slowly and clearly, and look directly at the person. Be prepared to repeat what you say without irritation until the elderly person has taken it in, and listen to what he or she says. If the person's hearing is significantly reduced, he or she may need a hearing aid.

If the person cannot manage a hearing aid, the modern ear trumpet with a flexible tube or microphone, small amplifier and earphones may be the answer. Help him or her to learn how to lip read; this is a skill that can be learned at any age. The telephone is a very important means of maintaining contact with the outside world, especially for someone living on their own: people who are hard of hearing can have special adapters fitted to enable them to hear the person on the other end of the line. Equally important is a light that flashes on and off when the door bell rings: the elderly person may be unable to hear the bell ringing, but will see the light. Your doctor or the audiology department of your local hospital will advise you on how to obtain these devices.

Blindness

Although blindness is isolating and distressing, and causes many practical difficulties, there is no need for a blind person to lose interest in the world or to become entirely dependent on others. You will need professional advice and support in enabling a blind person to cope with everyday life. Your doctor will be able to suggest sources of help.

A blind person living alone is particularly vulnerable and cut off from the world around. Various aids are available: there are talking books for him or her to listen to and devices to help make the home environment safe. If you have a blind person living with you, make sure that the furniture and familiar landmarks are not changed around. Keep the passages, corridors and pathways used by the person through the various rooms clear, taking special care with stairways.

Living with the elderly

Loneliness is perhaps one of the greatest hardships of old age. Being wanted and needed and being important to the family are high priorities for the elderly. Some prefer to live with their families but this is not always possible. Moreover there is no denying that several generations living together can give rise to problems. The elderly person coming to live with a son or daughter finds his or her position changed from that of a carer or equal to that of a dependant and this reversal of roles is sometimes difficult: it may, for instance, make an elderly relative want to be stubbornly independent.

An elderly relative can be a great support to a parent with young children.

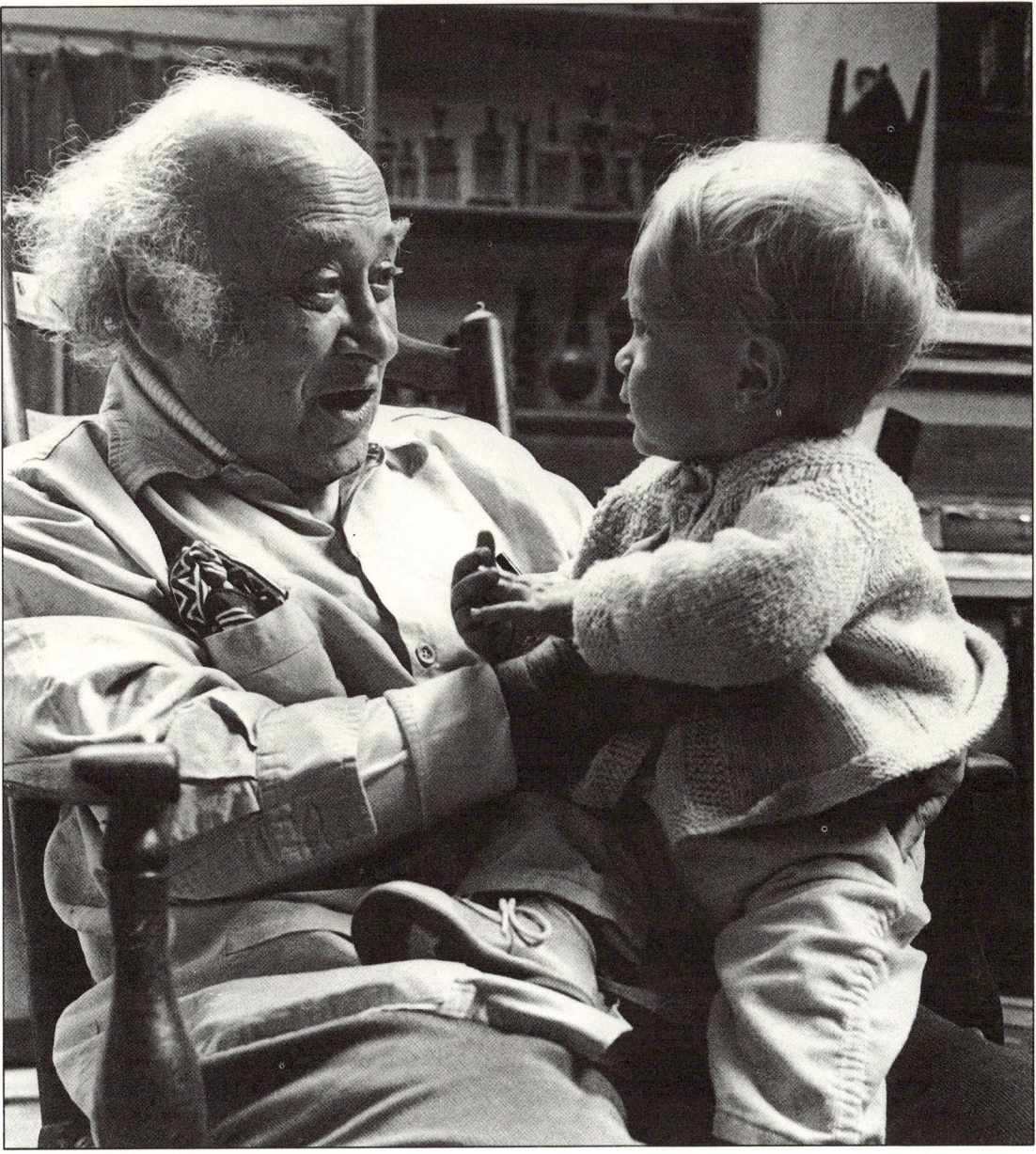

An elderly relative's difficulty in accepting that times have changed may also cause problems. Maybe it is the woman of the household who goes out to work, leaving home and caring to her partner. Or maybe the children are brought up differently, and seem to the older person to have too much independence too soon. In the case of a grandparent coming to live with the family, the authority of the head of the household may be threatened. A strain may be placed on the marriage, with the couple feeling that they are never alone and cannot say what they really feel or have a really good argument without being overheard. Living together like this needs a lot of give and take on both sides if it is going to work. If possible, the elderly relative should have a sitting and sleeping area where he or she can keep personal belongings and be alone. This helps everyone concerned to retain a sense of independence.

Nevertheless, elderly people often have a very special relationship with the younger generation and are able to bridge the generation gap. The young may well feel able to discuss a problem with and ask advice from a grandparent when they cannot talk to a parent.

Maintaining a sense of dignity at all times is vital. Never treat an elderly person like a child even if he or she seems muddled and confused. Everyone likes to feel useful and the elderly are no exception – make a point of asking him or her to help you in some way. Invite the elderly person to join in whenever you can, for what he or she needs is to feel part of a family, a part of society.

If the time comes when you feel you can no longer cope, for whatever reason, you should not feel guilty. In some situations, it is better for professionals or people outside the family to care for your elderly relative, not only for your sake but for his or hers.

CARE OF THE DISABLED

The terms 'handicapped' or 'disabled' can be applied to people suffering from a wide range of conditions which prevent them from living their lives as independently as normal. They are terms usually used to describe physical problems, ranging from arthritis to almost total paralysis. However, handicap can also have its roots in emotional or psychological problems, or in social deprivation, in which case it may be known as 'environmental handicap', although it is often accompanied by physical problems. This section focuses on coping with physical disabilities, as these require most home care.

The handicapped child

If your child is born with a handicap, the news is usually devastating and very difficult to take in. Feelings of disbelief that this has happened to you are common. You may feel resentful or hostile toward the staff at the hospital, or you may feel guilty, particularly if the disorder is inherited. Some parents feel that they just cannot cope and find themselves totally rejecting the child. All these are quite normal reactions. Fortunately, most parents of children who are born handicapped come to love them and are somehow able to give them the best quality of life possible in the circumstances.

In the very early days, try to discover the exact extent of the handicap and ask your doctor to explain what the future might hold for your child. Find out the address of a local support group that specializes in the type of handicap affecting the child. Talk to parents of similarly affected children and ask how they managed and what help they received. As well as gathering information, give the whole family time to take in what has happened: the mother, in particular, needs time to accept the situation and to recuperate after giving birth to the child.

If your child is born with a handicap, the handicap can be accepted by all concerned as a part of that person as he or she grows up. If, on the other hand, the child is born perfectly normal and becomes handicapped through illness or injury, the problems of accepting what has happened are often greater, not only for the child but for the parents and the rest of the family.

Caring for a handicapped child

The parents of a handicapped child tend to be naturally overprotective, but they should understand how important it is that he or she learns to be as independent as possible and that he or she develops confidence. A good understanding of all the available information about the child's future development is crucial in helping him or her achieve this goal. For example, you need to know whether the child will:
○ ever be able to stand
○ ever be able to walk, with or without artificial aids
○ always need a wheelchair
○ learn to talk
○ learn to read

The answers to questions like these will help you and the family make the right decisions in the years before the handicapped child goes to school, a time of rapid physical and mental development when treatment is likely to be most effective.

The education of the baby and the young child, whether handicapped or not, is very much in the hands of the parents. Young children learn through play, meeting new people, going to new places and listening to people talking. Help the child to meet and mix with other children. If the handicap is not too severe, he or she may be able to join a local playgroup or nursery school. Alternatively, it may be necessary for the child to attend a special school, where the staff will encourage as much independence as possible. Ask your doctor or health professional to suggest activities and toys to encourage the development of a handicapped child.

Teaching acceptable social behaviour, if this is possible, starts early. Within the limits of the child's disability, aim to help him or her to communicate, to be easy to get on with and not to be an attention-seeker. To encourage speech, talk to the child with simple words, not only when you are doing something for him or her, but whenever you are together. You will need expert assessment to help you decide, for example, when to start toilet training, when to expect the child to feed or dress independently, and how to cope with temper tantrums, destructiveness and so on. Once you know what progress to expect, you will be less likely to become frustrated or dispirited. Although there will almost certainly be times when you feel like giving up, try to measure the child's achievements in his or her own right rather than against the achievements of other children. Do not expect too much too soon, be kind and patient but firm, and give lots of praise when the child does well by his or her own standards.

Coping as a family

Achieving a good balance between the needs of the handicapped child and the rest of the family may be problematic. Brothers and sisters often seem to be particularly good at getting the best out of a handicapped member of the family. Sometimes, however, a brother or sister feels resentful of all the attention being centred on the handicapped child. Also, a child with disabilities may be well accepted by brothers or sisters when young but may be felt an embarrassment to them as he or she grows older.

Make sure that your handicapped child has plenty of opportunities to make friends – he needs social contact as much as any other child.

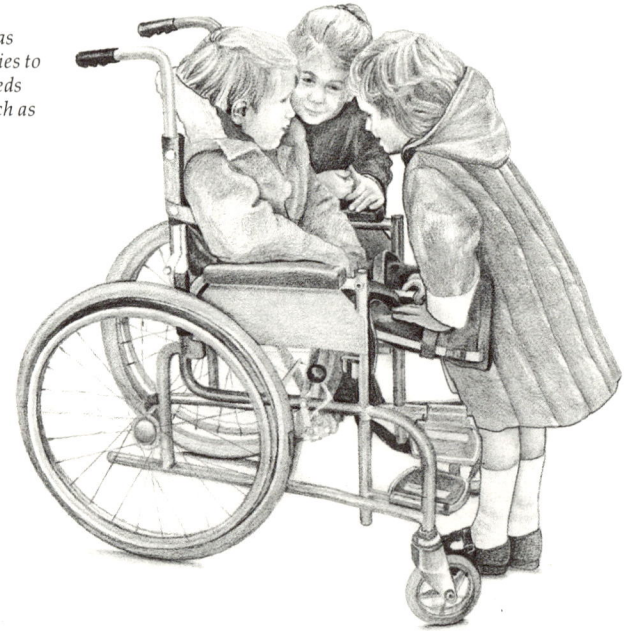

The handicapped adolescent

Adolescence brings new challenges for disabled young people. The normal teenage desire to be just like other friends may make the handicapped teenager painfully aware of his or her differences. The growing need for independence may also be thwarted by physical difficulties: however, with some thought, you may be able to come up with new ideas for enabling the teenager to become more self-sufficient than was possible when he or she was younger.

Sexuality can also be a difficult area for disabled adolescents and their parents: remember that a handicapped teenager will develop sexual feelings just like any other teenager, and that he or she will need tactful help in resolving the problems that this may present.

Finding a job

For the handicapped adolescent, finding a job is difficult and often frustrating. Even if he or she has good qualifications, certain types of work may be ruled out because of the handicap. Yet making a contribution to society and holding down a job is a great boost to a person's self-respect.

During the last few years at school, the young handicapped person should visit a variety of suitable places of work that appeal to him or her and discuss the routine and requirements of working in those environments. He or she should also get accustomed to using some form of transport for travelling to and from work. All this may well be part of the curriculum at the school he or she attends but it is certainly worth checking. Perhaps the handicapped person is able to go on to further education or training. If so, seek advice from the school.

Long-term prospects

Many parents with handicapped teenagers are understandably anxious about the future. What happens when they, the parents, die? Is it fair to expect other members of the family to shoulder the responsibility? Perhaps there are no brothers or sisters and the only prospect is some kind of institutional care.

Nowadays, there is much more emphasis on the handicapped living as part of the community, so parents need not fear that their son or daughter may be shut away in isolation. However, it is a good idea to look at all the choices available for the future, and to consider these well ahead of time.

Helping a disabled adult

An adult may be disabled as the result of a long-standing illness, such as multiple sclerosis, or as a result of an accident. Severe accidents may leave a person with paralysis, or loss of movement and sensation: both the upper and lower halves of the body may be paralysed (quadriplegia), or the lower half of the body only may be affected (paraplegia). For a normal healthy adult who becomes disabled through disease or an injury, the greatest problem is loss of independence.

If you are worried about the return home of a person who has been in hospital following an accident or illness that has left him or her disabled, talk to the staff at the hospital or contact an organization or support group. It is helpful to talk with someone who has experienced the same problem. Try not to worry when things go wrong and above all try to keep a sense of humour and positive attitude.

Wheelchairs

A person who uses a wheelchair may be unable to stand at all or may simply have difficulty in moving so that a wheelchair is an easier way to get about. Someone who has become confined to a wheelchair needs a great deal of support from relatives and friends. He or she may find it very difficult to accept the prospect of never being able to walk again and may resent the inactivity and lack of independence. Electric wheelchairs offer great advantages for ease of mobility, and enable the disabled person to get out without being dependent on the caregiver.

Emotional adjustment

Whatever the handicap, you will need to understand the feelings of frustration, anger and uncertainty that the invalid may be experiencing – you may well share these feelings. If he or she appears angry or resentful and takes it out on you, try to have patience and realize that this is merely a way of coping with the present situation. Offer positive suggestions and encourage the invalid to concentrate on those aspects of the illness or disability that can be improved.

Fear of losing friends and being left out of the social aspects of life and family occasions may cause considerable anxiety. The more social contact with other people that can be kept up, the better. If you are unable to take the invalid out to visit friends, encourage them to come to see him or her. It is important to get out and mix with other people, even if you do nothing more than wheel the invalid out into the park or down to the shops.

Encouraging independence

If someone who becomes disabled previously held a job, every effort should be made to get him or her back to work, either in the same or in another more suitable job. Failing this, encourage him or her to take up a new hobby or to resume an old one: an interest in something is essential. A specially adapted car, if this is a possibility, gives considerable independence. If this is not possible, help the invalid to practise getting in and out of a car belonging to a friend or relative willing to drive him or her around.

Adaptations in the home help to make life easier for everyone, if they can be afforded. This may mean rearranging the downstairs rooms to provide a bedroom, washing facilities and a toilet all on the same level, or installing a shower instead of a bath so that the disabled person can shower him- or herself, or lowering the level of the kitchen units or adapting the kitchen to enable the person to cook and work there. There are many aids available, including hoists and bathroom equipment (see pages 52 and 63). If the person uses a wheelchair, you will need doors wide enough for the chair, ramps instead of steps and room enough to manoeuvre the wheelchair indoors.

Encourage the disabled person to dress him- or herself independently: replace zips and buttons with Velcro and throw out or adapt clothes whose fastenings are difficult to reach.

Someone who has been paralysed from the waist down as the result of an accident will be taught how to move from bed to chair, and from chair to toilet seat, using the strength of his or her arms. The chapter on **Lifting and Moving** gives more ideas on how to help anyone who has difficulty moving without assistance.

Physical care

Pressure sores are a potential problem for anyone who cannot move about in bed (see page 78). They may also be a problem for someone confined to a chair or wheelchair: encourage the sick person to raise his or her buttocks off the seat every 15 minutes to relieve the pressure. A foam rubber cushion, 5 to 10 cm (2 to 4 in) thick, placed in the chair and covered with a sheepskin, also helps prevent pressure sores.

If the handicapped person has lost sensation in any part of the body, he or she should not be given a hot-water bottle or allowed to sit too close to a radiator, fire or unlagged hot-water pipes, as the invalid will not know if he or she is being burnt. You should also check that washing water is not too hot.

Control over the bladder may be lost. The chapter on **Day-to-day Care** gives advice on caring for someone who is incontinent or has a catheter. Some people paralysed from the waist down are able to empty their bladders by straining and pressing down. In general, anyone with these problems should be encouraged to drink plenty of fluids in order to prevent urinary infection.

A disabled person who has lost control of the bowels should have professional advice on how to ensure regularity, and the routine suggested should be strictly followed at home. It may be necessary for the person to take laxatives or suppositories on occasions. Drinking plenty is helpful: it is also important that the diet includes enough fibre.

Anyone who is handicapped needs a diet high in protein and fibre, and low in carbohydrate and calories – high protein to keep the skin in good condition, high fibre for the bowels, and low carbohydrate and calorie to help keep the weight steady. It is also important that any exercises recommended by the doctor or hospital are continued.

Sexual activity

Sexual feelings are rarely lost and, if the disablement is severe, professional advice should be sought on how to continue a sexual relationship. Counselling may be helpful, whatever the degree of disablement. The problems vary from case to case. In the case of paraplegia, for example, women can conceive and bear children but do not have the normal sensations during intercourse, while some men still get erections but only a few ejaculate, so the chances of their fathering a child are low.

Professional help

Whatever the cause of the handicap, and whether the handicapped person is a child or an adult, what matters is the quality of life both of the affected person and of the family. For the handicapped person, the need to learn and to experience a sense of achievement is always present, and as an adult the need to feel useful is also important. This is often the cause of problems, and the caregiver should seek help from the experts:

○ the physiotherapist, for help with mobility, posture, balance and exercises to increase independence
○ the occupational therapist, for help with the skills of everyday living, such as feeding, washing and dressing

Depending on what the handicapped person's individual needs are, it may be necessary to see any of the following:

○ a speech therapist
○ an audiometrician (hearing)
○ an orthoptist (sight)
○ a psychologist (emotional problems)
○ a social worker (financial problems, housing)
○ a dentist (teeth)

Take advantage of these services if they are available. You may well need help not only with physical problems related to the disability but with emotional problems arising out of it.

Other sources of help include self-help groups, voluntary associations, friends and neighbours. Never turn down an offer of help, particularly if it gives you and the rest of the family a break in which to lead your own lives.

The severity of the handicap may mean that the person needs to be cared for in a special home. In some cases when a handicapped person has been looked after at home, the problems become too great for the family to cope with adequately and the handicapped person may then benefit from the care of professionals. Or it may be that the caregiver falls ill and is unable to look after him or her. Or perhaps the family needs a holiday or a break. You should not see the need for the handicapped person to move to a residential home or a hospital either permanently or temporarily as a failure on your part.

CARE OF THE DYING

Death and the dying are subjects that many people feel uncomfortable talking or even thinking about. The very words and all that they imply inspire fear, although these days we seem to be becoming more open about our feelings on the subject.

Most health professionals feel that the dying should be cared for in their own homes if this is at all possible and what all concerned want. Home is where the person is likely to feel happiest and most secure in familiar surroundings, and where care can be given by the people who know and love him or her best. More often than not, this loving care from the family needs to be supplemented with professional help from the family doctor and other visiting health professionals.

Emotions associated with dying

Commonly, both the dying person and those who love him or her experience a particular sequence of emotions as death approaches. Not everyone goes through all the stages described below, nor are they necessarily in this order.

This sequence starts with feelings of denial, of not allowing yourself to admit the reality of what is happening. This can produce anger, rage and hostility. The person dying may take out his or her feelings on those around or on the doctor or hospital staff. Parents of a dying child may also become aggressive toward other members of the family or the professionals caring for their child.

The next stage for the sick person and for those who love him or her involves trying to put off the inevitable by bargaining with God or fate, in order that he or she may be allowed to live longer.

This is often followed by a state of depression. The dying person may be preparing to accept the loss of everything and everyone that he or she loves. A sense of great sadness may make the person withdraw into him- or herself, preferring not to talk about feelings yet needing reassurance that the people around understand. Just as deep are the caregivers' feelings of depression.

Eventually there comes a stage of acceptance. The anger and depression have passed. The person dying is more likely now to want to sort out practical details, such as writing a will. Although perhaps seeming calmer this does not necessarily mean that he or she has given up the fight against death. At this time, the caregivers may also start to come to terms with the inevitable separation.

The dying child

Accepting the news that someone you love is going to die is always hard, but particularly so in the case of a child. Reactions vary from tears shed in anger and sadness to aggression and disbelief mixed with the fear of not knowing how you will cope. Parents may feel that it is their fault in some way: they may ask 'What have we done to deserve this?' or 'Could it have been prevented if we had done this or that?'. There is rarely anything that parents could have done to change the situation, but it is quite normal to react in this way. Try to talk to someone about these feelings, preferably a health professional or someone who can give spiritual support. Or contact a support group (see page 220) and find someone who has been through the same or a similar experience.

A child's understanding of death

Caring for a dying child places great strains and demands on the caregivers. It is difficult enough to cope with your own feelings, let alone those of the child. In order to help the dying child, some understanding of his or her view of death is important. Children's ability to comprehend what is happening and their reactions vary as they get older.

☐ Under the age of 4 years, a child may see death as equivalent to being asleep for a long time, as a reversible state, and as a separation from the people who love and care for him or her. The idea of being parted from these people may make the child feel insecure and frightened.

☐ Between the ages of 5 and 9 years, the child may see death as something that happens only to other people or as a punishment for something that he or she has done wrong, whether real or imaginary.

☐ From the age of 9 until adolescence, the child generally sees death as final and realizes that eventually everyone will die. He or she will have experience of it from watching television or hearing about the death of someone in the family. At this age the child may no longer see death as sleep but may be afraid that it might be uncomfortable and painful and may also have a fear of the unknown.

☐ The adolescent and young adult see death as being final; there is no coming back. The person in this age group may also see it as preventing all the things that he or she had planned and wanted to do so much, and feel cheated of his or her chance at life. Various aspects of the care may be resented, including having to depend on other people just when he or she was gaining independence.

When your child asks questions, try to answer them honestly, according to the child's age and understanding – the best help that you can give is to show that you can cope with the reality, despite your feelings.

Friends and family

Brothers, sisters and school friends of the dying child must be told, in terms they can understand, that the child is ill and unlikely to get better. Once the patient has died, these children need to have the situation explained to them. They may be worried that they have the same symptoms or have caught the illness that caused the death.

You may also need to offer help to adult friends and relatives who are affected by the tragedy: grandparents, for example, may be just as upset as parents or brothers and sisters.

Physical care

As the dying person's condition deteriorates, try to give the special sort of care that he or she as an individual needs. This will include nursing in whatever position is most comfortable for him or her. Whether sitting in a chair or lying in bed, the patient should be warm and comfortable, and well supported with pillows, and if immobile should be turned frequently to prevent bedsores: the chapter on **Day-to-day Care** gives more advice on this.

If sleeping a great deal, semi-conscious or even unconscious, the patient should be laid on his or her side, with the pillows arranged in an inverted V-shape and at least two pillows between the head and shoulders to prevent the shoulders from being squashed. Gently pull the lower arm free so that it does not become uncomfortable. Cross the upper leg over the lower leg and place a pillow between the two. This helps the person feel more comfortable and prevents the legs from rubbing together and becoming sore. Support the patient's back with a pillow. Take great care when changing his or her position to make the movement gentle: the chapter on **Lifting and Moving** tells you how.

Physical care remains very important and may become increasingly demanding as the sick person's condition deteriorates.

□ Keep the dying person washed, his or her teeth cleaned and hair combed: this helps the invalid to feel comfortable and well cared for. In the case of a man, give him a facial shave if he wants one or if he usually shaves every day. The dying often breathe through the mouth, which then becomes dry and sore: regular mouth care (see page 65) is therefore important. You should also change the bed linen frequently.

□ Although the invalid may seem nearly unconscious, he or she may be more aware than you realize, so explain what you are doing to the invalid, avoid talking as if he or she is not there and try to keep the sickroom light and airy.

□ Eventually the sick person may be able to tolerate only a liquid diet. If you are giving a milk-based liquid feed, it is a good idea to follow it with a few sips of water to keep the patient's mouth fresh.

□ Incontinence may become a problem and your doctor may suggest a catheter and urine bag (see pages 74-77).

□ There may come a time when someone must sit with the patient at night and carry out any care that may be needed. If possible take turns with others, so that you regularly have a good night's sleep.

**Pain and
pain-relief**

One of the main fears of someone who is dying is of pain. The control of pain is usually possible provided that it is carefully managed. The first step is to assess the pain: where it is, how severe, when it starts, how long it lasts and how it is related to the person's emotions; also, how it is affected by movement, meals, bowel movements and passing of urine. Your doctor needs to know the answers to such questions in order to prescribe the right medication.

In the case of severe pain, medication should be given regularly in order to control the pain. The effects of any medicine given to relieve pain should always be checked about 30 minutes after the dose and then again 30 minutes before the next dose is due. If the medicines are not controlling the pain, the doctor must be informed so that something more effective can be prescribed. Make it clear to the dying person that he or she is not expected to put up with pain; encourage the invalid to tell you of any pain without fear of being thought cowardly or ungrateful.

When death is near, the patient may be semi-comatose, but this is no reason to stop controlling the pain. He or she may now need to be given opiates: strong drugs such as heroin or morphine. These drugs can be given by mouth, by injection or into the rectum as suppositories. These medicines must be continued, once started, to prevent withdrawal symptoms which the dying person may otherwise suffer, though perhaps unable to tell you about them. Some of these opiate-type drugs do have side-effects so it is important to ask your doctor what these are likely to be. If they trouble the invalid, tell the doctor as soon as you can – he may be able to change the medication.

**Emotional and
spiritual care**

Good physical care makes a great difference to the comfort and dignity in which a person dies. However, spiritual and emotional needs should not be neglected. If the sick person has a religious faith, someone from his or her church may be of great comfort to the patient and a tremendous support to the family.

The caregiver can help by just sitting at the bedside and holding the patient's hand. The sick person may experience mood swings, confusions of fear, anger and self-pity, and a sense of having lost control over his or her own life. Uncontrollable emotions may frighten the patient, and may also frighten you and lead you to feel that it is safer not to talk about them. However, even if it is painful to you, it is of the utmost importance for both you and the patient that you discuss these feelings openly, particularly when the patient is first told that he or she is dying. Listen to what the sick person says and do not discourage him or her from expressing fears, as sharing them will help the invalid to feel less isolated. Listening is at least as important as talking. Let the patient finish a sentence, listen carefully and, if anything seems unclear, repeat it back for confirmation of what he or she has asked or told you.

Listening is probably the most important thing that you can do, but relaxation and distraction also help by relieving some of the tension. Ask your doctor for advice on relaxation techniques: one simple exercise is to encourage the patient to breathe rhythmically and deeply, focusing on his or her breathing. Playing soft music, reading aloud or simply talking may all serve as a distraction.

At this time, the patient may like to talk about the past and about pleasant memories. He or she may want to have letters, and perhaps visits, from old friends, or to look at old photographs and momentoes. This is a time, too, for laying to rest old quarrels with relatives. Parent and child may have had differences over the years, or even have become estranged. It is important for both the dying parent and his or her child that such differences should be sorted out now so that there will be no regrets, and that they should talk about their love for one another.

People who are dying may show bitterness, ingratitude or resentment toward those who are going to be alive after their death. This can be very hurtful and upsetting but should be seen as their way of handling their own death. The worst way you can respond to this is by withdrawing, hurt and angry. Far better to tell the patient that you are aware of his or her anger and frustration while making it clear that you are hurt.

Caring on your own

It may be that you are caring for a person who is dying on your own. Quite naturally, you may be frightened of finally being left on your own. You may also feel inadequate, unable to cope competently with the pain, nausea or other symptoms that the person in your care is suffering. If so, talk to your doctor or the community nurse about your worries and fears.

This kind of intensive caring on your own is exhausting and time-consuming: you probably have time only for snacks, not meals; you may be confined to the house; and you may get very little sleep. Try to make sure that your snacks are nutritious and that you use any time available for rest. If the patient is waking in the night, it may be pain that is the cause: do not hesitate to ask your doctor for advice.

Hospital or hospice?

It may not be possible to continue caring for your loved one at home and if he or she does have to be admitted to a hospital or hospice, there is absolutely no reason why you should feel that you have failed in any way. Go with the patient to the hospital or hospice and see that he or she is settled in. Ask to be involved in the patient's care: offer to feed and help him or her take drinks. Sit with the person just as you did at home and offer reassurance that you are still there.

A hospice is a hospital designed especially for the care of the dying. Hospice care concentrates on providing the dying with mental and physical comfort and on enabling death with as much dignity and happiness as possible. The emphasis is on giving the dying time to talk and express their fears to people who are able to help by meeting their spiritual needs, who can help dispel their fears and who can control any pain, all within a homely atmosphere which encourages friends and relatives to be involved.

Bereavement

For most people, the most natural thing to do when someone has died is to express their grief by crying, but some people find themselves unable to cry. Perhaps they have had to put on a brave face throughout their loved one's illness and now that it is all over they simply cannot let go. Men may be particularly inhibited about showing their emotions, though encouraging words may be all that is needed.

Just as in accepting the news of impending bereavement, so in bereavement itself a person may experience anger or the need to blame someone else for the death. You may suffer a sense of guilt because you feel relief that the dead person is no longer suffering, because the person died when you were not there or perhaps because you spoke sharp words to him or her in a moment of tension.

This may be followed by a feeling of depression and emptiness. The hustle and bustle of the busy day caring for a loved one is gone, friends and relatives feel that the worst is over and no longer show their former concern, and life may seem purposeless and lonely, especially for someone left on their own. As time goes on, your interest in life will re-awaken, although there are bound to be moments of great sadness for many months or years, particularly on occasions such as Christmas or other family festivals. If your relationship to the person who has died was close, it will probably take about a year to get over the initial grief and from 2 to 3 years to completely accept the death.

Coping with grief

When a person dies, friends and relatives tend to avoid discussing the subject; they may even avoid mentioning his or her name in case this might upset you. Take the initiative, talk about the person and recall the happy times you had together, even if others do not raise the subject: they will probably be delighted in your trust in sharing the memories.

In general, the recently bereaved gain comfort from their own home and a regular routine, even if it does seem quiet and strange at first. Sometimes well-meaning friends and relatives try to persuade the mourner to move house or take a holiday. However, the bereaved should give themselves the chance to come to terms with what has happened and to plan their own future. Having a friend to stay some-times helps, particularly if you have been left on your own.

Children and bereavement

When a child experiences the loss of a parent, he or she may feel frightened, insecure and worried that other people in his or her world may die as well. The bereaved child may even fear that he or she is somehow to blame for the death. What this child needs more than anything is plenty of love and affection, to be cuddled much more than usual and to be given the chance to express his or her anxieties. In fact, a child often copes better with death than an adult.

Coming to terms with the death of a child may take longer than any other bereavement. One reason for this may be that the grieving is not only for a life lost but also for the future and all that that life might have been. Try talking to people who have suffered similarly.

Professional help

For those bereaved who are left without a family, or those who feel the need for more support than friends and family can offer, there are organizations that specialize in helping the bereaved. Their addresses may be found at the end of this book. Bereavement counselling services are beginning to grow; ask your doctor whether he has any information.

Medical and Surgical Problems

This chapter describes the illnesses that commonly require home nursing and the type of care that may be needed. The demands made by different conditions vary greatly. You may be looking after a person with a short-term illness – a child with a bad attack of tonsillitis, perhaps; or you may have to nurse a person who has recently been discharged from hospital following an operation; or you may have taken on the exacting job of nursing someone with a chronic disabling disease. Although the demands vary, in any of these situations you will need to know how best to care for the sick person.

The chapter is not meant to be a do-it-yourself guide to medicine, and it is important that you do not try to diagnose an illness and treat it on your own. Always seek qualified medical advice if you are worried about your own or someone else's health, and do not hesitate to ask your doctor about anything that puzzles you.

QUESTIONS TO ASK YOUR DOCTOR

Time with your doctor tends to feel short and pressured: it is so easy to forget all you wanted to ask during the consultation, and to remember as soon as you get home. Writing the questions down beforehand can save a lot of frustration, and ensures that you get the much-needed information. The list below is only intended to give general guidelines. In any particular case you will probably need to ask only some of the questions listed, and there will be questions not included that you want to ask.

Questions concerning the illness
☐ How will this illness affect the person concerned?
☐ What is the expected course of the disease?
☐ What will be done to treat the problem? Get the doctor to explain any treatment in detail.
☐ Is there anything that the person can do to help him- or herself, for example, stop smoking, follow a special diet, take more rest or start a special programme of exercises?
☐ Should the person stay off work or school, and if so, for how long?
☐ When does the doctor want to see the person again?
☐ If the disease is a long-term one, ask the doctor for the address of a local self-help group.

Questions concerning any medicines to be taken
☐ What effect will the medicines have?
☐ How many times a day should the medicines be taken, and in what amounts?
☐ How long should they be taken for?
☐ Are there any foods or drinks that should not be taken with these medicines?
☐ Are there any side-effects?

Questions to ask before surgery
☐ Why is this operation necessary?
☐ What exactly will be done?
☐ Could this problem be treated in any other way and, if so, what would be the disadvantages of the alternative treatment?
☐ Is there any special preparation the person should make before the operation? For example, it might be advisable for someone who is overweight to lose weight.
☐ Are there any special tests that will be done before or after the operation?
☐ Will there be any other treatment after the surgery?
☐ How much pain will there be, and for how long?
☐ What will be done to control pain?
☐ How long will the person be in hospital?
☐ How long will it be before he or she can expect to be fit again, and to return to work or school?

Questions to ask before going home after surgery

☐ Who will remove any stitches, if they have not already been removed, and when?

☐ Will the wound need dressing at home? If so, who will do it? (If you are expected to dress the wound, make sure you know exactly what to do.)

☐ Will any special care be needed at home?

☐ Should any special diet be followed? Are there any foods that should be avoided?

☐ Is it safe to take a bath?

☐ What exercise is allowed? Are there any activities which should be avoided?

☐ Is lifting allowed? This can be a particularly important question for mothers of young children.

☐ Are there any special exercises that should be practised?

☐ May the convalescent drive a car? (Check the small print on the insurance policy to see when it is permissible to drive following a general anaesthetic.)

☐ When may the convalescent resume normal sexual activities?

☐ Should crowded places be avoided, and if so for how long?

☐ Are there any signs or symptoms that should be reported to the doctor?

☐ When may the person return to work or school?

☐ When does the surgeon want to see the convalescent again?

The Brain and Nervous System

HEADACHES

Occasional mild headaches that are not accompanied by other symptoms are usually nothing to worry about. More severe, frequent or persistent headaches may be caused by any of a variety of conditions, but most are either tension headaches or migraine headaches.

Tension headaches
These are usually felt at the front and sides of the head and tend to occur when the person is under particular stress.

Home care
Encourage the person to spend 10 minutes relaxing and offer a gentle massage of the back and neck, shoulders and temples to help relieve the headache. If necessary, give a painkiller such as paracetamol.
Consult your doctor:
○ If a bad headache persists for more than 2 or 3 days
○ If a headache is accompanied by stiffness and pain in the neck
○ If a headache is accompanied by diarrhoea or vomiting

Migraine headaches
Migraine headaches are severe and throbbing, usually affecting one side of the head or one eye only. They are often accompanied by feelings of nausea or even vomiting. There may also be disturbed vision for a short period before the headache begins, which may take the form of visual 'auras', flickering vision or a partially blank image. Bright light and loud noises make the headache feel more painful.

Home care
Encourage the person to rest in bed in a darkened room until the migraine has gone. A cold compress (see page 100) placed on the forehead may give some relief. Give a painkiller such as paracetamol.

You should also consult your doctor – he may well be able to prescribe medication that will help. He may also be able to help you identify factors that may trigger off the migraines: common factors include foods such as cheese and chocolate, glare, cold weather or release of stress.

EPILEPSY

This is a term given to a group of disorders characterized by recurring fits. The fits usually occur suddenly and last a few minutes. There are two main forms of epilepsy: petit mal (minor epilepsy) and grand mal (major epilepsy).

Petit mal epilepsy begins in early childhood. The child momentarily loses contact with the surroundings. He or she may stop talking in the middle of a sentence and, after a few seconds, continue again, quite unaware of having stopped; or just stare into space blankly; or suddenly stop walking. These attacks may happen several times in one day. Petit mal attacks rarely continue beyond puberty.

Grand mal epilepsy usually begins between the age of 7 and 17. A person having a grand mal fit suddenly falls unconscious to the ground and usually remains quite still and rigid for a moment before beginning to jerk convulsively. After a few minutes the jerking stops and the person then usually sleeps for an hour or so and wakes fully recovered.

Home care
Epilepsy can be well controlled by medication and
there is nothing to stop an epileptic leading a normal
life. However, it is important to make sure that any
drugs prescribed are taken in the correct dosage at
the right time, and there are one or two restrictions
that should be observed. If you are caring for an
epileptic, check whether he or she is allowed to drive
a car. Anyone suffering from epileptic fits should
also avoid swimming alone. And if there is anything
that the individual knows is likely to provoke a fit –
for example, television, flashing disco lights or
alcohol – this should of course be avoided. If
someone in your household is a newly-diagnosed
epileptic it is well worth contacting a support group
(see page 220).

An epileptic should carry a card or wear an
identity disc or bracelet, to inform anyone who
might try to help during a fit that he or she has
epilepsy.

In the event of a fit:
- Do not try to control the jerking, but clear a space
  around the person so that he or she does not come
  to any harm
- Do not put anything into the mouth
- When the fit has stopped, put the person into the
  recovery position (see page 198)
- Do not try to wake the person but stay close until
  he or she has fully recovered. There is usually no
  need for medical help but contact a doctor
  immediately if convulsions continue for more
  than 10 minutes or if several fits occur one after
  the other, or if you are worried about the person's
  condition

MENINGITIS

Meningitis is an inflammation of the meninges (the
membranes surrounding the brain), caused by
bacterial or viral infection. It is most common in
young people. The symptoms of meningitis are
headache, pain and stiffness in the neck and a
dislike of bright light. There may also be nausea and
vomiting. The person is likely to be drowsy, irritable
and unresponsive, or even confused.

Home care
If you suspect that someone may have meningitis,
obtain medical advice at once. The sick person will
probably be treated in hospital.

On return from hospital, the patient will probably
feel quite well but tired. He or she will need plenty of
rest and sleep, and a well-balanced diet (see page
110) for energy. A person recovering from
meningitis may find it difficult to concentrate for
several weeks or even months, so bear this in mind.

STROKE

A stroke occurs when the blood supply to part of the
brain is reduced or cut off. This may be caused by a
blood clot in an artery supplying blood to part of the
brain; the narrowing or blockage of an artery to the
brain; pressure on an artery by a tumour; or
bleeding into the brain from a ruptured artery.

The effects of a stroke vary depending on its
severity and on which part of the brain has been
affected. If you liken the brain to a telephone
exchange and imagine that part of the exchange
becomes damaged, then all those subscribers
controlled by the damaged part will find that their
telephones are out of order. If the part of the brain
that is damaged governs speech, say, or movement
on one side of the body, then the person's ability to
speak or to move that side will be impaired.
Someone who has had a minor stroke may suffer
from mild temporary clumsiness of hand, leg or
speech. A more severe stroke may mean complete
loss of movement on one side and inability to speak.

Levels of consciousness vary according to the
severity of the stroke, from slight confusion to
unconsciousness.

Home care
If a slight stroke occurs, put the person to bed and
send for the doctor. Stay with the patient in case
there are successive strokes.

In the case of a severe stroke, put the patient in the
recovery position (see page 198). Seek medical
advice urgently.

Most stroke patients will be nursed in hospital
initially. Hospital staff will concentrate on helping
the patient to regain movement and speech with
physiotherapy, occupational and speech therapy.
When the person returns home, make sure he or she
has plenty of rest, but also continues the therapy.
The hospital staff may suggest that the person
should return on an outpatient basis for therapy, or
you can ask your doctor to arrange for a therapist to
visit the patient at home. Do help and encourage the
patient with any exercises a therapist suggests.
Make sure also that he or she brings home the
appropriate equipment, such as a wheelchair, stick
or walking frame.

You can also help by letting the person do as much
as possible, if necessary adapting equipment to
make it easier for a disabled person to cope (see
pages 63 and 163). Consider putting handrails in the
bathroom and toilet. You may like to provide a long-
handled brush and comb, and to attach a soft nail
brush to the side of the wash basin with suction
cups, so the patient can wash his or her hands
without help. Replacing buttons and zips on
clothing with an adhesive fastening, such as Velcro,

makes dressing easier. To make eating unaided easier, place a non-slip mat under the plate and buy a knife and fork combined, or adapt the handles of cutlery to make them easier to grasp (see page 115).

A person who is recovering from a stroke may cry very easily, or become confused, forgetful and withdrawn or even difficult and unco-operative. He or she needs your support and understanding but there will probably be times when you have to be firm. You will need plenty of patience and so will the sick person, to adapt to a different way of life. However, even a patient suffering from a severe stroke may make considerable improvement over the following weeks or months.

Depending on the degree of disability following a stroke, you may become tired and depressed and wonder why you have all this to cope with. Both you and the patient may become frustrated at lack of progress. Try setting small, easily attainable goals to work to.

Ask your doctor if there is a local support group you can contact (see page 220)

Aids for stroke sufferers

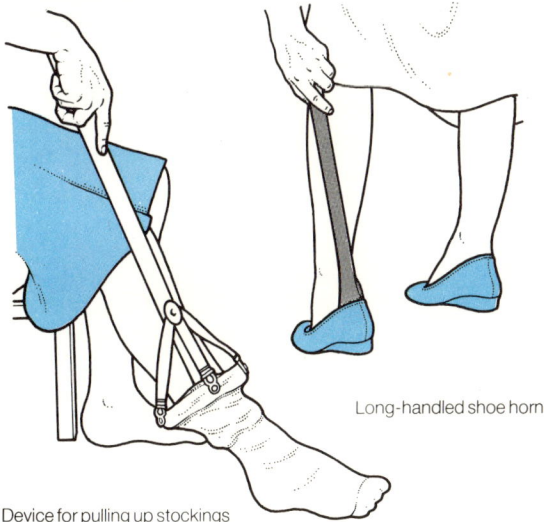

Long-handled shoe horn

Device for pulling up stockings

MULTIPLE SCLEROSIS

This is a disease of the nervous system. The symptoms are varied, as different parts of the nervous system are affected. A symptom may appear and then disappear for good, or reappear weeks, months or even years later. There are periods of remission, when there are no symptoms at all and the affected person feels quite well. In severe cases, however, as time goes on, additional symptoms appear more frequently and the disabilities tend to become permanent.

Home care

Good nursing care can make a lot of difference to the life of a person with multiple sclerosis. The aims should be to seek relief for the symptoms and to help the person to stay as active as possible. Always help and encourage the sick person to keep up involvement with friends, hobbies and outside interests.

Consider adaptations to the home (see pages 63 and 144) and any equipment (see pages 115 and 163) which will help the person remain independent.

It is particularly important for someone with multiple sclerosis to eat a well-balanced diet with plenty of fibre, a high vitamin content and lots of fluids: the chapter on **Diet and Nutrition** gives advice on this.

Fresh air and sunshine are good for the person's physical well-being and morale, but do not allow him or her to become too hot or too cold, as either may aggravate the symptoms of multiple sclerosis. For the same reason, hot baths or saunas are not advisable.

A person with multiple sclerosis should also avoid fatigue. He or she needs a good night's sleep and may need a rest during the day. Try to provide a peaceful, relaxed environment. A person with multiple sclerosis should never be hurried or expected to respond quickly either physically or mentally. This slowness can sometimes be very irritating for those who have to live with the person concerned. You may well find that you need help in coping with this. A support group (see page 221) can offer useful advice, and help.

The specific care needed varies according to the particular disabilities of the person you are caring for. It is important to emphasize that not everyone with multiple sclerosis will suffer from all of the same problems.

□ Ask the doctor or physiotherapist to show you how you can assist the person with any exercises that have been prescribed to help strengthen the muscles.

□ Encourage him or her to keep mobile for as long as possible, if necessary with the help of crutches or a walking frame (see pages 53 and 156). To help overcome problems caused by lack of co-ordination, encourage the person to walk with his or her feet wider apart to give more stability.

□ If the person has problems in co-ordinating arm movements, wrist supports or specially adapted cutlery (see page 115) may help.

□ A person with multiple sclerosis may lose bladder or bowel control. For information on how to care for someone with these problems, see page 71.

□ Some people have speech difficulties. If this is the case, ask the doctor to arrange for help from a speech therapist.

☐ The person may have double vision. Again, talk to the doctor, who may arrange for the person to wear a frosted lens to block the visual impulses of one eye.

☐ If he or she needs a wheelchair, make sure that it is the correct size and meets the person's requirements (see page 48).

☐ If the person is immobile or confined to a wheelchair, special attention to pressure areas will be needed (see page 78).

☐ Someone with the disease may well become depressed, withdrawn or resentful, or behave in some other way that is out of character. At these times, he or she will need a great deal of help, support and encouragement. And of course it is at these times that it becomes hardest to remain understanding and supporting. It may help to set short-term goals that you know the person can, with an effort, achieve. When these goals are reached there is a sense of success for everyone concerned.

Walking with a stick or crutch
The sick person should hold the stick in the hand opposite the affected leg. He should bring the bad leg and the stick forward at the same time, putting most of his weight on the stick and the good leg. He should keep the stick and bad leg in place while he steps forward with the good leg.

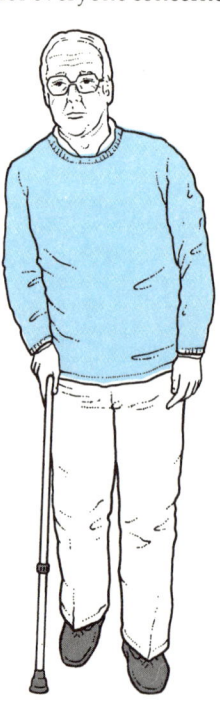

PARKINSON'S DISEASE

This is a progressive disease which affects parts of the brain. There are wide variations in the severity of symptoms. Characteristically, a person with Parkinson's disease walks with short, shuffling steps. There is trembling or shaking of the hands. The face tends to be mask-like, showing very little emotion, and speech is slurred and monotonous.

Home care
The treatment of Parkinson's disease is based on drugs, which will be prescribed by the doctor, and physiotherapy. You need to ensure that the medicines are taken in the correct amounts at the right times and that exercises are done regularly.

There are various drugs that can be very effective, for a time at least, in alleviating the symptoms of Parkinson's disease. These drugs are powerful, and they do tend to have side-effects. Ask the doctor to explain how the particular medicines prescribed will help the person you are caring for, and also how they will affect him or her.

Physiotherapy plays a very important part in helping a person with Parkinson's disease to stay mobile. The right kind of exercise increases muscle strength and helps with co-ordination and the problem of muscle rigidity. Ask the doctor to arrange for the sick person and yourself to have help and instruction from a skilled physiotherapist. You can then assist the person to do the exercises. You can also help in the following ways.

☐ Encourage daily exercise in a form the person enjoys – perhaps walking, riding an exercise cycle, gardening or swimming.

☐ Encourage the person to swing the arms and lengthen the stride when walking.

☐ Stretching exercises may help to loosen up the joints: get the sufferer to stretch a limb, hold it in position for a moment, then relax.

☐ Sometimes a person with Parkinson's disease gets the feeling that his or her feet are glued to the floor. If this happens, get the sufferer to lift his or her head, raise the toes and then rock from side to side with the knees slightly bent; or to lift the arms up in one short, sharp movement.

The sick person may well tire easily, and if he or she is over-tired the symptoms will tend to be more pronounced. A bath followed by a massage and exercises help to relieve painful muscle spasm.

A person suffering from Parkinson's disease may find it difficult if not impossible to express any feelings, and there is a tendency for sufferers to become depressed and withdrawn. He or she will need lots of emotional support, from you and from other people, and you yourself will need support, too. The following measures may help to combat depression.

☐ Try to reassure the person that the disabilities associated with the disease can be prevented or delayed.

☐ Encourage the sick person to be actively involved in his or her own treatment and day-to-day care and to set short-term goals for improvement.

☐ Plan the day to include periods of interesting activity as well as rest: make sure the person retains some interest in life – some reason to keep mobile.

The Heart, Blood and Circulation

VARICOSE VEINS

Varicose veins in the legs are very common, especially among women. The veins become engorged and enlarged and can be seen on the surface of the skin. There may be pain in the feet and ankles and a tired, heavy feeling in the legs.

Wearing support stockings helps to take some of the strain off the legs, as does sitting with the legs raised on a chair or stool. However, if varicose veins are causing discomfort or are getting worse, a doctor should be consulted. The doctor may suggest one of the following procedures.

☐ The varicose veins may be removed under general anaesthetic. The patient will usually come out of hospital 2 or 3 days after the operation.

☐ More rarely, the veins may be injected with a substance which causes the blood to clot and block off the veins. The injection is given on an outpatient basis and a general anaesthetic is not required.

Home care
Elasticated stockings stretching from toes to thigh must be worn for several weeks after surgery or injection. These stockings should be put on in bed before getting up in the morning (see page 159).

Standing or sitting in one position for long periods should be avoided, as should sitting with the legs crossed or dangling. When the person is sitting, his or her feet should be raised on a stool. Keeping body weight within normal limits, and not wearing tight girdles or garters, may help to prevent varicose veins.

HIGH BLOOD PRESSURE (Hypertension)

Normal blood pressure is described on page 88. A high blood pressure is a pressure over the accepted norm for a particular age group. Unless blood pressure gets very high indeed, when it may cause blurred vision or headaches, there are usually no symptoms and hypertension is often discovered only when a routine blood pressure reading is taken. So everyone should have their blood pressure checked from time to time. Ask your doctor for advice on frequency of testing.

Home care
If anyone in your care has high blood pressure, encourage him or her to:
○ Stop smoking
○ Lose weight if the doctor thinks this is advisable
○ Cut down on salt intake in the diet

○ Try to reduce the amount of stress by allowing time to relax, getting plenty of sleep, working reasonable hours, and, as far as possible, avoiding situations that are known to be stressful or to provoke anxiety

The doctor may prescribe medicines, which must be taken exactly as prescribed. It is also important to maintain any diet that the doctor or dietitian prescribes.

CORONARY ARTERY DISEASE

In coronary artery disease there is thickening and narrowing of the coronary blood vessels (arteriosclerosis) and plaques of fatty material are deposited in the lining of the arteries (atheroma), causing further narrowing. This all leads to a reduced blood supply to the heart. When the coronary arteries become very narrowed the flow of blood through them becomes sluggish and small clots tend to form in the arteries. Coronary artery disease may lead to angina, heart attacks (see page 159) and eventually to heart failure.

Home care
Anyone who has been diagnosed as having coronary artery disease or whose lifestyle puts them at risk should be encouraged to take the following steps, after seeing a doctor:
○ Stop smoking, or at least cut it down
○ Eat less sugar, salt and animal fat
○ Reduce weight if the doctor thinks that this is advisable
○ Take regular exercise: if the sufferer is not used to exercise, then check with the doctor first that there is no reason why he or she should not start gently and work up to a more vigorous programme – brisk walking is often an ideal form of exercise to begin with

ANGINA

Angina is a heart condition marked by attacks of sudden severe pain in the centre of the chest. This pain may pass into the arms, especially the left arm, the neck and the lower jaw. Sometimes the sufferer may complain of a tight feeling around the chest and difficulty getting breath. Angina occurs when there is a lack of blood and oxygen to the heart muscle, possibly because of narrowed coronary arteries (see Coronary artery disease). In some people attacks may be brought on by exercise, heavy meals, emotional reactions or even cold weather.

Home care
A person suffering from angina should be
encouraged to:
○ Stop smoking
○ Lose weight if the doctor thinks it necessary
○ As far as possible avoid any activities that tend to
   bring on the pain
○ Take prescribed medicines as directed
○ Take a moderate amount of exercise
○ Avoid pushing himself or herself beyond the
   point of tiredness
○ If possible take things rather slowly for a couple of
   hours after a full meal
○ Avoid going out in cold weather. If he or she must
   go out, then it is important to wrap up warmly
   and walk more slowly than usual

In the event of an attack
Get the person to sit or lie down, whichever is more
comfortable, to reduce the strain on the heart. If
appropriate, give any prescribed medicines. He or
she may well have some tablets to take in the event of
an attack. Read the instructions carefully to find out
how the tablets should be taken. Often the tablet is
placed under the tongue and allowed to dissolve. If
the attack lasts for more than 20 minutes, or you are
worried about the patient, seek medical advice.

THROMBOSIS

A thrombosis is a clot of blood inside a blood vessel,
either an artery or a vein. These clots are most
commonly found in:
○ the coronary arteries of the heart (a coronary
   thrombosis or heart attack, see page 159)
○ a brain artery, causing a stroke (see page 154)
○ one of the deep veins in the leg (deep vein
   thrombosis – DVT), usually in the calf but
   sometimes in the femoral vein in the thigh

Deep vein thrombosis
A deep vein thrombosis may occur when someone is
confined to bed, immobilized, particularly in the
case of the elderly, the overweight or a person who
has recently undergone surgery. They may also
occur in women taking the contraceptive pill. Any
woman taking the pill should discuss all the
implications with a doctor. In particular, she should
mention if she has ever had a deep vein thrombosis,
or if there is any history of arterial disease in her
family.
   When deep vein thrombosis occurs there is slight
pain and tenderness or a feeling of heaviness in the
affected limb. There may sometimes be a slight rise
in temperature. There may be oedema (fluid in the
tissues causing swelling) around the leg and ankle.

   If you suspect that a deep vein thrombosis is
present it is very important that you seek medical
advice. A deep vein thrombosis is not a serious
illness in itself, but, if untreated, part of the clot may
detach itself and move off into the blood stream. It
then flows along the veins, passes through the heart
and may finally obstruct a blood vessel in the brain,
heart or lungs.

Home care
Prevention is the priority.
□ Anyone confined to bed should move about in
the bed and do regular leg exercises (see page 79).
□ If possible, get the person up and sitting in a chair
with his or her legs raised on a stool (see page 56).
□ Discourage the sufferer from sitting on the bed
with his or her legs hanging over the edge.
□ Discourage sitting with the legs crossed.
□ Never place a pillow under the knees of a person
who is in bed or sitting in a chair as this restricts the
blood supply.
   If someone with a deep vein thrombosis is being
looked after at home, he or she should be in bed until
the prescribed medicines have had a chance to work.
If the person has been in hospital, some care will still
be needed on return home.
□ Treatment is likely to be with anticoagulants,
which prevent the clot from becoming larger. The
dosage will probably be changed according to the
results of blood tests, which will be taken frequently.
It is important to check with your doctor that any
other medicines being taken do not interact
adversely with the anticoagulant. For instance,
vitamin tablets, aspirin, cold medicines and
antibiotics should be avoided. Ask your doctor how
much alcohol is allowed. Anyone taking
anticoagulants should carry a warning card.
□ Any bleeding or extensive bruising, for example
nose bleeds, gum bleeding and injury following
teeth brushing, blood in urine or stools (see pages
94-95), should be reported to the doctor. If you have
difficulty in stopping bleeding, apply the principles
described on page 203 and seek medical advice.
□ While the patient is confined to bed, use a bedcradle (see page 56) to keep the bedclothes off the leg.
□ Do not massage or rub the limb: handle the limb
very gently.
□ Take care of the patient's skin, pressure areas and
mouth (see pages 57, 65 and 78).
□ Give plenty of fluids to make sure that he or she
does not become dehydrated, as this would
aggravate the condition.
□ Encourage the person to do deep breathing
exercises (see page 79).
□ For as long as the doctor thinks it necessary, the
affected leg should be raised, in bed or supported on
a footstool.

□ An elasticated stocking should be worn. This will reduce the swelling and support the leg. The stocking must be well-fitting, smooth and wrinkle-free. If it is too loose it will be ineffective, if too tight it will constrict and impair the blood flow. The stocking must not be left at knee level, as it would then constrict the blood flow.

□ When the person is allowed up, get him or her to do a little gentle walking, increasing it each day.

Putting on an elasticated stocking

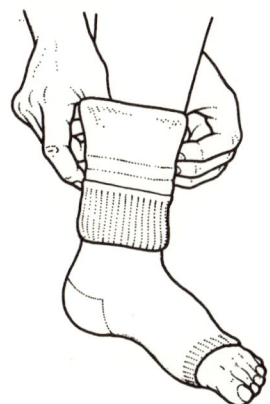

Putting on and taking off one of these stockings for someone else can be quite a struggle. Let the person sit or lie down, then stand as nearly as possible in the same position as you would if you were putting the stocking on yourself. Roll the stocking right down and ease it over the toes. Keeping your thumbs inside the stocking on either side of the leg, gently but firmly pull it up the leg.

HEART ATTACK

A heart attack occurs when the coronary arteries are narrowed and thickened and one of the arteries becomes blocked by a clot. The part of the heart supplied with blood by that artery is damaged. If a minor artery is blocked and only a small part of the heart is affected, the dead heart tissue is eventually absorbed and all that is left is a scar. If the clot blocks one of the major arteries then the heart is unable to continue working.

When a heart attack occurs there is chest pain which may spread into the neck or left arm. The pain may be no more than an ache and may be mistaken for indigestion, or it may be very severe. It lasts much longer than an attack of angina (see page 157). There may also be vomiting, wind and belching. The affected person may be restless, sweating, pale and cold and the skin may feel clammy.

Immediate home care
Follow these immediate steps:
○ Loosen clothing and let the patient choose the best position for breathing – usually sitting up
○ Keep calm and reassure. Minimize shock (see page 200)
○ Call for medical help
○ If unconscious, put the sick person in the recovery position (see page 198)
○ If heartbeat and breathing stop, resuscitate (see pages 194-197)

If someone has had a heart attack and is being nursed at home instead of going to hospital, the procedures described below should be followed.
□ The sick person should be nursed in bed in the position that feels most comfortable, usually propped up with pillows and a backrest. If the patient becomes breathless, sit him or her up a little. Bed-rest is essential and the patient should be disturbed as little as possible in the first few hours.
□ It is a good idea to have a board under the mattress, as this makes it easier to give heart massage, if necessary (see page 196).
□ Ask the doctor if he wants you to record the patient's temperature, pulse and blood pressure, or to measure urine output (see pages 84 to 92).
□ Give drugs as prescribed by the doctor, and also oxygen if it has been prescribed (see page 103).
□ Diet should be suited to the patient's condition. Get advice from your doctor as to what sort of diet the patient should follow. He may suggest restricting the invalid's salt and fat intake (see page 160).
□ A man should use a urine bottle and a woman a bedpan for passing urine. For bowel movements it is better to help the person onto a commode as this actually causes less strain than perching on a bedpan. Discuss this with the doctor.
□ It will probably also cause less strain for a man if he shaves himself, with your help, when necessary.
□ If the patient is sweaty then washing his or her face is refreshing – but only do what is really essential. The damaged heart should be put under as little strain as possible.
□ Even once the immediate attack has passed, visitors should be restricted to close family. The patient must not be over-tired.
□ A person who has had a heart attack will be very frightened and need a great deal of emotional support. He or she may, in addition, be worried about work or other responsibilities. You can help most by organizing someone else to take over. Tell the sick person what you have done and insist that the work be handed over to others. If there is a telephone in the room it may be necessary to have it temporarily removed so that proper rest is possible.

Usually the sick person gets much better within a few days. The doctor will tell you when the patient is well enough to get up for a short time, perhaps for less than an hour. The time can be increased each day depending on condition and providing that there is no further chest pain. The doctor will decide the regime. You should, however, keep a very close eye on a person in the early days after a heart attack in case of another attack or cardiac arrest, in which the heart stops beating. Be prepared to use emergency cardiac massage or artificial respiration if necessary.

Care on recovery
Someone who has been in hospital will probably be ready to come home about 2 weeks after an uncomplicated heart attack, if there has been no more chest pain after the onset. He or she will gradually become able to lead a normal life. More severe cases will take a little longer and the person may need to modify his or her lifestyle, perhaps taking a less demanding job. Each case must be looked at individually.

Encourage the convalescent to lead as normal a life as possible, and to:
○ Take regular moderate exercise, which can be gradually increased, providing that there is no chest pain
○ Take proper periods of rest
○ Stop smoking
○ Follow a diet low in sugar, salt and animal fats
○ Reduce weight, if the doctor thinks this is advisable
○ Take the doctor's advice about when to return to work – this will usually be at least 2 and possibly 4 months after the heart attack

Diet
If the convalescent is overweight, he or she will probably be put on a reducing diet. Losing the excess weight means that the heart is under less strain. Large amounts of fat around the abdominal area may restrict the breathing, which worsens the breathlessness associated with heart disease. Your doctor may advise the person to restrict the amount of salt eaten. If so:
○ Cook with the minimum of salt but ensure that the food is still palatable
○ Do not add salt to food at the table
○ Avoid salty foods, such as canned vegetables, tomato juice, canned meats, canned fish, chutneys, pickles, ketchup and sauces, canned or packet soups, bacon, ham, tongue, sausages, smoked fish, meat and fish pastes, meat and yeast extracts, stock cubes, and any foods that contain salt or monosodium glutamate.

Reduce the amount of saturated fats eaten by:
○ Using skimmed milk instead of whole milk
○ Cooking with corn oil and using margarines high in polyunsaturated fats
○ Offering lean cuts of meat, white meat and fish rather than fattier meats
○ Avoiding cheese, liver, kidney, pastry and cakes made with egg and butter, ice cream, chocolate and toffee
○ Restricting egg yolks to one per week

ANAEMIA

A person suffering from anaemia has insufficient haemoglobin, the oxygen-carrying pigment in the red blood cells. There are various possible causes. Two of the most common are loss of blood in heavy periods in women, or a deficiency of iron (which is needed for the production of haemoglobin) in the diet. Tiredness, weakness, pallor, nausea, loss of appetite, and consequent weight loss may all be associated with anaemia, but these symptoms develop slowly and are often ignored, as the sufferer becomes used to feeling vaguely unwell. Anaemia is often discovered incidentally, as a result of a blood test taken for some other purpose.

Home care
Seek medical advice – the treatment for anaemia will vary with the cause. Treatment will almost certainly include iron supplements.

The most important aspect of home care is providing a well-balanced diet, including plenty of foods rich in iron (see page 112).

Bones and Joints

BACKACHE

Backache is usually caused by tearing or straining the ligaments (bands of tough fibrous tissue) around the spine, resulting in inflammation and pain in the affected area.

Home care
The most useful home care is prevention. One of the most frequent causes of back injuries is lifting a weight in a way that puts undue strain on the back. And there is a warning here for you as a caregiver – if you are lifting and moving an invalid at home, you need to be particularly aware of the risk of hurting your back. Read and apply the general rules for lifting and moving on page 34.

A back which has been strained must be rested as much as possible. If the pain is severe the person should lie down, either in bed (with a board under the mattress if it is not a firm one), or on the floor. He or she should lie in whatever position is most comfortable. If he or she is more comfortable in an armchair, support the back with pillows or cushions.

Applying heat to the part that hurts helps to relieve the pain. Use a hot-water bottle or a heating pad or electric blanket. Aspirin not only relieves pain but also reduces inflammation. However, aspirin must be avoided in certain circumstances (see page 109). If you are in any doubt, give paracetamol for pain instead. You should also seek medical advice, as medication – for example, muscle relaxants – can be prescribed.

Until the back has completely recovered the person should not lift anything heavy. See your doctor if when the back was hurt there was pain, numbness or tingling in the legs; or if severe back pain persists for more than 48 hours.

SLIPPED DISC

The vertebrae of the spine are separated by discs of cartilage. Sometimes a disc cracks or becomes displaced and presses on a nerve. This causes pain, sometimes near the injury but more often in the muscles supplied by the nerve concerned. For instance, if a disc in the neck slips it may cause numbness and pins and needles in the fingers and sometimes shooting pains down the arm. A slipped disc lower down the back may cause pain which travels down the back, across one buttock and down the back of one leg.

Most slipped discs return to normal if the back or neck are rested. In the case of a neck injury this may include wearing a supporting collar. Sometimes, however, manipulation is needed, and in a few cases an operation may be necessary.

Home care
Home care is basically the same as for backache, but medical advice should be sought. This is particularly important in the case of an injured neck.

FRACTURED LIMBS

For the immediate care of a person with a broken bone, see page 207. After a broken limb has been set, plaster of Paris is often used as a cast to hold the bone in the correct position as it heals. The length of time that a plaster cast should be left in position depends on the extent of the damage, but generally a cast stays on for 6 to 8 weeks on an upper limb and for 3 months or longer on a weight-bearing bone. How long the person stays in hospital depends on which bone was broken and also on the extent of other injuries, if any. He or she may not need hospitalization at all.

Home care
When someone who has broken a bone comes home from hospital, provide a well-balanced, nourishing diet to encourage healing (see page 110). Make sure

that any exercises that are prescribed are continued, and that the convalescent takes as much general exercise as possible. Call your doctor if there is increasing pain at any time.

While you are looking after someone with a plaster cast, the following hints may be helpful.
☐ If the fingers or toes on a limb in a cast are blue, pale, cold, numb or tingling, it may be that the plaster is too tight. To test, press the fingernail or toenail: when you let go, the colour of the nail should change from white to pink at once. If the colour change is slow, inform your doctor.
☐ Never poke a sharp object under the plaster. If the limb itches, suggest scratching another part of the body – this sometimes helps.
☐ Do not get the plaster or the padding wet, as this can cause damage to the skin underneath. To clean the cast of superficial dirt, just wipe with a slightly damp cloth. You can use household scouring powder to get off more permanent marks.
☐ If the plaster becomes damaged, you should consult your doctor.
☐ When the plaster is taken off, there may be some aches and pains in the affected limb, and difficulty in using it. It may look mottled and feel cold or even swell. This is often rather depressing for the person concerned, who has been counting the days until the removal of the plaster and now finds that it was easier to manage with the plaster on. Reassure him or her that the limb will soon be back to normal.
☐ If physiotherapy is advised by your doctor or the hospital, make sure that any exercises taught by the physiotherapist are practised regularly.
☐ Sometimes the skin underneath a cast becomes scaly and yellow. This is best left alone: do not try to pick or pull off the scales, as this may cause bleeding and soreness. The scaliness can be gradually cleaned away with moisturizing cream over the days following removal of the cast, and the skin colouring will soon return to normal.
☐ If the convalescent needs to use crutches or a walking stick, it is important that they are the right height. Ask advice from the doctor or physiotherapist. A walking stick should be used on the side opposite the broken limb (see page 156).

ARTHRITIS

The term arthritis means inflammation of a joint. There are two common forms of arthritis, osteoarthritis and rheumatoid arthritis.

Osteoarthritis
In osteoarthritis there is degeneration of one or more joints, with a gradual wearing away of the cushion of cartilage that lines the joint, a loss of

lubricating fluid and the formation of rough deposits of bone. An affected joint is stiff and painful. The joints most commonly affected are the weight-bearing joints such as the hip, knee and spine. Sometimes the hands are affected. Osteoarthritis most commonly occurs in people over the age of 50 years old.

Home care
Exercise helps to keep the joints and muscles supple. The doctor may recommend physiotherapy, and in this case the person will probably be taught the exercises at the hospital and then be expected to carry on at home.

A walking stick may be helpful, to take some of the weight off an affected leg. If a stick is used it should be held opposite the affected leg (see page 156).

It is best to alternate periods of rest and activity and to keep the joints as comfortable as possible. Try to make sure the person does not stand for long periods, carry heavy weights, or climb stairs more often than is necessary, or do anything that involves much overhead stretching.

It is important for someone suffering from arthritis not to become overweight, as this will put more strain on the joints. The doctor may advise that the person should lose some weight.

Heat, either sitting in a hot bath or placing a hot-water bottle over an affected joint, helps to relieve pain. Cold applications (see page 100) may be helpful as well. Take the doctor's advice on this.

Sometimes an operation is necessary, to replace an affected joint with an artificial joint (see page 163). A person suffering from severe osteoarthritis needs a great deal of emotional support, especially at times when the pain is severe. A support group (see page 220) can provide useful advice.

Rheumatoid arthritis
With rheumatoid arthritis the lining of the joints and the surrounding tissues are inflamed and swollen, causing pain. Rheumatoid arthritis tends to affect younger people, often those under 40, and it is more common in women. The smaller joints – fingers, toes and wrists – are usually the first to be affected. Later the elbows, shoulders, ankles and knees may become affected as well.

The disease can be mild, affecting one or two joints, or it can be more severe and widespread. Sometimes it comes and goes, so there may be periods when there is no pain. Joints may become very swollen and painful and then improve considerably. Sometimes the joints are damaged and after the swelling has subsided they look out of shape and cannot be moved properly. No two patients are alike, so the treatment and outcome vary from person to person.

Home care
The most important aspects of caring for a person with rheumatoid arthritis are to follow the medical treatments prescribed by the doctor, to help prevent the deformities that may occur; and to encourage the person to remain independent.

Make sure any medicines are taken as prescribed, and that hot or cold treatments for muscle relaxation and relief of pain are given (see page 100), if they have been prescribed by the doctor. If the person is in pain go back to the doctor to see if the medication can be changed or if there is anything else that can be done to help.

Special exercises help to maintain the joints' full range of movement and to improve those with limited movement. They also help to strengthen the muscles. The sufferer will probably be taught these exercises at the hospital by a physiotherapist, and they should be continued at home. Make sure that the person does not overdo exercise: any physical exertion that increases pain and swelling for more than an hour or two afterwards is too taxing. However, if a joint is not moved for long periods it will become stiff and painful, so you need to strike a happy medium.

Your doctor may suggest the use of splints to correct the position of a joint or to help use a joint (working splints). But by no means everyone with rheumatoid arthritis needs splints.

It will help the person to remain independent if you can adapt equipment in the home to make it easier for him or her to use.

If the person has difficulties with sexual activities, perhaps because of an arthritic hip, professional advice should be sought. Ask your doctor where you can get help.

The following points may be helpful.
☐ A person with rheumatoid arthritis should always lower him- or herself gently into a chair, holding onto the arms of the chair. If the hips and knees are affected, provide a raised chair.
☐ The person should always straighten up before starting to walk.
☐ He or she should avoid carrying heavy objects, especially when walking upstairs.
☐ The person should be careful not to become overweight, as this puts an added strain on the weight-bearing joints. The doctor may suggest some weight reduction.
☐ It is particularly important to avoid putting strain on the small joints of the fingers and thumbs if the hands are affected (see page 115 for equipment that can help here).

A person suffering from rheumatoid arthritis may become depressed and anxious because of the pain and disability it causes: it is well worth contacting a support group (see page 220).

Aids for arthritis sufferers

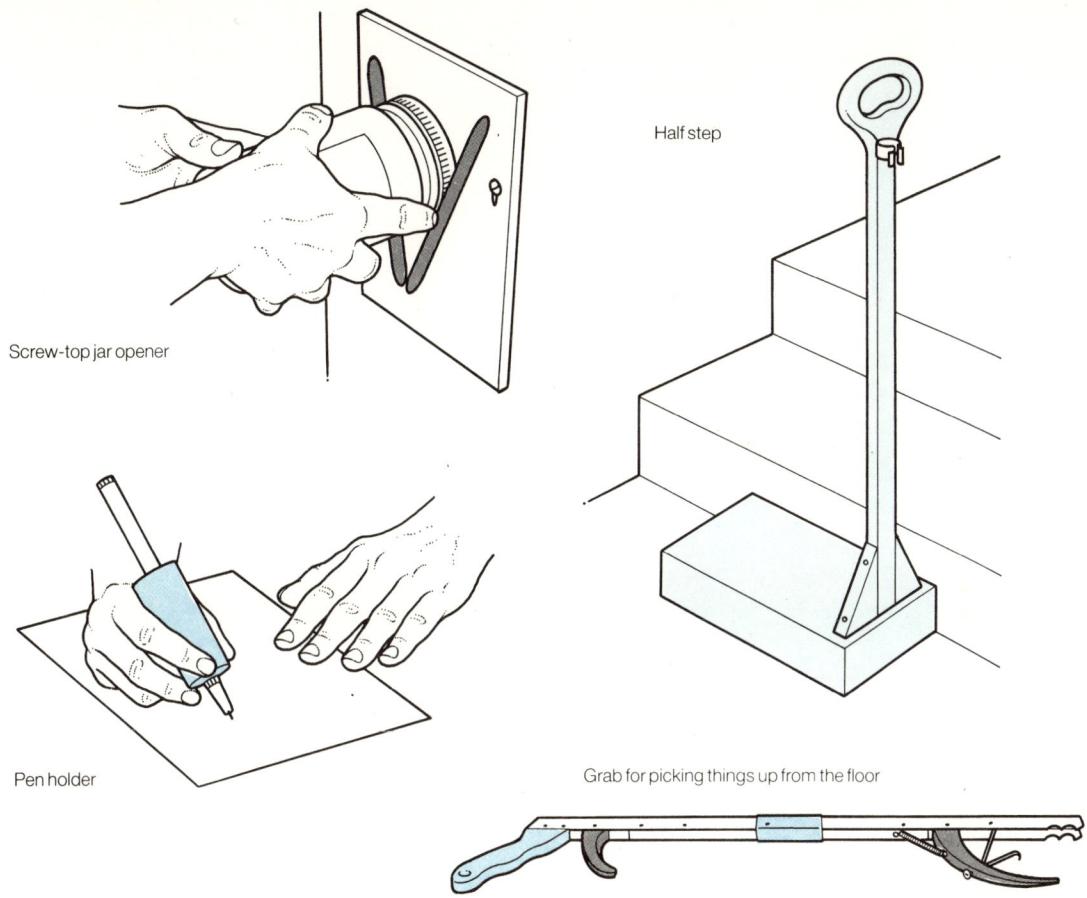

Screw-top jar opener

Half step

Pen holder

Grab for picking things up from the floor

HIP REPLACEMENT

The joint at the top of the long bone in the thigh (the femur) and the socket in the pelvis can be replaced by an artificial joint. Usually the operation is performed on people severely disabled by painful arthritis of the hip or who have had severe hip injuries.

After the operation, pain-relieving medicines may be needed for 2 to 4 days. The person should be up and walking about 24 to 48 hours after the replacement of a hip joint.

Home care
The person usually comes home about 2 to 3 weeks after the operation. The following points should be borne in mind when caring for someone who has had a hip replaced.
☐ Make sure he or she always sits in a fairly high chair and sits with the knees apart. Crossing the legs should be avoided, as should sitting for more than 30 minutes without getting up and walking around.
☐ If elastic stockings have been used in hospital the convalescent should continue to wear them. (For advice on putting on elastic stockings, see page 159).
☐ He or she will need to lie flat for about 30 minutes, twice a day. Ask the surgeon how long this practice should be continued.
☐ Help the person to continue any exercises taught in hospital.
☐ If there are problems in getting on and off the toilet, you can either put a rail beside it or raise the seat (see page 134).
☐ The convalescent will probably need the support of a walking stick for a while, when going for walks. The stick should be used on the side opposite the affected joint (see page 156).
☐ It is usually possible to go back to work 3 to 4 months after this operation, depending on the type of work.

KNEE REPLACEMENT

This is the replacement of the knee joint with an artificial joint.

Home care
Home care is the same as for a patient who has had a hip replacement operation (see page 163), with two additional points.
☐ The person must use a walking stick to help keep the weight off the new joint. The walking stick should be held on the side opposite to the affected leg (see page 156).
☐ The surgeon may like the patient to use a splint at night to maintain the full extension of the knee joint. Check how long this should continue (it is usually about 3 to 4 weeks).

AMPUTATION OF A LIMB

A limb may be so badly damaged, for example in an accident or by a condition such as gangrene or cancer, that it has to be removed.

Physiotherapy plays an important part in rehabilitation following amputation, and it is usual for a physiotherapist to visit the patient and start exercises even before the operation. These exercises are essential to preserve and improve the function of the muscles in the affected limb.

After the operation, the physiotherapist will continue the exercises and will also teach the person how to manage a prosthesis or false limb. Usually a temporary prosthesis is fitted immediately after the operation and fitting the permanent prosthesis is delayed until the stump has healed and the stitches are out. This is normally about 3 months after the operation.

Inevitably the patient must dread the disability which follows the amputation of a limb and he or she will need lots of encouragement. Quite often the hospital will introduce someone who has overcome the problems of amputation. This gives the patient and you, the caregiver, the chance to ask any questions and get plenty of advice from someone who has been through the same experience. It is also very encouraging to see someone coping well after an amputation.

Home care
Home care after an amputation is very specialized and will depend on which limb has been amputated and why. The hospital will make sure that you have contact with all the rehabilitation services; see also the Appendix: **Where to Find Help**.

The hospital staff will have shown you how to take care of the end of the stump. Report any soreness or

breaks in the skin to the doctor. There may be a small amount of pain from the operation. This will be relieved by a painkiller such as paracetamol. The person may also complain of pain in the amputated limb – phantom limb pain.

It is most important that the exercises that were taught in hospital should be continued. After a leg amputation, if there are no complications, the person may be able to walk on the prosthesis without crutches about 6 weeks after the operation.

Someone who has had a limb amputated needs a great deal of love, support and reassurance that this has not changed the way his or her family and friends feel. The family can do a great deal to help the person back to independence by helping him or her to face any grief, fear or embarrassment and by refusing to allow the amputation to change their relationship to the person concerned. They can also hold out the highest expectations that he or she will continue to lead a normal life.

Amputation is most common among people between 60 and 70 years old who have diabetes or vascular disease, and an elderly person may have particular problems getting mobile again; but physiotherapists are specialists in this type of rehabilitation and will do everything they can. The caregiver can play an important part by encouraging the person and helping with any exercises.
It is very important that someone who has had a limb amputated should become as independent as possible. This is especially so in the case of a child, adolescent or young person. Being treated like an invalid by caring parents will not help. Plenty of time to play with other children will probably help to restore the child's confidence.

A growing child will need to have the prosthesis changed, so regular check-ups are necessary to see that it still fits and is comfortable. If the child is very active the stump is likely to become sore and there may be breaks in the skin: in this case, seek medical advice. The child is likely to become tired more quickly than other children, so it is especially important to see that he or she gets a good night's sleep and eats a well-balanced diet which will give plenty of energy but keep weight within normal limits (see page 110). If the child becomes too heavy, his or her mobility will be impaired.

The experience of losing a limb is always traumatic, and for an adolescent or young person, anything that makes him or her feel different is going to be difficult to cope with, particularly with all the other bodily changes which are occurring at this time. Parents need plenty of patience, tact and understanding, but above all a very positive outlook. Encourage the young person in what he or she can do and do not dwell on what has happened or what might have been.

The Skin

PSORIASIS

Psoriasis is a skin condition which usually takes the form of a rash of red patches with silvery scales. These are most obvious on the front of the knees or on the elbows but can affect any part of the skin. The rash can last for up to 3 months. It may then fade, but it tends to recur. Psoriasis varies greatly in its severity, from a few patches to a widespread rash.

Home care
A person with psoriasis should see a doctor. Moisturizing creams or coal-tar preparations may be prescribed, and you should make sure that these are applied regularly. Sunshine may help clear the psoriasis and so may ultra-violet light from a sunlamp, but ultra-violet lamps should be used only under medical supervision. You should also be careful that the person does not become sunburned, in sunlight or from a sunlamp.

The person may find the psoriasis very embarrassing and depressing, and need a lot of morale-boosting and general emotional support. If stress makes the psoriasis worse, help the sufferer to avoid stressful situations.

ECZEMA (Dermatitis)

The terms 'eczema' and 'dermatitis' are often used interchangeably. There are several forms of eczema, but characteristically the skin becomes dry and red, then cracked, weepy, scaling and itchy. The extent and severity of eczema varies widely.

Home care
Take the person to see the doctor. Various moisturizing creams, or creams containing zinc and castor oil or even steroids may be prescribed, and should be applied as directed.

Try to discover if there is anything that triggers the eczema. It can be difficult to find anything specific but eggs and milk do sometimes make eczema worse.

The following measures may also help.
☐ Washing with soap and water often makes eczema worse; try using an emulsifying cream or lotion instead.
☐ It is best to avoid clothes made of rough or scratchy materials. The clothes worn next to the skin should be made of cotton.
☐ Many detergents cause irritation. Use only mild detergents for washing clothes, and make sure the clothes are very thoroughly rinsed. Some detergents are specifically recommended for use by people with sensitive skin. An eczema support group (see page 220) will let you have a list.

Scratching the eczema should be strongly discouraged, as it can cause bacterial infection. But eczema is very itchy, and it can be difficult to stop a person, particularly a child, from scratching. Moisturizing creams will soothe the rash to some extent. And, at any rate, do make sure that the fingernails are kept short and very clean, to minimize the harm done by scratching.

This type of skin problem can be very distressing, so try to give the person plenty of emotional support. In particular, babies and children with eczema can often be very upset, and need a great deal of love.

The Eyes

CONJUNCTIVITIS

Inflammation of the conjunctiva, the thin membrane lining the eyelids and covering the front of the eyeball, caused by infection or allergy, is known as conjunctivitis. The eye looks red and waters, and there is a yellow discharge. The eyelids are stuck together in the morning. The eye feels as if there is something in it.

Home care
Someone with conjunctivitis should be seen by a doctor. Whatever the cause there are medicines and eyedrops that can be prescribed (see page 98). In the case of an allergy the doctor will also want to discuss any possible cause.

CATARACT

A cataract is opacity of the lens of the eye. As the lens does not allow enough light through, vision becomes blurred, as if the person were looking through a mist. The treatment for cataract is an operation to remove the lens. A replacement lens may be implanted at the time of the operation.

Home care
If the patient comes out of hospital a few days after the operation, it may be necessary to wear a metal or plastic shield over the eye at night, to protect it from being accidentally damaged during sleep. Check with the surgeon when the use of the shield can be stopped.

Give any eyedrops as prescribed and ask the hospital staff to show you how to give them. Avoid using eye baths or irrigations unless they have been prescribed by a doctor.

For at least 6 weeks after the operation, the following precautions should be taken:
○ The patient should avoid sunlight and wear dark glasses if the light is bright
○ He or she should not rub the affected eye
○ The person should not bend, stoop or lift anything heavy
○ As far as is possible, sneezing and coughing should be avoided

If the person is worried that he or she may have damaged the eye in any way – during a sneezing or coughing fit, or for any other reason – contact the hospital, or get in touch with your own doctor.

The eyes are usually tested 6 weeks after the operation and then, if necessary, a prescription for glasses or contact lens will be given. Until these are supplied there may be only limited vision, so it is important that the convalescent's surroundings are familiar and that the person concerned knows exactly where things are. This will encourage him or her to regain independence safely.

If the patient is worried about a cataract recurring, he or she should be reassured that once the lens has been removed from the eye no further cataract can occur in that eye, because there is no lens. The risk of a recurrence is slight even if a replacement lens has been implanted.

GLAUCOMA

Glaucoma is caused by increased pressure of the fluid in the eye. If left untreated, the optic nerve may be damaged, causing deterioration, and even loss, of vision.

Depending on the type and severity of the glaucoma, there are various treatments available. Drops that unblock the drainage channels in the eye can be given, there are medications and drops that will reduce the fluid pressure, and an operation can also be performed to create an artificial drainage channel. Very rarely, an operation to drain the fluid may be necessary.

Home care
Home care is as for cataracts (see above). However, after an operation, the person concerned will be given a special prescription for glasses or contact lenses immediately, instead of having to wait for 6 weeks.

The Ears, Nose and Throat

EARACHE

Many different conditions can cause pain in the ear: the most common cause is an infection of the middle ear. Other causes include a cold wind in the ears; a cold, a sore throat or mumps; a foreign body in the ear canal; a boil in the ear canal; or pain from a toothache in the back teeth, which may be felt in the ear as well as the tooth. Children are particularly prone to earache.

Earache may be accompanied by nausea and vomiting, and the sufferer's temperature is often raised.

Home care
Regular doses of painkillers, such as paracetamol, will probably be needed. A cold or hot compress (see page 100) may help to relieve pain. If the earache is very severe or continues for more than 24 hours, and especially if there is a raised temperature, you should consult a doctor.

If antibiotics are prescribed it is important that the whole course should be taken even if the pain has gone. Failure to complete the course may mean the return of the infection and the earache.

COLDS

A cold is a viral infection of the nose and throat. It causes a congested or runny nose, a sore throat, a generalized aching and feeling of being unwell and frequently a slightly raised temperature. Most colds last about 7 to 10 days.

Home care
Give plenty of fluids. Steam inhalations (see page 102) will help to clear the nasal passages. You can give paracetamol to relieve the symptoms.

If a baby with a cold cannot feed properly because of difficulty in sucking, clean the nostrils with moist cotton-buds. If this does not help, the doctor may prescribe nose drops containing a decongestant. But do not continue to give them to the baby for more than 3 or 4 days.

There is generally no need to see a doctor about a cold. However, you should get medical advice if there is earache; or a wheezy cough, which brings up yellow or green mucus; or a *significantly* raised temperature – 37.4°C (99.5°F) in children or 37.7°C (100°F) in adults – that persists for more than 3 or 4 days; or if a baby with a cold has feeding difficulties.

SINUSITIS

Sinusitis, or inflammation of the sinuses, often follows a cold. There is pain over the infected sinus – under the eye, along the cheekbone or over the eye – which is usually worse when the person leans forward or lies down. There may also be a raised temperature, watering eyes, a yellow or green discharge from the nose or a blocked nose.

Home care
Steam inhalations (see page 102) may help the sinuses to drain more freely. Paracetamol helps bring the temperature down and gives some relief from pain.

See the doctor if the face is very painful, or there is a significant fever.

LARYNGITIS

Laryngitis is inflammation of the larynx (voice box) and vocal cords, resulting in a sore throat, coughing and hoarseness, or even temporary loss of the voice. It usually lasts 3 to 10 days.

Home care
Steam inhalations (page 102) help clear the airways. If the person is feverish or feels very unwell, you can give soluble paracetamol. A cough medicine or, preferably, a glass of warm water and honey taken at night may soothe a dry, irritating cough.

See the doctor if a young child has laryngitis, especially if there is any difficulty in breathing, or if it persists for much longer than a week in an adult or older child.

SORE THROATS AND TONSILLITIS

Sore throats vary a lot, depending on whether the cause is a bacterial or viral infection, which part of the throat is affected and how severely. A mild sore throat may cause nothing more than a little discomfort. A bad sore throat, especially one that involves infected and swollen tonsils, can be very troublesome. The sufferer may have a high temperature and enlarged neck glands, as well as a sore throat and difficulty in swallowing.

Home care
Give plenty of fluids and if necessary a painkiller such as soluble paracetamol.

See your doctor if a sore throat gets worse after 48 hours, if the person's temperature rises above 39.5°c (103°F) or if you are worried about his or her condition.

TONSILLECTOMY AND ADENOIDECTOMY

A tonsillectomy is an operation to remove the tonsils. These days surgeons take out tonsils only when the operation is felt to be absolutely necessary after repeated attacks of tonsillitis.

The adenoids are situated at the back of the nose in children. After the age of 5 years, they gradually start to shrink and disappear by puberty. Enlarged adenoids may be removed (adenoidectomy) if they are thought to be involved in causing recurrent ear infections or sore throats. Children may have the tonsils and adenoids removed at the same time.

After a tonsillectomy pain relief is usually required for 2 to 5 days. There is usually very little pain following an adenoidectomy performed without removing the tonsils.

Home care
When the person returns from hospital, encourage him or her to eat a balanced diet, with regard for his or her preferences, and to take lots of fluids.

Plenty of rest is needed. A child should have a daily rest period in bed for about a week after the operation.

Following a tonsillectomy, the surgeon may recommend taking soluble paracetamol for the pain. Although it is safe to use a mouthwash, it is better not to gargle with it, as this might cause bleeding. The mouth should be rinsed out, and as soon as possible the teeth should be brushed frequently, at least three times a day, to ensure that the mouth is clean and to prevent any infections in the healing tonsil beds.

If it is warm enough, encourage the convalescent to get out in the fresh air, but avoid crowded places where there is a likelihood of coming into contact with infection. There should be no swimming until after the follow-up appointment at the hospital when the surgeon checks on progress.

Call your doctor if there is any sign of bleeding – in children this should be suspected if the child is swallowing frequently. You should also ask for help if there is earache with a raised temperature, or if you are worried.

Following a tonsillectomy, the person will usually be fit to resume normal activities in about 2 weeks, but ask your own doctor or the surgeon for advice on when to go back to work or school. An adult can usually expect to return to work 3 weeks after the operation. Children can usually go back to school in about 2 to 3 weeks. In the meantime it may be a good idea to get some school work sent home for the child to do when he or she feels better. Following a simple adenoidectomy, consult your doctor about how soon the convalescent should return to work or school.

The Lungs

COUGHS

Coughing is a reflex action stimulated by irritation of the lungs or air passages. Repeated coughing may indicate an infection, such as a cold (see page 166) or bronchitis (see page 169), or any one of several other conditions.

Home care
Give plenty of fluids to loosen the cough. Steam inhalations (see page 102) help to clear the airways. If the cough is troublesome at night a hot lemon drink with a teaspoon of honey or, for a dry cough, a cough medicine may help the person get some sleep.

A baby or child with a cold may be troubled at night by a cough caused by mucus trickling down the back of the throat. In this case a child might be more comfortable propped upright in bed with pillows. A baby should be put to lie on his or her side, without a pillow.

See the doctor if:
○ A cough persists 2 to 3 weeks after a cold has gone
○ The cough produces blood, or mucus which is becoming darker or greener in colour
○ There is chest pain or difficulty in breathing
○ The person is feverish and feels very unwell
○ You are worried about the sick person's condition

ASTHMA

Asthma is a respiratory condition characterized by attacks of difficulty in breathing and of wheezing. In a susceptible person, asthma attacks may be brought on by:
○ Breathing in, touching or eating something the sufferer is sensitive to – examples include the tiny house-mites found in dust, feathers, cat, dog or horse hair, pollens in the spring and summer, plants, shellfish, chocolate and eggs
○ Emotional upsets or crises – for example, anger, frustration, fear of exams or interviews
○ Infections, such as colds or chest infections
○ Exposure to cold air
There may in some cases be no obvious cause.

Home care
If certain things are known to precipitate attacks, home care largely consists of helping the asthmatic person to avoid those things.
☐ If the sufferer is allergic to dust, the bedroom should be vacuum-cleaned and damp-dusted regularly. House-mite dust can be reduced by enclosing the mattress in a plastic bag and by changing bedclothes frequently.

☐ If feathers or animal hair are a problem, feather or horsehair bedding and pillows should be replaced with synthetic materials, such as foam rubber.
☐ If sensitive to pollen, a person who suffers from asthma should stay indoors as much as possible when the pollen count is high and should avoid flowers and plants.
☐ If the person is really allergic to a cat, dog or horse you may have to find another home for the animal concerned.

In addition you should:
○ Strongly discourage smoking
○ Make sure all drugs are given as prescribed
○ Encourage correct breathing, from the diaphragm (for breathing exercises, see page 79)
Treatment may involve the use of an inhaler. If so, ask the medical staff to show you how to use it correctly.

In the event of an attack:
○ Loosen any tight clothing
○ Get the person into the position he or she finds most comfortable

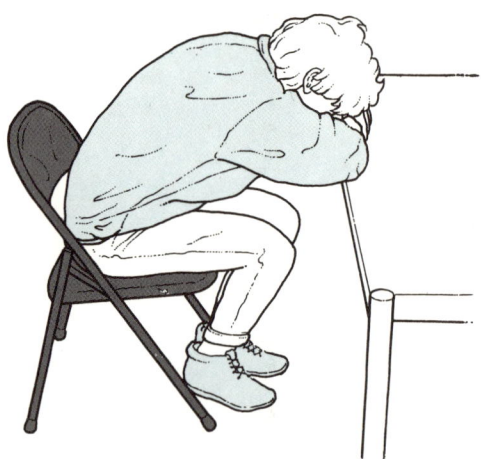

Position during an asthma attack
The most comfortable position is often sitting down, leaning forward slightly onto a table or the back of a chair.

○ Keep calm yourself: talk calmly and firmly, and encourage the person to breathe in and out, using the diaphragm
○ If the sufferer has an inhaler to be used during attacks, help him or her to use it effectively (see page 102)

BRONCHITIS

Bronchitis is inflammation of the bronchi, the large tubes which lead from each lung into the windpipe. There are two types of bronchitis, acute bronchitis and chronic bronchitis.

Acute bronchitis

Acute bronchitis is usually caused by a virus infection – it often occurs after influenza or a cold. The affected person has a raised temperature and a cough which produces thick and sticky mucus. There is often wheeziness. There may also be a headache, loss of appetite and discomfort or soreness beneath the breastbone. Attacks of acute bronchitis usually subside in a few days. They are usually serious in young children and the elderly, in which case antibiotics and medical supervision will probably be needed.

Home care
□ The person should rest in bed in a warm atmosphere. He or she will probably be more comfortable in a fairly upright position, supported with pillows or a backrest.
□ Give lots of fluids to help loosen the cough.
□ Steam inhalations may help to clear the airways (see page 102).
□ Painkillers such as paracetamol may be given for headaches and to relieve discomfort or soreness.
□ Give a light diet which looks attractive and is easily digested.

Chronic bronchitis

In chronic bronchitis there is a chronic swelling of the lining of the bronchial walls and the bronchi tend to become clogged with mucus. This causes obstruction of the airflow through the lungs. Breathing out can be especially difficult. Factors associated with chronic bronchitis are: cigarette smoking; breathing in coal-dust over a lengthy period; and living in an atmosphere which is damp and foggy, or polluted with smoke.

The first indication of the development of chronic bronchitis may be breathlessness while walking or running and a 'smoker's cough'. Over months or years the cough worsens and the person becomes more breathless and wheezy. As the disease progresses, the airways become increasingly obstructed and breathing becomes more difficult. The sufferer may reach a stage where he or she is breathless even when at rest.

Established chronic bronchitis cannot be cured, but the symptoms can be alleviated, and the progress of the disease slowed or even halted. Home nursing can play an important part in improving the outlook.

Home care
If you are looking after someone with chronic bronchitis, encourage the sufferer to do as much as possible for him- or herself, and try to persuade him or her to:
○ Stop smoking
○ Reduce weight, if necessary
○ Avoid smoky or polluted atmospheres, if this is at all possible
○ Avoid going out in very cold weather: if it is essential to go out, he or she should keep a scarf over the nose and mouth, so that the air breathed in has been warmed a little
○ Take a moderate amount of exercise – but avoid becoming overtired as this aggravates breathing difficulties
○ Sleep propped up with pillows in a warm bedroom, with the windows closed if the night air is cold. A humidifier, or a bowl of water over a radiator, helps to keep the air moist, which may make it a little easier to breathe
○ Take any drugs or oxygen (see page 103) exactly as prescribed

Ask the doctor or physiotherapist to teach you how to help the person with breathing exercises. These exercises strengthen the muscles used in breathing and help with breathing out, so it is important that the person should do them regularly, and a good deal of encouragement may be needed to enable daily practice.

The physiotherapist will also show you how to help the person cough effectively to clear the airways. Chronic bronchitis involves a great deal of coughing and bringing up of phlegm, which can be distressing for you as well as for the person concerned. It is important to realize that it is very necessary. If you feel nauseated listening to the cough, take some slow, deep but quiet breaths. You can then continue to help the person, and he or she remains unaware of how you feel.

Chronic bronchitis is a serious illness. Ensure that the sick person sees the doctor regularly. In particular, seek medical advice if there is any sign of chest infection, such as increased shortness of breath, a raised temperature or a change in the character of the mucus coughed up. Ask the doctor if the person should be immunized against influenza.

A person with chronic bronchitis may well become very depressed and anxious. You, the caregiver, can help a lot if you find time to listen, and give the person the opportunity to talk about his or her fears and anxieties. It may help, too, if you can look together at the sort of life the sick person has been used to and see if, between you, you can sort out a way that he or she can live a satisfying life within the limits of the disability.

EMPHYSEMA

In emphysema, which is also known as 'chronic obstructive airways disease', the air sacs or alveoli which make up the lungs are destroyed, leaving distended spaces so the area available for the taking in of oxygen and the breathing out of carbon dioxide is reduced. The lungs lose their elasticity and become stiff. This means that the chest does not move very well, so breathing out becomes difficult and prolonged. Emphysema most commonly occurs in association with chronic bronchitis.

A person suffering from emphysema will display the signs and symptoms of chronic bronchitis and in addition the chest may become barrel-shaped because of the abnormal way in which the person now takes every breath.

Home care
Home care for emphysema is the same as for chronic bronchitis.

PNEUMONIA

Pneumonia is inflammation and infection of the air sacs (alveoli) of the lungs. The lungs are divided into lobes, the right lung into three lobes, the left into two. If the pneumonia is confined to one lobe of a lung, it is usually called lobar pneumonia. This is now rare. If the infection and inflammation affect both lungs in different areas the disease is termed bronchopneumonia.

Pneumonia varies greatly in severity. It usually affects people with lowered resistance to infection, the very young and the elderly. With both lobar and bronchopneumonia, there is a cough, producing infected yellow or green mucus, breathlessness, a raised temperature, a feeling of tiredness and loss of appetite. There may also be chest pain.

Home care
Except in the very young, the old or the frail, pneumonia is usually treated at home.
☐ Nurse the patient in bed, sitting upright and well supported with a backrest and pillows.
☐ Encourage the person to cough. Give plenty of fluids to help loosen the cough and provide lots of tissues and a pot to spit into.
☐ Provide a light, easily digested diet.
☐ Help the person to do deep breathing exercises (see page 79).
☐ Ensure that any drugs prescribed are given in the correct amounts at the right time. Give oxygen if it has been prescribed by the doctor (see page 103).

As the sick person recovers, keep the surroundings warm but introduce short trips out into the fresh air, unless the weather is damp, foggy or wet. It is quite usual to feel tired, weak and depressed after pneumonia, so do not allow the convalescent to do too much, or he or she will become overtired and strained.

Gradually over the next few weeks the convalescent can get back to normal activities. Ask the doctor for advice on when he or she should return to work.

The Digestive System

VOMITING

In adults and older children
There are many possible causes of vomiting, most of them not serious. Vomiting in adults is most often associated with a reaction to food or drink, travel sickness, or an infection. Migraine is another possibility. Many women vomit in early pregnancy.

Some children vomit very frequently, whenever they are at all ill, from excitement or stress, in any moving vehicle, or for no reason that can be discovered; but vomiting in children is most often a reaction to something they have eaten, or a sign of illness.

Home care
While vomiting continues the sick person should eat nothing, but drink a small quantity of water, in little sips, every 2 hours or so.

As the vomiting stops, start to give a little solid food in the form of bread, dry biscuits or dry breakfast cereal. The person can gradually return to a normal diet.

Consult your doctor if:
○ Vomiting continues for more than 24 hours
○ There has been a recent head injury
○ A vomiting child has a temperature of 38°c (100.4°F) or above
○ A young child has a severe bout of diarrhoea as well as vomiting
○ You are worried about the person's general condition

In babies
Babies often bring up a little milk with their wind. This is perfectly normal. Even if a baby brings back quite a lot of milk, the cause is likely to be only a minor feeding problem – the baby may simply be

taking too much milk, or sucking in too much air with the milk. In the first few months of life, projectile vomiting, when the milk shoots out with force, may be associated with an obstruction of the stomach outlet known as pyloric stenosis: this is more common in boys. This can be remedied by a minor operation. If you suspect your baby may have pyloric stenosis, tell the doctor at once. The defect is not dangerous in itself, but regular projectile vomiting will deprive the baby of essential nourishment. Profuse or prolonged vomiting also carries a risk of dehydration.

Sometimes vomiting may be caused by an infection, such as gastroenteritis. In this case, the baby usually seems definitely unwell.

Home care
As long as the baby seems well, there is no diarrhoea and he or she is growing and thriving, there is probably nothing to worry about. Give feeds as usual and just keep an eye on the baby in case there is any deterioration. If you are disturbed about a feeding problem, ask your doctor's advice.

However, you should consult your doctor immediately if:
○ Vomiting is profuse or prolonged
○ There is diarrhoea as well as vomiting
○ The baby is unusually drowsy and unresponsive
○ The baby seems unwell, especially if there is any fever

A small baby who is not keeping down enough liquid can become dehydrated and very ill in just a few hours. If any of the following signs become apparent, get the baby to a doctor or a hospital at once. They indicate a serious degree of dehydration.
○ Sunken fontanelles (the soft areas on the top of the head)
○ Sunken eyes
○ Dry tongue and mouth
○ Inelastic skin

DIARRHOEA

Diarrhoea is the frequent passage of loose, runny stools. It may be accompanied by cramp-like stomach pains.

Home care for adults and older children
A person with profuse diarrhoea should eat nothing and drink only clear liquids, such as water or squash, for 24 to 48 hours. An adult may take a kaolin mixture (available from a chemist) to reduce the diarrhoea, but do not give a child any medicine to control diarrhoea except on a doctor's advice. When the diarrhoea subsides, it is better to take only easily digested foods, such as clear, fat-free soups, for a

time before returning to normal food. Milk, cream, butter and eggs should be avoided for a few days.

To prevent the spread of diarrhoea, sufferers should be especially careful to wash and dry their hands after each visit to the lavatory. No one with diarrhoea should ever be allowed to cook or prepare any food.

See the doctor if:
○ Pain becomes continuous
○ The attack follows a trip abroad
○ A person is having repeated attacks
○ There is blood in the stools
○ Severe diarrhoea persists for more than 48 hours, or more than 24 hours in a child
○ A child with diarrhoea is also vomiting

Home care for babies
If a small baby has profuse diarrhoea you should consult your doctor at once. A baby with diarrhoea can become dehydrated very quickly. The doctor will probably advise you to give the baby oral rehydration solutions (ORS), powders of glucose and salt to be added to sterile water. Or you can add 4 level teaspoons of powdered glucose or sugar and a pinch of salt to 600 ml (1 pt) of cooled boiled water. Give as much of this solution as the baby will take. If the baby is breast-fed, continue feeds: a breast-fed baby is not likely to get diarrhoea caused by a bacterial infection, but it can happen. Otherwise, do not give any milk or solids for up to 24 hours.

If the baby shows any signs of dehydration, go to a doctor or a hospital immediately.

Bottle feeds should be reintroduced gradually over the 36 hours after the diarrhoea has stopped. Your doctor is likely to advise you to give half-strength, then three-quarter-strength feeds, before returning to normal-strength. If the diarrhoea recurs at any stage of this process, consult the doctor.

CONSTIPATION

Constipation is the infrequent, straining passage of hard stools. Infrequency of bowel movements alone does not mean that a person has constipation. For some people it is quite normal to have a bowel action only three or four times a week. Constipation may be caused by lack of fibre or fluids in the diet. A lack of exercise – perhaps because the person is confined to bed – can also cause constipation, and so can failure to empty the bowels when the need arises. The habitual use of laxatives followed by their withdrawal is another possible cause – the bowel may become dependent on the laxatives and be unable to work without them. Occasionally constipation is an indication of a more serious disorder.

Home care

A simple and effective way to prevent or treat constipation is to give a diet which is high in fibre (see page 120). Anyone who is constipated should increase his or her consumption of fluids, and, if possible, the amount of exercise taken, as well as gradually increasing fibre intake. Do not give laxatives except on medical advice.

See your doctor if:

○ There is a marked change in regular bowel habits
○ There is any bleeding from the rectum
○ The passage of stools causes severe pain
○ Constipation is accompanied by other symptoms, such as fever or vomiting
○ A person remains constipated even after changing to a high-fibre diet and increasing fluid consumption and exercise

PILES (Haemorrhoids)

Piles are enlarged veins just inside the anus. They may protrude when stools are passed and cause considerable pain. Usually piles are caused by constipation over a prolonged period.

Home care

The most effective way of preventing piles is to provide a diet rich in fibre. If piles do develop, avoiding constipation becomes very important.

Provided that further constipation is avoided, small piles will often subside with the use of ointments or suppositories which can be obtained from a chemist. If piles become troublesome, your doctor may suggest that they should be injected in hospital with a fluid which causes scarring that blocks off the enlarged vein.

Larger piles are sometimes removed under a general anaesthetic (an operation known as haemorrhoidectomy). The patient usually comes home from hospital 7 to 10 days after this operation.

Following a haemorrhoidectomy, the hospital may give a mild laxative to be taken at home until regular bowel habits have been established. Rubbing the area with toilet paper should be avoided: pat it dry instead. Daily or even twice-daily hot baths with some salt added will encourage healing and prevent infection. It is a good idea to have a bath after the bowels have opened.

A convalescent may suffer quite a lot of pain after this operation. A painkiller such as paracetamol should help. Call your doctor if the pain gets very bad or if there are any other signs of possible infection, such as a raised temperature.

He or she should be back to work in about 3 to 4 weeks, depending on the type of work. Ask for advice from the surgeon.

HERNIA (Rupture)

A hernia is a place where an organ or part of an organ has come through a weak part of the muscle which normally holds it in position. Hernia most commonly occurs in the lower abdomen and appears as a swelling in the groin. An abdominal hernia is often called a rupture.

An operation may be performed to strengthen the muscle wall and keep the organ in the abdomen.

Home care

The patient usually comes home about 5 to 10 days after the operation, although some hernia repairs are done during a single day's stay in hospital.

If the doctor advises, the person should have a daily bath to keep the area of the operation clean. Clothes which rub this area should be avoided. A painkiller such as paracetamol may be taken to relieve discomfort.

Call your doctor if there is any swelling or discharge from the operation site.

To avoid the hernia recurring through the newly repaired spot it is important that there should be no sudden increase in pressure in the abdomen. This can be caused by lifting, strenuous exercise, sneezing, coughing and vomiting or even laughing too heartily, or braking suddenly when driving a car. The wound should be supported with the hand if the convalescent is coughing or sneezing or vomiting. Any strenuous activity should be avoided for about 8 weeks: check this with the surgeon. Check, too, when it is advisable to drive a car again.

Once the hernia repair has healed, the convalescent should still avoid heavy lifting if possible, but if lifting is essential, should learn to lift correctly (see page 34). The person should usually be back to work in about 3 to 4 weeks, depending on the kind of work, and should be able to resume full activity within 2 to 3 months.

APPENDICITIS

The appendix is a small, blind-ended tube attached to the large intestine. If the appendix becomes blocked and inflamed, this is known as appendicitis. In the early stages, there is usually pain in the middle of the abdomen, around the navel. This later moves to the right side of the lower abdomen.

Home care

If you think someone may have an appendicitis, seek medical advice at once. An inflamed appendix, if not removed, may burst.

After an appendicectomy most people recover quite quickly and come home within about 5 days.

The stitches are usually removed 5 to 9 days after the operation. A dry sterile dressing may still be needed: ask your doctor about this.

If the doctor advises, the person should have a daily bath to keep the area of the operation clean. Make sure that clothes do not rub the scar line.

A well-balanced diet is essential to prevent constipation, so provide lots of vegetables, fruit, wholemeal cereals and fluids.

Rest and sleep are important and the person must avoid heavy lifting, although he or she should take some gentle exercise, such as short walks.

Call your doctor if there is any swelling or discharge from the area of the operation.

In about 2 to 4 weeks the person should be able to resume normal activities, but check this with your doctor, and ask when it will be possible to return to work or school. In the case of a child it may be a good idea to get some school work sent home: when the child feels better, he or she can do a little at a time. The convalescent should not take part in active sports or other strenuous activities for 2 to 3 months after the operation.

CHOLECYSTECTOMY

A cholecystectomy is an operation to remove the gall bladder. It is usually performed because gallstones – pebble-like formations in the gall bladder – are causing pain or other symptoms.

Home care
The person is usually allowed home 10 to 14 days after the operation.

Ensure that the patient continues to take any medicines that have been prescribed since the operation.

If the doctor advises, he or she should have a daily bath to keep the area around the operation site clean. Make sure that clothes do not rub this area.

It is not unusual for there to be runny or loose stools perhaps two or three times a day after this operation. Gradually, over weeks or in some cases months, the stools will return to normal.

It is advisable to restrict the amount of fat in the diet for some time after the operation, perhaps even for life.

Inform your doctor if:
○ The skin or whites of the eyes take on a yellow tinge – this may be caused by jaundice
○ The stools are pale
○ The skin starts to itch
○ There is an increase of pain
○ The temperature rises
○ There is any swelling or discharge from around the operation site

A person who has had this operation is usually able to go back to work in about 6 to 8 weeks, depending on the type of work. Any lifting must be avoided for another 2 months after this. The convalescent can return to full activity within about 3 to 4 months.

STOMACH ULCERS (Peptic or gastric ulcers)

These ulcers may be found in the stomach or in the duodenum – the part of the small intestine immediately below the stomach. The pain caused by an ulcer usually takes the form of a burning sensation in the middle or upper part of the abdomen. The pain tends to come and go: it may be present for a few days or a week, then disappear for weeks or months before it occurs again.

Home care
If you suspect that someone has a stomach ulcer, seek medical advice and treatment.

Anyone with an ulcer should stop smoking. As far as possible stressful situations should be avoided, because stress stimulates the secretions in the stomach, which may hinder the healing of the ulcer. Plenty of rest and sleep are also important.

Establish a regular eating pattern, with regular meals and snacks such as milk and biscuits between meals. Milk often relieves the pain: make sure that there is plenty of it to drink between meals and during the night. Any necessary medicines should be taken as prescribed. Alcohol, coffee, and any foods that are known to cause pain, as well as medicines containing aspirin, should be avoided.

HEPATITIS

Hepatitis means inflammation of the liver. Two distinct types are recognized: infective hepatitis (A) and serum hepatitis (B).

Infectious hepatitis is caused by a virus which is found in the carrier's stools and is passed on by the contamination of food or water.

Serum hepatitis is also caused by a virus, but this one is most commonly carried in the blood. Infection may be spread through blood transfusion, or it may be communicated by contaminated syringes and needles, so drug addicts are particularly at risk. In some countries, including the UK and the US, blood for transfusion is screened to check that it does not carry the virus.

The first symptoms of hepatitis are loss of appetite, nausea and vomiting, and a general feeling of tiredness, with aches and pains. This is followed a few days later by jaundice.

Home care

Severe cases are usually nursed in hospital, but mild cases may be nursed at home.

In the case of infectious hepatitis the stools are infectious before the person becomes jaundiced, so other members of the family may well be infected already. Everyone should pay particular attention to hygiene, especially handwashing after using the toilet. The doctor may suggest that all the family have an injection of immunoglobulin, which may prevent them from developing hepatitis or reduce the severity of the disease.

The important aspect of home care for either type of hepatitis is to rest the liver and give it time to recover naturally. The sick person needs lots of rest. He or she should have plenty of fluids, but no alcohol for several months. Provide a light diet, high in carbohydrate and low in fat.

Get advice from your doctor on when the sufferer can resume normal activities. In the case of infectious hepatitis, this may be about 3 weeks after the jaundice has gone. With serum hepatitis, it will vary with the severity of the disease. You can expect the sick person to feel tired and even depressed at times for about 3 weeks to 3 months, or even longer.

COLOSTOMY

A colostomy is an opening of the colon (part of the intestine) through the abdominal wall, so that faeces can pass out of the colon through the abdomen. The part of the colon that is brought through the abdominal wall is called a stoma. A colostomy may be performed because there is an obstruction in the bowel that prevents the normal evacuation of waste through the anus, or because part of the bowel has been removed. The colostomy may be temporary or permanent. If it is temporary, the person may stay in hospital until it is reversed. A person with a permanent colostomy will be able to go home as soon as he or she or the caregiver is able to manage the care involved.

Home care

The person concerned and his or her family will be visited by a stomatherapist, a nurse who has had special training to help people with this problem. The stomatherapist will make sure that the convalescent and you, the caregiver, know exactly what to do and are familiar with all the equipment and techniques you will need to use.

The most important aspect of management of a colostomy is to achieve a bowel action at a regular time and to avoid an unexpected bowel action. Balanced meals eaten at regular intervals and a regular time for emptying the bowel are essential.

Some people manage such a regular bowel habit that they can simply go to the toilet at the same time everyday and hold a bowl under the stoma until the bowel action is complete.

Another method of ensuring that the bowel is emptied regularly is to use a washout. A specially prepared irrigation set is available, consisting of an irrigating bag containing washout solution and a pouch to receive the bowel movement.

After an effective washout there should be no likelihood of another bowel action for quite a while. Washouts are usually performed every other day.

After a bowel action or a washout the area around the stoma should be washed carefully with warm water and soap, rinsed and patted dry.

Whichever method of emptying the bowel is used, the stoma needs to be covered. At night a small pad of cotton-wool may be placed over the opening and held in place by a crepe bandage, or an abdominal support belt, or even a home-made belt. During the day, most people wear a disposable plastic bag attached to the stoma to catch any leaks. But sometimes the stoma is covered by a dressing of cotton-wool and a thick plastic disc (a colostomy shield) held in position by a belt. The stomatherapist will give advice on the most suitable method to use.

There is no reason why a person with a colostomy should not lead a normal active life. He or she can travel, take part in any form of sport, including swimming, wear any type of clothing so long as it does not constrict the stoma. A woman with a colostomy can have a normal pregnancy, though she will need careful attention from her doctor.

A person with a colostomy will need a lot of loving and caring support. They need to know that they are accepted just as they were before and that their family and friends feel the same about them. You as the caregiver will need support too.

A support group (see page 220) will offer useful advice and can help you through difficult times.

Diet

In the first 6 weeks after the colostomy operation, the convalescent's diet should be slightly constipating to help regulate the bowel movement. Once the bowel movement is regulated the aim is balance – the person should not have diarrhoea but equally should not be constipated. Different foods can be introduced on a trial and error basis. If something causes an upset leave it out of the diet for a period.

It is usually best to avoid very fibrous foods such as wholegrain cereals and raw fruit, which can cause diarrhoea, and beer and fizzy drinks and highly spiced foods, which may cause wind. The stomatherapist will be able to give you more detailed advice.

The Kidneys and Urinary System

CYSTITIS

Inflammation of the bladder lining, usually caused by a bacterial infection, is known as cystitis. A person suffering from cystitis feels the need to pass water frequently but is able to pass very little at a time. There is a stinging or burning feeling or discomfort on passing water. Women are much more prone to cystitis than men because their urethras are shorter.

Home care
At the start of an attack, get the affected person to:
○ Drink lots of water, milk or weak tea, at least 280 ml (½ pint) every 20 minutes for the first 3 hours
○ Take a solution of potassium citrate or bicarbonate of soda in water to make the urine alkaline
○ Take paracetamol to relieve discomfort
Consult your doctor if symptoms persist – he may prescribe an antibiotic.

To prevent further attacks
A person with a tendency to cystitis should be encouraged to take the following precautions:
□ Drink plenty of water.
□ Wash the genital area well, using baby soap or plain unscented soap and a special flannel, which must be boiled daily.
□ After going to the lavatory, always wipe from front to back, to avoid carrying bacteria from the bowel to the bladder.
□ Use soft toilet paper.
□ Do not use bath oils, bubble baths, talcum powder, genital deodorants or antiseptics.
□ Shower rather than bath, if possible. If not, bath in shallow, luke-warm water.
□ Before intercourse, both partners should wash the genital area with plain water. A special lubricant (obtainable from the chemist) can be used to prevent soreness and bruising. The woman should pass water after intercourse.

PYELONEPHRITIS

Pyelonephritis is inflammation of the kidney. It may be acute (the result of an active bacterial infection) or chronic (a slow progressive disease).

With acute pyelonephritis there is frequently pain or a burning sensation on passing urine. There may also be a dull aching or pain in one or both loins and tenderness over the bladder. The sufferer's temperature is raised.

The symptoms of chronic pyelonephritis are tiredness, headaches, a dull aching pain in the loins and loss of appetite but extreme thirst. There is usually a history of attacks of acute pyelonephritis.

Home care
Seek advice from your doctor. Make sure any prescribed medicines are taken as directed.

The sick person should drink plenty of fluids and, if he or she has a fever, should rest in bed.

Care for prevention of infection or inflammation is the same as for cystitis.

KIDNEY FAILURE

The normal functions of the kidneys are: to excrete waste products; by excreting certain minerals and retaining others to maintain a normal balance in the body; and to manage the balance of body fluid. If a person takes in more fluid than the body needs, then the kidneys excrete more in the urine. In very hot weather or if the person has a fever, the kidneys excrete less urine.

If the kidneys fail, the body's normal balance is disturbed. Waste products and other substances start to accumulate and the levels of these substances in the blood rise too high. There are two kinds of kidney failure, acute and chronic.

Acute kidney failure
This occurs when the kidneys suddenly and temporarily fail. There are various possible causes, but two of the most common are excessive blood or fluid loss, resulting in shock; or a blockage of the flow of urine down the ureters, or from the bladder. The person is acutely ill and will be admitted to hospital to be looked after until kidney function returns to normal.

Chronic kidney failure
Chronic kidney failure is the final result of many diseases of the kidney. Early symptoms are vague: they include tiredness and lack of energy. The sick person may pass large amounts of urine and have to get up several times during the night. As the disease progresses, there will be symptoms which affect every system of the body. In most cases these symptoms are quite mild and the progressive course of the disease can be slowed down over many years by medically supervised diets and drug treatment. But if the kidney failure worsens, the symptoms become more severe and dialysis or a kidney transplant will be necessary.

Haemodialysis

Very simply, haemodialysis means taking the blood out of the body, removing the toxic substances and excess water, and then pumping the clean blood back into the body. The blood is taken from an artery to the kidney machine where it passes over a cellophane or similar type of membrane. On the other side of the membrane there is a solution of dialysing fluid which is warm and contains the correct proportions of various salts and other substances normally found in the blood. The high levels of these substances in the blood of the person with kidney failure move across the membrane and into the dialysis solution. This continues until the patient's blood levels are back to normal. Once the person is off dialysis and begins to take in food and water, so the levels of waste substances start to rise again and soon dialysis is required once more. There are several different kinds of haemodialysis, which can be performed in hospital or in the sick person's home. The whole process is monitored by a kidney machine which ensures that the procedure is carried out safely.

Most people with kidney failure dialyse for a period of about 4 to 8 hours and repeat the procedure three times a week.

Peritoneal dialysis

The alternative is peritoneal dialysis, in which fluid is passed into the peritoneal cavity in the abdomen, and allowed to absorb the waste products built up in the blood. The fluid is then drained out and the cycle begins again until the blood levels are back to normal.

The patient has a small tube permanently inserted into the abdomen, although dialysis is carried out only every few days. The tube is covered with a dry dressing when not in use.

Home care
If dialysis is to be performed at home the sick person and you as the caregiver will be given careful instruction in the use and maintenance of the machine.

Once on a dialysis programme, the person concerned should try to live a normal life, go to work or school and gradually get back to normal activities. Encourage the person to manage and control his or her own treatment.

The sick person may feel depressed, useless and anxious. There may be a loss of sexual drive which can lead to marital problems. You, the caregiver, may well harbour feelings of resentment as a result of the personal sacrifices that have been made because of the illness and its treatment. All these problems need to be discussed openly. If the dialysis makes you or the person concerned feel restricted and tied to the house, talk to the experts at the hospital: they may be able to help. It is important to plan your lives so that there is time for activities that you enjoy.

A local support group (see page 221) should be very helpful.

Kidney transplant

A kidney transplant is the transfer of a healthy kidney from a living donor or from someone who has just died to a person whose kidneys have failed. There is a risk that the body will reject the new kidney, but these days kidney transplants are often very successful.

Nursing a transplant patient is a highly specialized business. If you have to care for someone who has had a transplant you will be given very detailed and precise instructions by the hospital and you will need the support of visiting health professionals when the convalescent returns home.

The Reproductive System

CIRCUMCISION

This is the removal of the foreskin from the penis. It may be done for religious reasons, for hygienic purposes, or because of a medical problem.

Home care
Babies and young children heal very quickly after circumcision and there is rarely any infection. An adult may have a lot of swelling at the operation site, but this usually subsides in a few days. The wound should be kept dry for the first 24 to 48 hours after the operation. If there is a dressing, do not pull it off but allow it to soak off gradually in the bath: ask the

surgeon when this should be done. Some surgeons prefer not to use a dressing but simply dust the area with antibiotic powder.

It is better if a child does not wear nappies, pants or trousers for 48 hours after the operation.

The convalescent should have plenty of rest and sleep. Children should not ride tricycles or rocking horses (and an adult should not ride a bicycle) until after the outpatient appointment to see the surgeon, which is about 2 weeks after the operation. Adults should ask when sexual activities can be resumed.

Call the doctor if the person is not passing urine, or if the wound starts to bleed, becomes smelly or produces a discharge.

VASECTOMY (Male sterilization)

A small part of each of the tubes which carry the sperm from the testes to the penis is removed and the two ends are tied. The operation is usually done under local anaesthetic, but occasionally under general anaesthetic. The whole operation takes about 15 minutes and if he has had a local anaesthetic the man is able to go home afterwards. After a general anaesthetic he will be kept in hospital or at the clinic for a few hours to recover.

Home care
The man should take things easy for about 48 hours to prevent any discomfort and should not undertake any very active exercise for the next few days.

Sexual intercourse can be resumed as soon as he likes but he should continue to use a contraceptive until a sperm count has been taken and the results are known. He is not immediately sterile after the operation.

He should be able to go back to work within a couple of days if he feels well enough.

FALLOPIAN TUBULAR LIGATION (Female sterilization)

In this operation the Fallopian tubes, which carry the egg (ovum) from the ovary to the womb, are either clipped or cut and tied. Either method prevents the egg from reaching the womb and the body safely reabsorbs it. The operation may be performed through two small incisions just below the navel, or through a cut along the lower abdomen, across the bikini line.

Home care
A woman is usually discharged from hospital 1 to 3 days after this operation. If the doctor advises, she should have a daily bath to keep the area of the operation clean and avoid wearing clothes which rub the area.

There is usually a lot of wind in the abdominal area, which causes pain. The best way to relieve it is to move about – this will help the body to pass the wind. There may also be some pain over the operation site. A painkiller such as paracetamol will help to relieve this.

Call the doctor if the wound becomes red and inflamed or there is a discharge.

This operation is immediately effective but most women do not feel like resuming sexual intercourse for a week or so because of the abdominal discomfort. There should be no heavy lifting or strenuous exercise for about 6 to 8 weeks. Check when the woman can return to work.

D AND C (Dilation and Curettage)

This operation may be carried out to investigate the cause of a problem, such as heavy, irregular or painful periods, to correct a problem or to remove the contents of a pregnant uterus, in an abortion or following a naturally occurring abortion. It is sometimes necessary to perform a D and C after the birth of a baby to remove a part or the whole of the afterbirth which has not been expelled naturally during labour.

The neck of the womb (cervix) is dilated or gently widened and an instrument called a curette is passed through it to scrape the lining of the womb. If a problem is to be investigated, a small amount of the scraping will probably be sent to a laboratory for examination.

Home care
How long the woman has to stay in hospital will partly depend on the reason for having the D and C. When this operation is done to investigate some menstrual abnormality the person is often only in hospital for a day and can go home when she has recovered from the very light anaesthetic. Following childbirth or a miscarriage, the woman will normally stay in hospital for longer.

She should take things easy and rest for the remainder of the day. A painkiller such as paracetamol can be taken to relieve any low back pain or general discomfort she may feel.

Some bleeding from the vagina is to be expected, but the doctor should be informed if there is any heavy bleeding.

Check with the doctor when she should go back to work and normal activities.

HYSTERECTOMY

In a hysterectomy the womb (uterus) is removed. It may be removed through the vagina or through an abdominal incision. Sometimes, the ovaries and fallopian tubes may also be removed.

Normally recovery after the operation is quick. The pain over the operation site usually settles, but pain-relieving medicines will be given if required. Most women are up and walking about 24 to 48 hours after the operation.

Home care
A hysterectomy is a major operation and a woman can feel exhausted and depressed afterwards. This may be particularly the case if she is young and the operation has been carried out before she has had a chance to have children. A woman in this position needs a great deal of help and understanding from

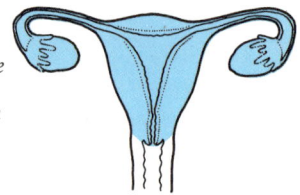

A hysterectomy may involve removal of the uterus, cervix, ovaries and fallopian tubes.

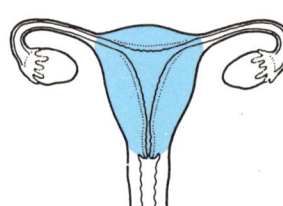

Alternatively, only the uterus and cervix may be removed.

her family and may need professional counselling in addition.

Following the operation there will be some vaginal bleeding and discharge which may persist for a few weeks, gradually lessening. She will no longer have menstrual periods. If the ovaries were removed at the same time the doctor may suggest hormone replacement therapy.

Encourage the woman to continue any exercises she was taught in hospital.

Call your doctor if:
- There is heavy vaginal bleeding
- There is a discharge that smells unpleasant
- The woman feels unwell
- She has a raised temperature

She will be restricted in what she can do for about 6 weeks. She must be careful to avoid lifting and stretching. For the first 2 weeks after the operation, she can undertake light jobs, such as dusting or typing, but she should reduce standing to a minimum and sit down whenever possible. Until 4 weeks after the operation she should not lift anything heavier than a full kettle of water. After about 4 weeks she should be able to tackle household jobs such as using a vacuum cleaner (with feet apart in a walking position), cooking and ironing. She should not drive a car for about 6 weeks after the operation, as this may cause pain in the lower abdomen. It is better not to be driven long distances either, as this involves sitting in one position for lengthy periods, which can be uncomfortable.

After 6 weeks she should be able to cope with most things, except for heavy lifting or prolonged stretching, but she should not attempt to lift or move heavy furniture until at least 3 months after the operation. If in doubt, she should leave any job until there is someone to help her. Normally, a woman should be able to go back to work about 6 to 8 weeks after the operation, depending on the type of work and what her doctor advises. She should be able to be fully active within 3 to 4 months.

Ask the surgeon when sexual activity can be resumed. Some women worry that they may have lost their ability to enjoy sex or to please their partners, but they should be reassured that there is no reason why this should be so. If there is pain during intercourse, a woman should tell her doctor or the surgeon.

PROSTATECTOMY

The prostate gland is situated directly below the bladder in males. It surrounds the outlet of the urethra – the tube through which the urine passes on its way from the bladder to the penis – and produces a fluid which mixes with the sperm cells to form the ejaculate, semen.

As a man gets older, from middle age onward, the prostate gland becomes larger. In some men it becomes excessively enlarged and affects the flow of urine. The man may have to get up frequently at night to pass urine, and he may have discomfort or difficulty when passing urine. He may also feel generally rather unwell. In this case, part or the whole of the prostate gland may be removed by surgery. The operation does not necessarily make the man infertile, nor does it affect potency.

Home care
How long the patient stays in hospital depends on his general condition, bearing in mind that this operation is most often performed on elderly men. But most men are able to come home 5 to 10 days after the operation.

There may still be a slight burning sensation on passing urine, or a need to pass urine frequently, or some dribbling on finishing passing urine, but this should clear up over the few weeks following the operation and passing urine will become normal once again.

For at least 2 months after the operation the man should always pass urine as soon as he first feels the need, to prevent pressure from a full bladder on the operation site.

It is also important to avoid becoming constipated, especially in the first weeks after the operation, so his diet should be high in fibre (see page 120). The convalescent should also take plenty of fluids: offer at least eight glasses of water a day. The hospital may also give the patient some mild stool softeners and laxatives.

It is usually best to avoid spicy foods and alcohol, as they may aggravate any burning sensation on passing urine.

The man should not do any lifting or take any strenuous exercise for a few weeks. Long car journeys should also be avoided for the first few weeks after the operation.

Call your doctor if there is any bleeding (though mild bleeding at first is not unusual), or if the amount of urine passed gets less.

Sexual activity can usually be resumed in about 6 to 8 weeks. Check with the surgeon.

The person is usually fit to return to work about 4 weeks after the operation. But again, check with the surgeon or your own doctor.

MASTECTOMY

A mastectomy is an operation to remove a breast or part of a breast. It is performed to remove cancerous tissue, and is sometimes followed by a course of radiotherapy to destroy any remaining cancer cells.

Although the breast is sensitive, the pain after the operation is not usually severe and can be well controlled by pain-relieving medicines.

Home care
The woman will probably be able to go home 8 to 12 days after the operation. When she is first at home it may still be necessary for the scar to be covered with a light dressing. If this is the case then the dressing will need to be changed regularly. Arrangements for doing this will have been made by the hospital. Make sure that the person concerned is fully aware of the arrangements.

Be aware that the area around the healing wound will have less feeling because the nerves have been cut. If radiotherapy treatment (see page 188) is being given, the area should not be washed until the doctor has given permission.

The staff at the hospital will have made sure that the woman has seen the scar. The size and line of the scar will vary according to each individual case. It probably looks rather obvious at the moment, but she should be reassured that it will fade.

A mastectomy is a traumatic experience for anyone, no matter how well prepared she may be. There are bound to be days when she feels tearful and depressed and it will help if she can talk to someone in the family, or a friend. She may have a feeling of deep personal loss, and she needs time to adjust to the situation.

It is particularly important that her husband or boyfriend is understanding and supportive, and reassures her that this change in her body makes no difference to their relationship. If she is worried about her partner's reaction to the wound, ask him to help her get undressed the first night at home. She will probably find undressing difficult at first and need his help anyway, but it will also give them both a chance to get used to the change in her body. It is encouraging to know that many women have found very happy relationships and have married for the first time after having a breast removed.

Even before the operation, or at least while the woman is still in hospital, it is a good idea to contact one of the associations which specialize in helping women who have had a mastectomy (see page 220). These associations can offer an enormous amount of support and helpful advice.

When first at home she should take things easily and not do too much. Make sure she has plenty of rest and do not worry if she tires easily. This is perfectly normal. It sometimes helps to sleep with the arm on the affected side resting on a pillow.

She will have been taught exercises in hospital and it is very important that these are continued at home. They are designed to increase the movement in the arm. A few more should be done each day, but the woman should always stop if the exercise causes pain. Using the affected arm to brush and comb her hair will also help, and knitting provides good exercise for the arm as well. She should try to use the arm as much as possible – for example, doing a little light housework or swimming. (However, if she is undergoing radiotherapy she must not swim until the doctor has given permission.) She should not carry heavy things, such as large pots and pans.

She will probably leave hospital wearing a temporary breast form – a prosthesis – which can be slipped inside the bra. If the wound is tender then a prosthesis of cotton-wool can be used. This will give her a normal shape, and give her confidence as she leaves the hospital. Later on, when the wound has completely healed, she can be fitted with a permanent prosthesis, so that, when dressed, she will look just as she always did. Make sure that the prosthesis feels comfortable and that she is really happy wearing it. You can also get specially designed swimwear or improvise by shaping an ordinary piece of synthetic sponge to fit the cup of an ordinary swimsuit. To squeeze the excess water out discreetly she just presses her arm against the cup on getting out of the water. Try it in the bath for the first time and see how she gets on.

Inform the doctor if the wound is red, swollen or tender, or there is a discharge. This might mean there is some infection. You should also contact the doctor if the arm is swollen.

A woman can expect to be able to undertake her normal activities and go back to work in a few weeks' time, depending on how much movement is regained in the affected arm, and how quickly.

Following a mastectomy she can lead an active life. Sexual difficulties may occur, but these should not necessarily be blamed directly on the mastectomy – they may be caused by the associated stress and anxiety. If she has any problems, encourage her to seek advice from a support group or the breast clinic at the hospital, or to talk to her doctor. She may need expert counselling about her feelings; this can be arranged through your doctor.

Lumpectomy (quadrantectomy)

Sometimes an operation called a lumpectomy or quadrantectomy is performed instead of a mastectomy. In this operation the cancer is removed together with some of the surrounding tissue, but the majority of the breast is left. It is usually followed by a course of radiotherapy or chemotherapy to destroy any remaining cancer cells.

The woman will probably come home from hospital 1 to 3 days after the operation and she may be well enough to go back to her normal activities and be back at work about 2 weeks after the operation unless there is further treatment.

The Glands

DIABETES

In normal health, a substance called insulin is produced by the pancreas, which keeps the amount of sugar in the bloodstream within normal limits. In diabetes mellitus, often called sugar diabetes, there is either a shortage of insulin being produced by the pancreas or the insulin that is produced is not effective and so the level of sugar in the bloodstream starts to rise.

There are two types of diabetes mellitus: juvenile onset diabetes, which occurs in children and young adults; and mature onset diabetes, which usually occurs in the middle-aged and elderly, but can also occur in younger people, especially if they are obese.

Juvenile onset diabetes

A person with juvenile onset diabetes tends to become excessively thirsty, to pass urine frequently, to lose weight and to feel generally exhausted and lacking in energy. Someone showing these symptoms should see a doctor, who will probably arrange blood and urine tests. If the person does have diabetes, there will be glucose and acetone in the urine and an abnormally high blood glucose level.

Home care
Treatment for juvenile onset diabetes is based on a special diet and injections of insulin. The doctor and dietitian caring for the diabetic calculate the diet of the individual, taking into account factors such as the age and build of the person and how active he or she is. The diabetic will be given a comprehensive list of foods that can be eaten, and in what amounts. This will be based on the total amount of carbohydrate allowed per day. Meals should be frequent and regular and should be taken at the same time each day to help stabilize the level of sugar in the bloodstream. If the person is injecting insulin, meals should follow within half an hour of each injection.

Injected insulin is slowly absorbed over a period of hours and replaces the insulin that should be produced by the pancreas. The staff at the hospital will teach the diabetic exactly how to give the injections. You should ensure that at least one other member of the family learns the technique as well. It is important to vary the site of the injections to avoid problems of infection and to keep the skin supple and prevent scarring. Possible sites include the arms, the thighs, the buttocks and the abdomen.

The hospital staff will also teach the person how to test blood for sugar and urine for glucose and acetone. These tests must be done regularly at the intervals advised by the doctor.

A person suffering from diabetes needs to have regular health checks. Find out how often the doctor thinks this necessary. Regular eye tests are also essential, as diabetes may cause sight problems. The feet of a diabetic need special care as circulation tends to be poor and any sore spot may become infected, so he or she should see a chiropodist regularly.

A diabetic should always carry a card or wear an identity disc or bracelet stating that he or she is a diabetic. The person should also carry glucose tablets or sweets for emergencies.

Diabetic emergencies
Hyperglycaemia occurs when too much sugar accumulates in the blood. It may follow an infection, or it may develop because insulin or other medications have been forgotten or the diet has not been followed carefully enough. Gradually the person becomes increasingly drowsy and thirsty and feels unwell. With advanced hyperglycaemia, the tongue is dry, the breathing faster than normal and the breath smells sweet.

This situation usually develops slowly over a few days, so the diabetic has sufficient warning to seek medical advice or to recognize what is happening and correct the situation.

Hypoglycaemia, or a 'hypo', occurs when, as a reaction to insulin, the blood sugar level drops too low. This may happen after a missed meal, unusually strenuous activity or an accidental overdose of insulin. Hypoclycaemia can develop rapidly, and an untreated hypo can lead to unconsciousness, and may cause brain damage or even death. Most diabetics are allowed to experience a mild hypo while under medical supervision, so that they know how it feels and what to do about it before it becomes a serious problem. It is important that the family and friends of the diabetic should also recognize the symptoms and know what to do. The symptoms of hypoglycaemia vary from individual to individual, but hypos tend to follow a pattern something like that described below.
□ Early symptoms are a feeling of weakness and hunger, sweating, trembling and confusion.
□ Very soon the diabetic may begin to feel faint and dizzy or even start staggering about as if drunk. He may appear aggressive, unco-operative and disoriented. Unfortunately, hypoglycaemia may be mistaken for drunkenness.
□ If left untreated, the diabetic will become progressively more drowsy and unresponsive and will eventually go into a coma.

What to do
□ If the diabetic is still conscious and able to swallow, give glucose tablets, sugar lumps, a piece of chocolate or a sugary drink to raise the level of sugar in the blood.
□ If the person is unconscious, place in the recovery position (see page 198). Get the sick person to hospital or call for medical help immediately. Do not attempt to give anything by mouth.

Mature onset diabetes
With mature onset diabetes, the symptoms of thirst and frequent passing of urine often develop very gradually and go unnoticed for a considerable time. The diabetes may only be discovered when a routine urine test is taken and the urine is found to contain glucose.

Home care
Insulin injections are rarely required by this type of diabetic. Sometimes tablets are prescribed to lower the blood sugar, but not all mature onset diabetics need to take any medicines at all. The special diet may be all that is necessary to keep the blood sugar in the correct balance.

The doctor may think it advisable for the person to lose weight. If so, the diet will be adjusted accordingly.

Otherwise, home care is as for a juvenile onset diabetic.

Infectious Diseases

Home nursing plays a major part in the care of many common infectious diseases – as you will know if you have nursed your children through measles or chickenpox or, indeed, an adult through a bad bout of influenza.

There are many ways in which infections may be spread: by touch; through droplets sprayed into the air when an infected person talks, coughs or sneezes; through taking infected food or drink; or through contact with infected stools or urine. It is very difficult to stop an infection spreading through a household, but being very particular about hygiene may help. So when you are nursing an infectious person, be careful that:
○ When the person coughs or sneezes he or she always uses a tissue, which can then be burnt or flushed away
○ The person washes and dries the hands thoroughly after using the lavatory
○ The sick person's towel and washing things are kept separate from those used by the rest of the family

○ He or she uses separate crockery and cutlery
The cause of an infection may be bacteria, virus, parasites or fungi. Most of the common infectious diseases are caused by either bacteria or viruses. Many bacterial infections can be cured by antibiotic drugs. For most viral infections, there is no treatment which will shorten the course of the illness. However, a viral infection does give some protection against further attack by the same virus, and vaccination can protect against some viral infections.

CHICKENPOX (Varicella)

Chickenpox is a viral infection that affects all age groups, but especially children. Most affected children are only slightly unwell, but chickenpox can be a distressing complaint in adults.

The time between contact with the disease and the appearance of the first signs and symptoms is usually about 14 to 16 days.

The rash of chickenpox begins with a crop of small red spots. There may be a slightly raised temperature at this stage. The spots, which are very itchy, usually appear first on the front of the body and then spread to the face, neck and the tops of the arms and legs. Within a day or so of appearing they become little blisters filled with clear fluid, which gradually crust over. Spots usually come in crops over 3 or 4 days.

The disease is infectious from a day or so before the rash appears until the last blister has crusted.

Home care
Inform your doctor. If you are uncertain of the diagnosis or the person is very uncomfortable, ask the doctor to see him or her. But if a child is only mildly unwell and you are sure the illness is chickenpox, this may not be neccessary.

If the temperature is raised, keep the person in bed or at least warm and resting until the temperature returns to normal. You can give paracetamol to help bring down the temperature and reduce discomfort. Calamine lotion may give some relief from itching, and a warm bath with a cupful of bicarbonate of soda added to the water is also soothing.

Chickenpox is normally a mild illness, but call the doctor if the person has a high fever or if the spots look infected.

To avoid spreading infection, a child should stay away from school, or an adult from work, until about 14 days after the appearance of the rash. Check with your doctor.

SHINGLES

Shingles is caused by the same virus as chickenpox. It most commonly occurs in middle-aged or elderly people, but it can affect young people and children as well. Following chickenpox in childhood, the virus lies dormant in the nerves which lead from the skin to the spinal cord. It usually remains dormant, but occasionally it becomes active again.

When it becomes active it causes a raised temperature and severe pain in the skin along the line of the affected nerve, followed by a painful, itchy rash of small blisters in the same area. The rash usually occurs on the trunk, but it may appear on one half of the forehead, causing a painful red eye. Gradually the blisters burst and form a crust, as in chickenpox.

Shingles is not highly infectious and cross-infection from one person to another is uncommon, but children may develop chickenpox from contact with the virus in adults. It is infectious, to this degree, until the last blister has crusted.

Home care
Call the doctor, who will probably prescribe some medication to ease the pain and help the sick person to sleep.

Keep the person warm and resting in bed and give plenty of fluids. Calamine lotion may give some temporary relief from the irritation of the rash.

The person should not go back to work until the doctor says he or she is well enough: older people may suffer discomfort even after the rash has disappeared.

GERMAN MEASLES

German measles is a mild respiratory illness, usually with a rash. Although it is not serious in itself, if it is contracted by a woman in the first few months of pregnancy it may seriously affect her unborn child. So it is important for girls to be vaccinated against German measles.

The time between contact with the disease and the first signs and symptoms is usually 16 to 18 days.

The illness usually starts with a headache, runny nose, sore throat and general cold symptoms, with a slightly raised temperature. There may also be swollen glands in the neck. A rash of small pink spots appears on the face and neck, then spreads to the body and limbs.

The person is infectious from a few days before the appearance of the rash until a week after the rash appears.

Home care
Keep the person warm and resting until the temperature returns to normal. Give plenty of fluids. You can give paracetamol for a troublesome sore throat or headache.

The person should stay away from school or work and from anyone who may possibly be pregnant until at least 7 days after the appearance of the rash. Check with your doctor.

MUMPS

Mumps is a viral infection which affects the salivary glands. It is most common in children of school age and young adults.

The time between contact with the disease and the appearance of the first symptoms is usually about 16 to 18 days.

The symptoms of mumps are very variable, but there is usually a slightly raised temperature with a headache, pains around and in front of the ear and swelling in front of and under the ear. There may be swelling under the jaw as well. Eating, especially chewing, may be painful. The swelling may last from 3 to 7 days.

In the case of adults, the disease can be much more painful and debilitating than it usually is for children. Boys and men who contract mumps after puberty may develop inflammation of the testes. So it is better for boys to have had mumps or to have been immunized before puberty.

It is possible to be immunized against mumps. However, the vaccine will not protect anyone who has been in contact with mumps before the vaccination.

Mumps is infectious from several days before the person becomes ill until the swelling goes down.

Home care

Ask the doctor to confirm the diagnosis if you are uncertain. Keep the person warm and resting until the temperature has returned to normal. Give plenty of fluids and a soft diet that does not need chewing. If the invalid finds it difficult to open his or her mouth, give fluids through a straw. Regular cleaning of the teeth and rinsing the mouth with water or an antiseptic mouthwash helps to keep the mouth moist and clean and to prevent infection. Paracetamol may be given to relieve pain.

Call the doctor if the person has a severe headache or vomits, has a continuing high fever, or if one of the testicles becomes swollen and tender. Cold compresses (see page 100) help soothe sore testicles.

Make sure that the invalid avoids contact with boys and men who have not had mumps. Keep children away from school for a couple of days after the swelling has gone down.

MEASLES

Measles is a viral infection of the respiratory system, with a rash. It most commonly affects children between the ages of 8 months and 5 years. Children can be vaccinated against measles during the first years of life.

The time between contact with the disease and the appearance of the first symptoms is usually between 10 and 12 days.

The illness starts with the child feeling miserable, with a stuffy head, a runny nose, a cough and a raised temperature. A child with measles can develop a temperature as high as 40°C (104°F). The eyes are sometimes sore as well. After 3 or 4 days, the rash starts behind the ears and close to the hairline, and then spreads over the face and body. The spots are dusky pink and slightly raised. At first they are separate, but after a while they run together, giving a blotchy appearance. The child usually begins to feel better by the time the rash spreads to the lower limbs, and after another couple of days the rash begins to fade.

The child is infectious from 5 to 6 days before the rash appears until about 4 to 5 days after the temperature is normal.

Home care

A child with suspected measles should be seen by a doctor. Try to keep the child in bed, warm and resting, until his or her temperature returns to normal. Give plenty of fluids. Paracetamol helps make the child more comfortable and lowers the raised temperature. Tepid sponging (see page 101) also helps to bring the temperature down.

Call your doctor:
○ If the child seems to be getting worse, rather than better, 2 to 3 days after the rash develops
○ If the child has persistent earache
○ If the child has a cough and is breathless
○ If he or she has a headache with a stiff neck
○ If you are worried about the child's condition

Keep the child away from school for about 10 days after the rash appears. Check with your doctor.

WHOOPING COUGH

Whooping cough is a respiratory illness caused by a bacterial infection. It is most common among children but may occur at any age, and it is highly infectious. It can be a very dangerous illness for a small baby. In older children and adults it is not quite as serious, but it can be a distressing and prolonged illness. Doctors generally advise that babies should be immunized against whooping cough. The immunization does carry a very slight risk of a serious reaction, and certain children – for example, those who have had a fit or convulsion – may be at increased risk. But for most children the advantages of immunization far outweigh any risk. Discuss any worries you may have about immunization with your doctor.

The time between contact with the disease and the appearance of the first symptoms is usually between 7 and 10 days.

Whooping cough starts like a cold, with a runny nose, a cough and a raised temperature. This continues for about 2 weeks, with the cough getting worse until the characteristic coughing spasms of whooping cough develop. The person coughs several times in rapid succession and often, but not always, then makes a whooping sound as he or she gasps for breath trying to breathe in. The person is left breathless and exhausted and may even go blue or vomit.

Coughing fits gradually become less frequent but the cough may last for 3 months or even longer.

Whooping cough is infectious from the first appearance of symptoms until about 3 weeks after the development of the coughing spasms.

Home care
Call the doctor if a cough is getting worse instead of better after about a week, or if you hear the whooping sound after a fit of coughing, or if for any other reason you suspect that someone may have whooping cough.

Young babies who need constant nursing are often admitted to hospital, but most children and adults are nursed at home. Effective nursing plays a very important part in the management of whooping cough.

If coughing fits are frequent and followed by vomiting it may be very difficult for the person to keep down enough food and liquid. Children, particularly, are at risk of dehydration. Give lots of fluids, in the form of small, frequent drinks. Frequent, small snacks are also a good idea: give light, easily digested food, avoiding anything dry or crumbly that might bring on a cough. Nourishing fluids may be all the person can tolerate (see page 120). The best time to give food and drink – in small quantities – is often as soon after a fit of coughing and vomiting as the person can manage. Then at least some of it should be absorbed before the next attack.

If you are nursing a baby with whooping cough at home, abandon any attempt to stick to a feeding routine. Give a bottle or breast-feed whenever the baby will take it. Again, it will probably be best to give small amounts often. If the baby vomits soon after a feed he or she will have to be fed again to make sure enough fluid is absorbed.

Apart from the generally debilitating effects of illness, the coughing fits are exhausting, and a person with whooping cough needs a lot of rest. If sleeping lying down brings on the cough, sit him or her up in bed, well supported with backrest and pillows.

The doctor may prescribe cough linctus to ease the cough. Paracetamol will reduce fever. Antibiotics are not effective against fully developed whooping cough, but they may be prescribed if a secondary lung infection occurs. They are also sometimes given to young babies who have been in contact with the infection, as they may prevent whooping cough from developing.

A young child with whooping cough may panic when he or she has a coughing fit and this will exacerbate the problem of breathlessness, so it is essential that you are there to give reassurance. You will also need to hold a child's head tilted downward during a coughing fit to prevent the inhalation of vomit or mucus.

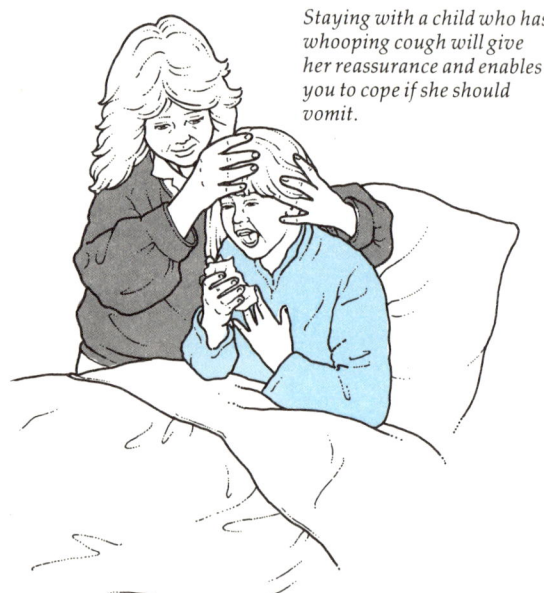

Staying with a child who has whooping cough will give her reassurance and enables you to cope if she should vomit.

Children tend to have fewer coughing fits if their attention is on something else. However, they need to be kept calm, as active play or much excitement may bring on the cough. So try to provide lots of peaceful entertainment in the form of books, television, and quiet games and toys.

If you are nursing a baby with whooping cough the doctor will need to see the baby frequently. With an adult or an older child, call the doctor:
○ If the cough is producing phlegm, and the person is breathless or increasingly unwell
○ If the person has a fit or convulsion
○ If the person is confused
○ If you are worried about his or her condition
Children should not go back to school, or adults to work, until the doctor says they may.

GLANDULAR FEVER (Infectious mononucleosis)

Glandular fever is a viral infection that is most common among young people in their teens and early twenties, but can also occur in children and in older people. It is sometimes called the 'kissing disease', as it is most frequently passed on by kissing or close contact. It can produce very variable symptoms, but usually the person feels unwell and tired, with no energy, and develops a sore throat, a fever and swollen glands.

Home care
Consult your doctor if you think someone might have glandular fever. The doctor may take a blood

sample to confirm the diagnosis.

The invalid will need plenty of rest. Give plenty of fluids, especially while the temperature is raised and the throat is sore. If the person finds it difficult to swallow food, provide nourishing liquids (see page 120). Ice cream is also soothing and easy to eat.

You can give soluble paracetamol to ease the sore throat and help bring down the temperature, or soluble aspirin may be used as a gargle and then swallowed. (But for circumstances in which aspirin should not be taken, see page 109.)

Close physical contact with other people should be avoided during the acute stage of the illness, but glandular fever is not very infectious, and it is usually fairly safe to have visits from friends.

Call the doctor if the person develops an increasingly sore throat and difficulty in swallowing, a severe headache with a stiff neck, or if you are worried about his or her condition.

Glandular fever is not usually a serious illness, but it does take a while to recover. A person who has had glandular fever may continue to feel unwell, tired and depressed and to have occasional fevers for several weeks or even months. To help him or her over this period a person needs plenty of rest, a nourishing, well-balanced diet, and also lots of encouragement and reassurance that he or she will soon feel better.

Young people can return to school, and adults to work, when the temperature and sore throat have subsided and they have been feeling better for a few days. This is usually 2 to 5 weeks after the start of the illness. Although young people may be very worried about missing school while studying for exams, it is often a good idea for the convalescent to go to school for half-days or work part-time initially, as he or she will probably still tire very easily.

INFLUENZA (Flu)

Influenza is a viral infection. It is not a serious illness in strong, generally healthy people, but it can be serious for the very young, the elderly, or anyone with a chest or heart problem. Immunization against influenza is available, but is generally given only to people who might be at particular risk if they had an attack, and has to be repeated each year. Consult your doctor if you think it might be advisable for anyone in your family to be immunized.

The time between contact with the disease and the first appearance of the symptoms is usually between 1 and 3 days.

A person with influenza may feel only slightly unwell, with what seems to be a cold; or the person may feel extremely ill, with a high temperature, sore throat, dry cough, soreness behind the breastbone,

headache and aches and pains in the limbs. Usually the fever subsides and the person begins to feel better after 3 to 4 days. However, he or she may feel generally low and exhausted for some time after the illness.

The person is infectious from just before the appearance of the symptoms until 5 to 10 days later.

Home care
Keep the person warm and comfortable, preferably resting in bed. Give plenty of fluids, but do not worry if someone with flu does not eat for a few days: his or her appetite will soon return.

You can give paracetamol to help bring down the raised temperature and relieve aches and pains.

Call the doctor:
○ If after 2 or 3 days the cough is producing yellow or green mucus
○ If the temperature remains high
○ If the symptoms are getting worse rather than better
○ If you are worried about the patient's condition
If you suspect that someone with a chronic heart or chest problem has influenza, call the doctor at once. Antibiotics may be prescribed – they will have no effect on the influenza, but may be effective in preventing a secondary chest infection. It is best for the person to be in a fairly upright position in the bed, comfortably supported by backrest and pillows. Encourage coughing.

Anyone who has influenza should stay away from work or school and as far as possible avoid contact with other people until he or she feels better. If in doubt, check with your doctor.

RINGWORM

Ringworm is a fungal infection of the skin or nails. It takes many different forms affecting different parts of the body, but it tends to appear as red, raised, scaly rings which are often very itchy. Scalp ringworm causes bald patches with broken hair stubs. Foot ringworm (athlete's foot) appears as white, sodden, dead skin between the toes. Ringworm is often passed from one person to another, or it may be caused by contact with an infected animal.

Home care
Athlete's foot can be treated with anti-fungal powder or cream bought from a chemist. With other forms of ringworm, or if athlete's foot does not respond to your treatment, consult the doctor. He will probably prescribe a special cream, which should be applied as directed. Tablets may also be prescribed by the doctor.

Except in the case of athlete's foot, all the family and anyone who may have been in contact with the infection and has a rash should be seen by their doctor in case they have been infected and need treatment. As far as possible, be careful to keep an infected person's washing equipment and towels separate from the rest of the family's. Make sure the basin, bath or shower is well cleaned after use by the infected person. Any animal with ringworm should be treated by a vet.

Children with athlete's foot do not have to be kept away from school, but they must not go barefoot for any activity until the athlete's foot has cleared up. Athlete's foot is often spread by way of infected floors, often in swimming pools, in school gyms or exercise studios. Children with other forms of ringworm should not go to school until the doctor says that they may.

WORMS

Threadworms are very common in children. These tiny white parasitic worms live in the digestive tract and can be seen in the stools. The eggs are laid on the skin in the area of the anus. This makes the skin itchy, the child scratches and the eggs are transferred to the fingers and later, probably, to the mouth, so reinfection occurs. Threadworm eggs may also get into the household dust and affect other members of the household.

Home care
See your doctor – there are various preparations that can be prescribed. All the family should be treated even if only one person has worms. And everyone must be very careful to wash their hands and brush their nails before meals and after going to the toilet.

Cancer

The word cancer is very frightening. It is important to remember that these days many cancers can be cured; with early treatment the outlook is good.

However, the early detection and treatment of cancer is vital. If cancer developing in one part of the body goes untreated it may well spread elsewhere in the body. Take note of the early warning signs listed below and if in doubt seek medical advice.

The early detection of cancer
See your doctor as soon as you can if any of the following signs or symptoms appear:
○ Any sore, especially a sore with raised edges on the face that does not heal quickly
○ Any unusual bleeding or discharge from any natural body opening
○ Any painless lump, especially on the soft tissue such as the breast, lips, tongue
○ Any persistent indigestion or unexplained weight loss
○ Any persistent hoarseness or cough or difficulty in swallowing
○ Any unexplained change in normal bowel habits
○ Any mole that enlarges, becomes irregular in shape, bleeds or itches

The treatment of cancer
Before it can be said that someone definitely has cancer, a biopsy is needed: a small piece of tissue is taken from the affected area and examined under the microscope. If the tissue is cancerous, a decision is made about what treatment will be needed.

Cancer can be treated in different ways and the type of treatment varies according to the type of cancer, the extent of the disease and many other factors. Treatment may involve surgery, special medicines (chemotherapy), X-ray treatment (radiotherapy), or a combination of these. Each case is assessed individually and the kind of nursing care needed at home will vary according to the treatment received in hospital. Any other, less conventional, treatment the sick person may consider should be discussed with the doctor.

Both having cancer and undergoing the various treatments can be very stressful for the person concerned. Caring for the person can be stressful for you. Either or both of you may have feelings of depression, fear, anger and even 'couldn't care less'. These are all normal reactions. You both need plenty of support from the medical professionals involved and from family and friends. A support group (see page 220) can also provide a great deal of help.

Surgery
Surgery was the first effective treatment for cancer and is still often the first line of attack. Following the surgery there is bound to be some pain, but the extent of the pain depends upon the type of operation. The use of pain-relieving medicines should control most pain.

The care the patient will need at home varies according to the type of operation. The hospital will give detailed advice on further care at home. The patient, or you, may also find it useful to ask the staff the questions listed on pages 152-153.

Chemotherapy and radiotherapy are more often than not given on an outpatient basis, so with these treatments home care is especially important.

Chemotherapy

The use of drugs or hormones to treat cancer is known as chemotherapy. It is often given in combination with surgery or radiotherapy. These drugs work by damaging or killing the cancerous cells. Unfortunately, they affect some healthy cells at the same time.

Chemotherapy may be given by mouth, in tablet or capsule form, or intravenously by injection. It is essential that these drugs are given exactly as prescribed. If you are responsible for administering any of them, be sure to get most precise directions from the doctor.

Side-effects and home care

Not everyone experiences severe side-effects to chemotherapy and certainly not all these listed below. Their effect may be comparatively mild.

Tiredness and lack of energy are very common side-effects of chemotherapy. They may get worse as each course of treatment goes on, but there is usually an improvement between courses. Encourage the person to rest as much as possible.

The person may suffer from decreased appetite, nausea and vomiting. For a few days following treatment encourage him or her to eat small, frequent meals, to eat slowly, chewing the food well so that it is easily digested, and to avoid spicy, fried or fatty foods.

The drugs may damage the cells lining the mouth, producing soreness and ulceration. Regular mouth-washes are important to keep the mouth clean and to ward off infection. After brushing his or her teeth, the person should use a mouthwash consisting of one teaspoon of bicarbonate of soda in a glass of warm water. Avoid commercial mouthwashes, which usually contain alcohol. Soft foods will be more comfortable to eat. If the mouth is very sore or white patches develop, seek advice from your doctor.

Diarrhoea can sometimes be a problem. The doctor will be able to prescribe medicine to help. In the meantime avoid foods that are high in fibre, such as raw fruits and vegetables and whole grain cereals.

Some chemotherapy may colour the urine for a few hours after treatment or even cause some bladder irritation. Increasing fluid intake to at least 2 litres (4 pt) a day for a couple of days following the treatment helps to flush the drugs through.

Hair loss may occur during treatment. This can be particularly distressing for women. Wearing a wig helps to lessen embarrassment: try to get it fitted and ready to wear before the hair loss is really noticeable. The hair sometimes begins to grow back in between courses of treatment and it will grow again when treatment is finished. Not all drugs cause hair loss – ask the doctor if this is a likely side-effect.

Sometimes the skin reacts by producing a red, raised itchy rash. The doctor will try to find out which drug is causing the problem and meanwhile he will be able to give something to reduce the irritation.

Some drugs cause muscle weakness and pins and needles in the fingers and toes.

Most of the drugs used in chemotherapy affect the bone marrow, where the body makes blood cells. The hospital staff keep a check by taking regular blood samples. If the level of white cells, which fight infection, or platelets, which help the blood to clot, drops too low, treatment may be stopped or delayed for a while to allow the cells time to increase. If the patient becomes anaemic because there are not enough red cells, a blood transfusion may be given.

Low white blood cell count

If the white count cell is low it is advisable to avoid crowded places and anyone who is known to have an infectious disease. Protective gloves should be worn for gardening or any dirty job. Seek medical advice if the person:

○ Develops a temperature over 38°c (100.4°F), and feels hot and cold and shivery
○ Has a burning sensation on passing urine – this may indicate a urinary infection
○ Develops a cough
○ Has diarrhoea for more than 2 days, combined with other symptoms

Low platelet count

If the platelet count is low, bleeding or bruising may result from a very minor injury. The person should not take any medicines containing aspirin, which may cause bleeding. You should also do what you can to help the person to avoid cuts. If a cut occurs apply firm pressure with a clean cloth for several minutes. If the bleeding does not stop quickly, seek medical advice.

You should also contact the doctor if:

○ The person has a nose bleed, bleeding gums, or blood in the urine or faeces (see pages 95-95)
○ Tiny red spots occur under the skin

Low red cell count

If the red cell count is low, the person will be anaemic and is likely to feel tired and irritable and to be short of breath. Seek medical advice if the sick person develops these symptoms.

Fertility

A woman's menstrual cycle may well become irregular, or she may stop having periods altogether. Sometimes in women over 30 years old, chemotherapy brings on an early menopause and the periods do not return after therapy has stopped, but this does not happen very often. Usually the menstrual cycle returns to normal once treatment has stopped.

As the contraceptive pill should generally not be taken during treatment a woman should seek medical advice on how to avoid becoming pregnant. Even if her periods become irregular during chemotherapy she may still become pregnant. If she thinks that she might be pregnant before or during treatment she must talk to her doctor so that he can arrange for a pregnancy test. She should discuss the implications of the effects of these drugs on the unborn child.

Some drugs used in chemotherapy may cause damage to a man's testes, resulting in sterility. Ask the doctor whether the drugs being used are likely to have this effect.

In either a man or a woman there may be a temporary loss of desire for sex. This is the result of stress and general tiredness rather than a direct effect of the drugs.

Some questions to ask about chemotherapy:
○ What will these drugs do?
○ Why are they necessary?
○ Is there any alternative treatment?
○ How are the drugs given?
○ How often is treatment given?
○ How long does each treatment take?
○ How long does each course of treatment last?
○ How many courses of treatment will there be?
○ How much time is there between courses?
○ Should any special precautions be taken before or after treatment?
○ Are there any side-effects?
○ How long will these side-effects last?
○ Are there any long-term side-effects?
○ Are the drugs used likely to affect the person's fertility?
○ Can the person concerned drive home after treatment, or will transport be needed?
○ If I am worried, whom do I contact and where?

Radiotherapy

X-rays and other forms of radiation are used to treat certain types of cancer or to prevent the reappearance of a cancer that has been removed surgically. Treatment is not painful but there are some side-effects. It is important that the patient and the caregiver should talk to the therapist about these side-effects, so that you know how to cope. You should also discuss any fears that you or the patient may have. For example, the person may well be anxious about the outcome of the treatment, the changes in lifestyle and the usual routine, and about whether he or she will feel pain or suffer from exhaustion and depression or any other side-effects mentioned by other people.

Side-effects and home care
The person undergoing radiotherapy will not necessarily be affected by all the side-effects listed below, and their effect may be only minor.

The skin over the area treated may become red, dry and peeling, so skin care is very important. No strappings or plaster should be put over the area that is being treated. No soap, talcum powder, creams, deodorants or perfumes should be used on this area. The person should be careful to avoid any injury or friction to the area and should try not to rub or scratch the skin. The area should not be exposed to sunlight or to winds.

A person having radiotherapy will probably suffer from tiredness and lack of energy. He or she may lose his or her appetite, or feel sick. If sickness is a problem the doctor may be able to prescribe some tablets that will help. Meals should be small and frequent.

Radiotherapy to the abdomen
Diarrhoea may occur as a side-effect of radiotherapy to the abdomen. The radiotherapist should be told about this. The person may be advised to take only liquids (but not milk or milk products) until the diarrhoea settles. Once the diarrhoea has subsided it may help to prevent a recurrence if high-fibre foods are avoided and milk and milk products are taken sparingly.

Radiotherapy to the head and neck
The throat may feel sore on swallowing after radiotherapy to this area. It is better to avoid spicy foods and alcohol. The person will find it easier to eat a soft diet of well-cooked foods which are cut up into small pieces and moistened with sauces. If even this soft diet is difficult to manage, then high-calorie, high-protein drinks may help (see page 120).

Anyone having radiotherapy to the mouth must take special care of their teeth (see page 65). Radiotherapy to the jaws may affect the salivary glands so that less saliva is produced. This makes the person more prone to developing a sore mouth. So give plenty of fluids and encourage the person to rinse his or her mouth out frequently to remove any food debris. Ice cubes can be sucked as an alternative to rinsing. The person may either lose the sense of taste or find that food tastes unpleasant. In this case, if you prepare food that smells good and looks attractive, and so appeals to the other senses, he or she may be encouraged to eat.

Radiotherapy to the testes or ovaries
This sort of treatment usually means that the person concerned will become sterile. However, some people who have had radiotherapy to these organs have later been able to have normal children.

Some questions to ask about radiotherapy:
○ Why is this treatment needed?
○ Is there an alternative?
○ Which part of the body will be treated?
○ How long will the course of treatment take?
○ How often will it be necessary to attend for treatment?
○ How long will each treatment last?
○ Can the person concerned drive home after each treatment, or will transport be needed?
○ Are there any special precautions required before or after treatment?
○ Are there any special side-effects which are relevant to this particular type of radiotherapy?
○ Will the person feel sick?
○ Will he or she feel tired?
○ How long will any side-effects last?
○ Are there any long-term side-effects?
○ Will the radiotherapy affect the person's fertility?
○ If I am worried, whom do I contact and where?

If treatment is unsuccessful

Sometimes any or all these treatments will fail to cure the person's cancer. As with any terminal disease there may be feelings of anxiety, fear, loneliness and depression – both for the dying person and for the family. Everyone concerned needs support, help and professional advice: the section on **Care of the Dying** discusses this in greater detail.

Mental Illness

Caring for someone who has a mental or emotional illness can be much more difficult, and less satisfying, than looking after someone who has a physical illness or disability. You may feel very isolated, reluctant to talk to or ask help from friends because of the wariness many people still feel about mental illness. If you have been close to the sick person, this loneliness will be even more pronounced. He or she may seem to have changed and withdrawn from you, and to be indifferent to all your efforts to help. The most important thing to remember is that the sufferer's whole view of the world is coloured by the altered state of mind. It may be hard for you to sympathize with what you regard as 'imaginary' symptoms, or to understand the sufferer's behaviour or inability to cope with normal situations. But it is important to continue to give support and understanding, and it will help once you realize that all these feelings are absolutely real to the person concerned – he or she is genuinely unable to 'snap out' of them and respond in a 'normal' way.

Mental or emotional illnesses are common, but only very rarely are they so severe that the person needs treatment in hospital. By far the most common are the 'neurotic' illnesses – periods of anxiety or depression, occurring in people whose personalities make them unable to cope easily with stress, and whose problems have temporarily overwhelmed them. Much less common are the psychotic illnesses, such as schizophrenia and manic-depressive psychosis, in which the person's thoughts become so disordered that he or she loses touch with reality, and thinks and behaves in a very bizarre way. Powerful drugs are needed to treat psychotic illnesses, and a period of hospital treatment is usually necessary.

DEPRESSION

Everyone has occasional periods of gloom, and there are times (after a bereavement, for example) when it is quite natural to feel depressed for a considerable time. But most people manage to cope with life normally even though they are sad, and gradually their mood lightens and they find they are enjoying life again. Some people, however, react to a stressful time or emotional blow in a different way; their depression does not pass, but persists and deepens until it disrupts their ability to lead a normal life.

A few people, often those who have a family history of depression, develop depressive illness, not as a reaction to stress but for no apparent reason. This is called 'endogenous' depression. Depression is also quite common after a viral infection such as glandular fever, and may result from the hormonal changes which follow childbirth. Depressive illness is common among the elderly, but people also seem to be particularly vulnerable during the often stressful years of late adolescence, middle age, and post-retirement.

Someone suffering from depression feels continually miserable and hopeless, cries a great deal and loses energy and appetite for life, food and sex. He or she may have difficulty going to sleep, or wake early and be unable to go back to sleep again, but lie feeling frightened and unable to get up and face the day. There are often physical symptoms too, such as indigestion, constipation or headache. People who have endogenous depression occasionally develop severe psychological symptoms, becoming deluded and losing touch with reality, believing that they are worthless or becoming suicidal: such seriously disturbed people need to be treated in hospital.

Home care

Make sure that the patient takes his or her medication regularly, and does not stop – despite feeling better – until the doctor gives permission. It will take 2 to 3 weeks for the medicine to take effect.

One of the most important things you can do is to try to help the sufferer to change the content of his or her thoughts. This involves making a conscious effort to 'think positive', to push out of consciousness any gloomy thoughts that arise. If you realize that the sick person is thinking negatively, divert the negative thoughts, forcing the sick person to think or talk about something else. Make sure that each day contains something, however small, which can be enjoyed – it need only be a new book from the library, a good meal or a favourite television programme. Persuade the sick person to go out if you can. Exercise is a powerful antidepressant, and so too is the company of friends. Give continual reassurance that, however bad he or she feels, it will pass. If, after a few weeks treatment with antidepressants, there is no improvement, sleep is still disturbed or weight loss is continuing, it is important that you should return to the doctor. Above all, always take any threat of suicide seriously.

ANXIETY

Anxiety is a natural response to a stressful situation. However, some people are so prone to anxiety that they become extremely anxious for trivial reasons, or feel continually apprehensive or tense for no apparent reason at all. Even someone who is not especially anxiety-prone may, if suffering very severe stress, develop this kind of 'anxiety state'.

Someone in an anxiety state will become irritable and unable to concentrate. He or she may suffer from insomnia and have sudden surges of fear, with palpitations, trembling, 'butterflies' in the stomach or diarrhoea, difficulty in swallowing or breathing, or sweating palms. There may also be sexual problems. Perhaps not surprisingly, some people tend to focus their anxiety on these physical symptoms and become hypochondriacal, convinced that they have some serious disease. Some anxiety-prone people suffer occasional terrifying 'panic attacks' when their feeling of terror becomes intense, their heart races and they can scarcely breathe, so that they believe they are having a heart attack or dying.

Home care

Relaxation techniques are probably the best way to cope with anxiety. Encourage the person to learn relaxation exercises, and to set aside a regular period to relax and unwind each day. This can take several forms – such as music, massage, yoga or meditation. Watch the person's posture, and if he or she looks physically tense, suggest a deliberate effort to relax. Physical tension can feed back and reinforce mental tension. Regular and fairly strenuous physical exercise can help relieve tension too. If an anti-anxiety drug has been prescribed, remember that these can become habit-forming. They should be taken simply to help the person over a bad patch and for no more than 4 months continuously.

People who have suffered a particular experience that has made them feel anxious will be helped to gain perspective if they are persuaded to talk about it. People usually become most anxious when they start to worry about things that might happen in the future, so encourage someone suffering in this way to turn his or her mind back to the present moment whenever thinking about the uncertain future becomes a worry. If anxiety is caused by a specific stress, discuss whether there is any way of removing this – it may be worth changing jobs, for example, if work is a continual source of tension. During a panic attack, all that the sufferer needs to do is to accept the feeling of fear and ride it out. Trying to fight the feelings only intensifies them.

Phobias

Some people feel intense and irrational fear only in certain, specific situations – when faced with a spider, for example. This specific anxiety is called a phobia. Most people manage to deal with a phobia simply by avoiding the feared object, but if it is centred around some normal daily activity – going outside the house for example (agoraphobia) – it can make it impossible for the sufferer to lead a normal life, and should be regarded as an illness. People who have crippling phobias need psychiatric help, but the treatment programme must be carried out at home, and will be much easier for the person to follow if he or she has the support and help of the person caring for them.

Home care

Treatment by professionals of a phobia usually involves desensitization – a process by which the person is made to face their fears in a 'hierarchy', first exposing themselves to the situation they fear least (for example, simply imagining it) then facing it in reality. Only a small step is taken each time, but gradually the fear becomes blunted. You can help someone suffering from agoraphobia, for example, by working through the 'hierarchy' with them, perhaps starting by making a brief visit to a friend, then to a small neighbourhood shop, and gradually going farther afield until he or she feels able to face what feels the most frightening situation of all.

Compulsive behaviour

A few people develop compulsive behaviour as a way of coping with irrational fears. They may become so obsessed with a fear of germs, for example, that they feel an overwhelming compulsion to wash their hands endlessly or clean the house ceaselessly. Even though they realize how absurd this is, they feel intensely anxious if they try to resist it. Medical treatment – usually the desensitization treatment described above – can help, and it is important to persuade anyone who does suffer from this kind of mental illness that he or she should see a doctor.

SCHIZOPHRENIA

Schizophrenia is a serious mental illness, with severe psychotic symptoms. People suffering from schizophrenia think in a way that seems illogical and disconnected. They may hear voices, and many lose touch with reality altogether, building up a fantasy world to account for their bizarre feelings and experiences.

Schizophrenia usually appears for the first time in late adolescence or early adulthood. Although it is a life-long condition, it is episodic, with attacks usually triggered off by emotional stress. Between these acute episodes, which must be treated in hospital, the patient may be able to lead a relatively normal life, either at home or in a hostel.

Home care
It is important to realize that even between acute attacks, when they are symptom-free, schizophrenics are still very vulnerable people, likely to become emotionally withdrawn and to have further breakdowns if they are put under stress. This can put enormous strain on a caregiver. Often all that can be done is to ensure that drugs are taken regularly (long-term medication will be necessary) and to provide as warm and relaxed a home environment as you can – family tensions are especially liable to provoke a breakdown. If the sufferer becomes increasingly withdrawn or starts to show other symptoms, make sure that he or she is put under medical care straight away – and above all, stay with the sufferer and offer reassurance.

Remember that it is just as possible for the person to become 'institutionalized' at home as in hospital; you will need to make constant efforts to socialize him or her – persuade him or her to go out, carry on whatever activities are possible, even to get out of bed in the mornings. Even though the sufferer may not be capable of holding down a job, regular attendance at a day centre is something you should encourage.

SENILE DEMENTIA

Senile dementia is a condition in which there is a progressive deterioration in brain function, especially in memory and intellect. It affects about 1 person in 10 over 65, and about a quarter of those over 80. Old people suffering from dementia are forgetful, particularly of recent events. They may become confused, and lack judgement, especially in new situations or environments; it is therefore always best to let old people stay in their own familiar homes as long as possible. They will slow down, both mentally and physically, and lose interest in the world around them. As the condition progresses, they find it increasingly difficult to express themselves. In the later stages of the disease there is a severe decay of the intellect and emotions. They will not know where they are or who is with them. Personality starts to die back, social and table manners deteriorate and the old person may start to neglect personal hygiene and be able to do less and less for themselves. In the final stages, sufferers occasionally become very unstable, alternating between apathy and uninhibited, even aggressive behaviour. These symptoms can also be shown by people suffering from Alzheimer's disease, a condition that can occur in people under 60.

Home care
The first rule, and often the most difficult, is to be patient. It will help to keep the person interested and alert if you can encourage independence. Help him or her to keep up hobbies, go for walks, see friends. A daily routine, with special high-spots – meals, a cup of tea, a television programme regularly watched, helps the person to feel less confused. Provide memory aids – lists, signs, reminders in large print and make sure that some identification is always carried in a pocket or handbag. Left to themselves many old people do not eat an adequate diet, so check that they have varied and nutritious meals. Old people who are beginning to lose some bladder control will be helped if you can remind them to go to the lavatory every 2 to 3 hours, or provide a commode (see page 70) which they can easily reach.

One of the pitfalls of caring for elderly people is that it is all too easy to attribute every problem to senile dementia, which cannot be treated, whereas it may well be due to some different, and treatable, condition. Many old people, for example, become slow and withdrawn not through dementia but because they have a treatable depressive illness. And incontinence should never be regarded as an inevitable consequence of senility; more often than not it has a physical cause, such as a bladder infection in women or an enlarged prostate in men.

First Aid

Situations which require first aid can range from the treatment of minor cuts and bruises to the use of life-saving techniques in the event of a more serious injury or accident. To be able to cope in an emergency, you will need to be familiar with basic first aid procedures and to keep calm so that you can assess the situation effectively. The instructions in this chapter give you the basic information that you need, but you will probably need to adapt them to fit the particular circumstances you find yourself in. Joining a first aid class will give you the opportunity to practise emergency first aid procedures on specially designed dummies and on other people in the class, which will help you gain confidence in your ability to cope.

WHAT TO DO IN THE EVENT OF AN ACCIDENT OR EMERGENCY

1 Move yourself and the injured person out of any immediate danger, taking great care if any fracture is suspected (see page 207).

2 Check that the injured person is breathing normally; if breathing has stopped, start artificial respiration (see page 194).

3 Check that the injured person's airway is clear of any obstructions (see page 194).

4 Check that the heart is beating; if heartbeat has stopped, start external chest compression (see page 196).

5 In the case of severe burns or bleeding, give immediate treatment (see pages 202 and 203).

6 If the injured person is unconscious, place in the recovery position (see page 198).

7 Prevent or minimize shock (see page 200).

8 Any wounds or burns should be dressed, and broken bones immobilized, if necessary (see pages 202, 207 and 214).

If the person is in urgent need of medical help and you are on your own, you will have to decide immediately whether to give any urgent first aid and then to call for help; or whether to get help right away. If possible, ask someone else to go for help while you give any urgent first aid.

If the injured person is conscious and needs medical help but does not require an ambulance, take him or her to the hospital or doctor's yourself. Always make sure that someone who is in shock or who has been unconscious, even for a few seconds, is seen by a doctor.

While waiting for help to arrive
☐ Note any changes in the injured person's condition and listen to what he or she has to say.
☐ Loosen any tight clothing around the neck, chest or waist but do not move the injured person or remove any clothing unnecessarily.
☐ Cover the injured person but do not apply heat or give alcohol or hot drinks as this will bring blood to the surface of the skin or to the stomach and deprive the heart and brain of the blood they need to keep functioning.
☐ Do not give anything to drink as the injured person may need to be given an anaesthetic later on, and any fluid taken may then be vomited.
☐ Do not give anything to eat or smoke.

How to call for help
☐ Find the nearest telephone and dial 999 for the emergency services.
☐ Give the phone number and address in case you are cut off and describe exactly where the injured person is.
☐ Say what you think is wrong with the person and what you think caused the problem.
☐ Speak clearly and precisely and do not put the phone down until the person on the other end says you may.

FIRST AID KIT

Keep the first aid kit in a clearly labelled container, locked and well out of reach of children. Make sure that all adult members of the family know where it is kept. Always replace anything that has been used. Any sterile packet which has been torn or damaged is no longer sterile and should be disposed of.

- Antiseptic cream – to help prevent infection of cuts and grazes
- Tin of adhesive dressings (plasters) – to cover small cuts and grazes
- Gauze dressings – to cover open wounds
- Sterile unmedicated dressings – six medium, two large and two extra large – to prevent infection developing in open wounds
- Adhesive dressing strip or adhesive paper strips – to hold dressings in place
- Two roller bandages – 5 by 5 cm (2 by 2 in) and 5 by 8 cm (2 by 3 in) – to secure dressings and immobilize broken bones
- Two crepe bandages – 5 by 8 cm (2 by 3 in) – to secure dressings and for broken bones
- Two triangular bandages – to secure dressings, for broken bones and for use as slings
- Tubegauz – to immobilize broken fingers
- 2 eye pads (sterile) – to cover injured eyes
- Packet of cotton-wool – to clean eyes, etc.
- Safety pins – to secure bandages
- Large safety pins – to pin sleeves to clothing when improvising slings
- A pair of scissors
- Disposable tissues
- A pair of tweezers – to remove stings and splinters

CONTENTS

ARTIFICIAL RESPIRATION

Breathing may stop after a serious accident for a variety of reasons, including choking, suffocation, drowning, strangling or poisoning. If breathing does stop, it is up to you to 'breathe' for the person, by giving artificial respiration, until he or she is able to breathe independently again; or until a doctor or another health professional takes over from you or tells you that there is no point in continuing as the person is not responding.

   Check that the person really has stopped breathing and has not just fainted or collapsed. Watch for chest movements and sounds of breathing; at the same time, feel for breathing by placing your hand on the person's chest and your ear close to his or her mouth and nose.

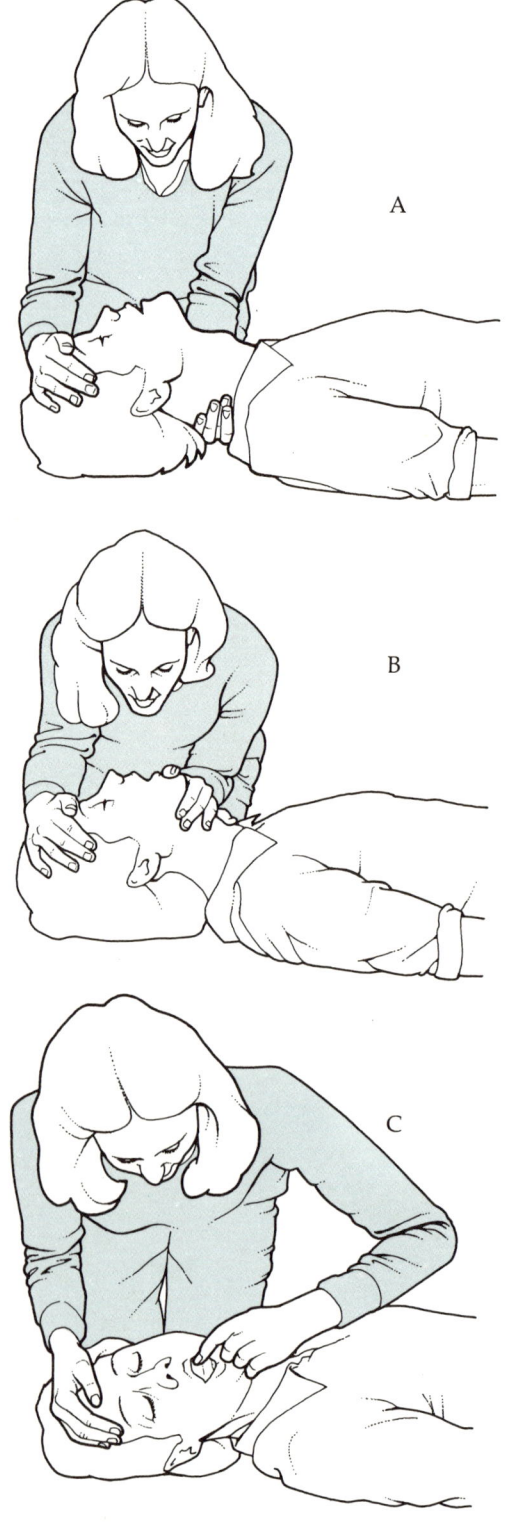

A

B

C

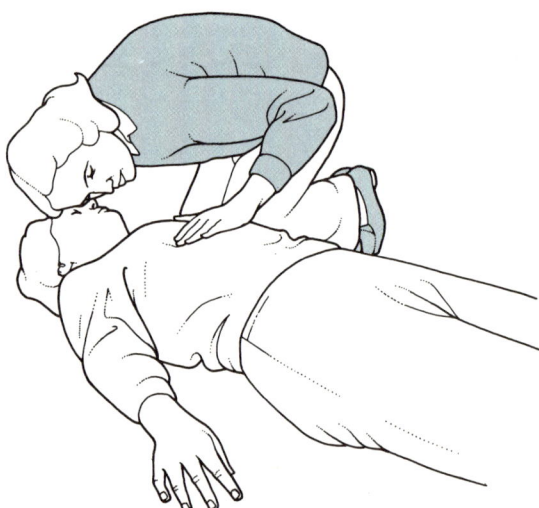

Opening the airway
If the person is not breathing, act quickly.

1 Lie the person on his back on a firm surface and loosen any tight clothing around the neck and chest areas.

2 Make sure the airway is clear: tilt the head back with one hand, lift the neck with the other hand (A), and pull the jaw forward (B). With the neck extended in this position, the tongue does not fall back and block the throat.

3 If breathing does not start, turn the head to one side. Hook your index finger and sweep round inside the mouth to remove any obstructions, such as dentures, food, vomit or loose teeth (C). Do not waste time searching for obstructions that are not immediately obvious.

Mouth-to-mouth

Once you have opened the airway and cleared the mouth of any obstructions, check again for signs of breathing. If the person is still not breathing, start giving artificial respiration immediately. Artificial respiration can be given mouth-to-mouth, which is the normal method, or mouth-to-nose. If the person is suffering from facial injuries or there is a risk of contamination, the Silvester method described overleaf can be used as an alternative.

1 Open the person's mouth and squeeze the soft part of his nose together (A).

2 Take a deep breath and cover his mouth with your mouth: blow hard enough to make the chest rise.

3 Remove your mouth and, as you take another breath, watch the chest fall. Give the first four full breaths rapidly without waiting for the chest to deflate completely (B). If you have to move the person, give these first few breaths before or during the move, if possible.

4 If the chest does not move, the airway may still be blocked. Turn the person onto his side and strike four times between the shoulder blades with the palm of your hand – this should dislodge any obstruction. Check again that the mouth is clear and replace the person on his back, taking care to open the airway, as before. Start giving artificial respiration again.

5 After the first four respirations, check the pulse in the neck to make sure that the heart is beating.

6 If the heart is beating, the person's colour should improve. Continue giving artificial respiration at a normal breathing rate of 16 to 18 breaths per minute. For a child, breathe more gently at a rate of 20 breaths a minute. Check the pulse every 2 minutes.

7 If the heart has stopped beating, the oxygen you are breathing into the person is not being circulated around the body. Start external chest compression (see page 196) immediately and combine it with artificial respiration.

8 Once the person is breathing normally, place in the recovery position (see page 198). This will ensure that if the person vomits, he will not choke. If he does inhale or choke on the vomit, turn him onto his side and strike four times between the shoulder blades with the palm of your hand. If breathing has stopped again, re-start artificial respiration.

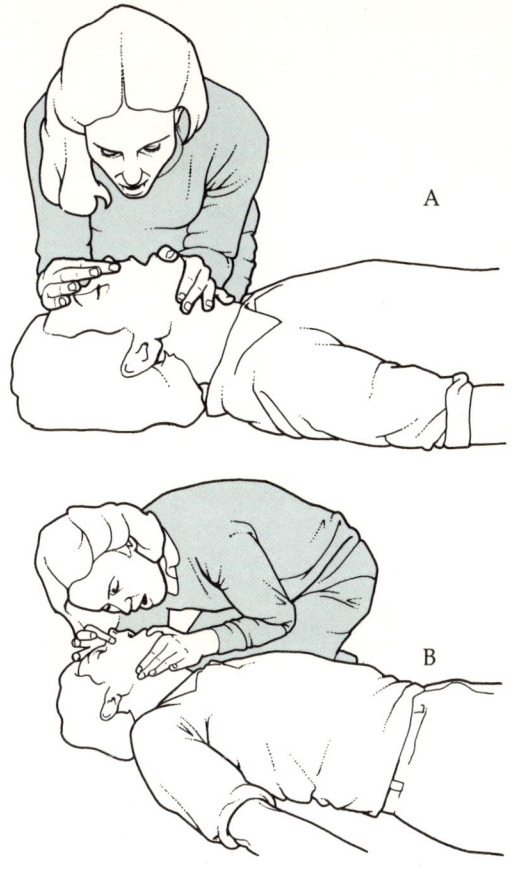

Mouth-to-nose

Clear the person's nose with your finger or a piece of cloth or tissue. Hold the mouth closed with your thumb and breathe into the nose. Open the mouth to allow each breath to be exhaled, while you take another breath ready to continue as for the mouth-to-mouth method.

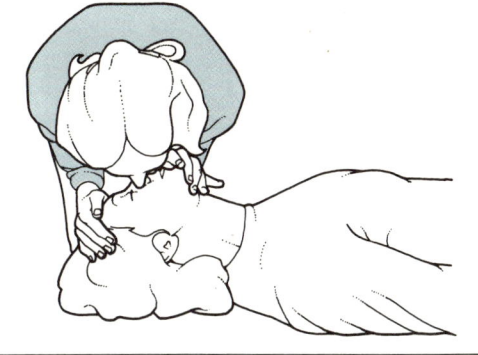

The Silvester method

This method of artificial respiration can be combined with external chest compression.

1 Lay the person on his back on a hard surface and raise his shoulders with a rolled-up coat or towel. Loosen any tight clothing and check that his airway is clear.

2 Kneel at his head and hold his wrists so that both your hands are over the centre of his chest. Keep your arms and back straight.

3 Rock forward and press down firmly on the lower part of his chest with a steady even pressure for 2 seconds (A). With a child, use less pressure.

4 Release by rocking back on your heels and sweeping his arms up and out (B).

5 Repeat this cycle of movements every 5 seconds.

6 Keep checking that the mouth is clear; if it fills with fluid, turn the person's head to one side so that it can flow out.

7 Check every four cycles that the heart is still beating. If it has stopped, give chest compression at the rate of 15 compressions to every two cycles. Compress the chest only when the injured person's arms are raised. If you have someone to help, give five compressions to every cycle.

8 As soon as the person starts breathing again, place in the recovery position (see page 198).

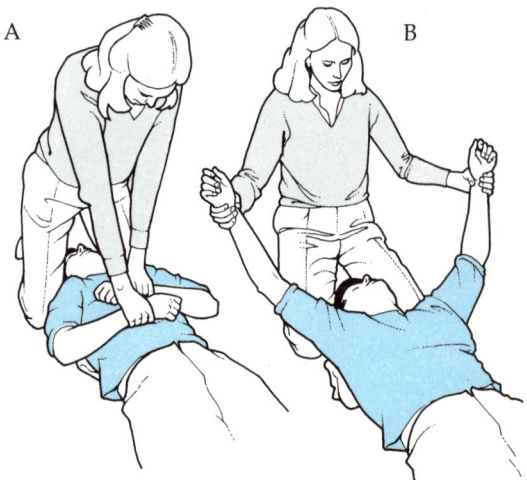

A   B

EXTERNAL CHEST COMPRESSION

It is important to ensure that the heart has stopped beating before starting external chest compression, as exerting pressure on a beating heart can cause damage. If the person is cold and grey and not breathing, and you cannot feel a pulse in the neck, the heart has stopped beating. Start external chest compression and continue with artificial respiration. You must act quickly as, once the heart has stopped beating, you have only 4 minutes before the brain, deprived of blood and therefore oxygen, becomes damaged.

Chest compression involves pressing the person's breastbone down onto the heart which in turn pushes the heart back toward the backbone. The heart is squeezed between the two bones and blood is forced out of it. When the pressure is released, the hearts fills with blood again. This process is called a compression and, when repeated at regular intervals, can take over from the heart and circulate blood around the body. As soon as the heart begins to beat again, the compressions must be stopped, although artificial respiration should continue until the person is breathing normally again.

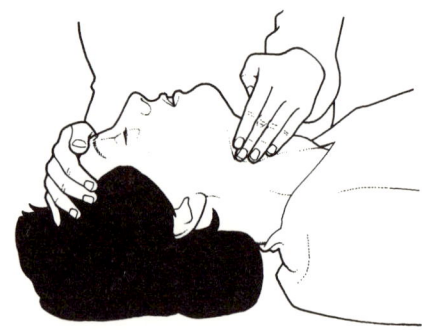

Artificial respiration and external chest compression with two people

If there are two of you, one should do the artificial respiration, the other the external chest compression. Never compress the heart at the same time as the lungs are being inflated, as this will prevent the person from getting adequate oxygen. Kneel, one on either side of the person's body. One of you gives the first four inflations and then checks for the pulse in the neck. If it is absent, one person gives five compressions and the other one inflation. Continue giving one inflation to five compressions at the rate of 60 compressions a minute.

1 Place the person flat on her back on a firm surface. Kneel beside her.

2 Feel for the top and lower end of the breastbone, and place the heel of one hand on the lower half of the bone. Place your other hand on top with your arms straight.

3 Keep your fingers and palm off the chest and apply pressure with the heel of your hand only.

4 Press down on the chest: rock your body forward and keep your arms straight. As you rock forward, the breastbone will sink as much as 5 cm (2 in): this is quite normal.

5 Release the pressure by rocking back and letting the breastbone rise, but leave your hands in position.

6 Repeat this movement 15 times at a rate of 80 per minute.

7 Move to the person's head, re-open the airway and give two breaths of artificial respiration.

8 Continue with the chest compression at the rate of 60 compressions per minute – give 15 compressions to every two artificial respirations. For children, use less pressure and only one hand, and give 15 compressions to every two artificial respirations at the rate of 100 compressions per minute.

9 Feel for the pulse in the neck after 1 minute and then every 3 minutes; as soon as you can feel it, stop the chest compression but continue with the artificial respiration.

10 When the person is breathing again, place in the recovery position (see page 198). Continue to check pulse and respiration rates and watch carefully until the person is fully conscious.

11 The person must be taken to hospital as, when breathing and heartbeat stopped, she was technically dead. She needs to be thoroughly checked by a doctor.

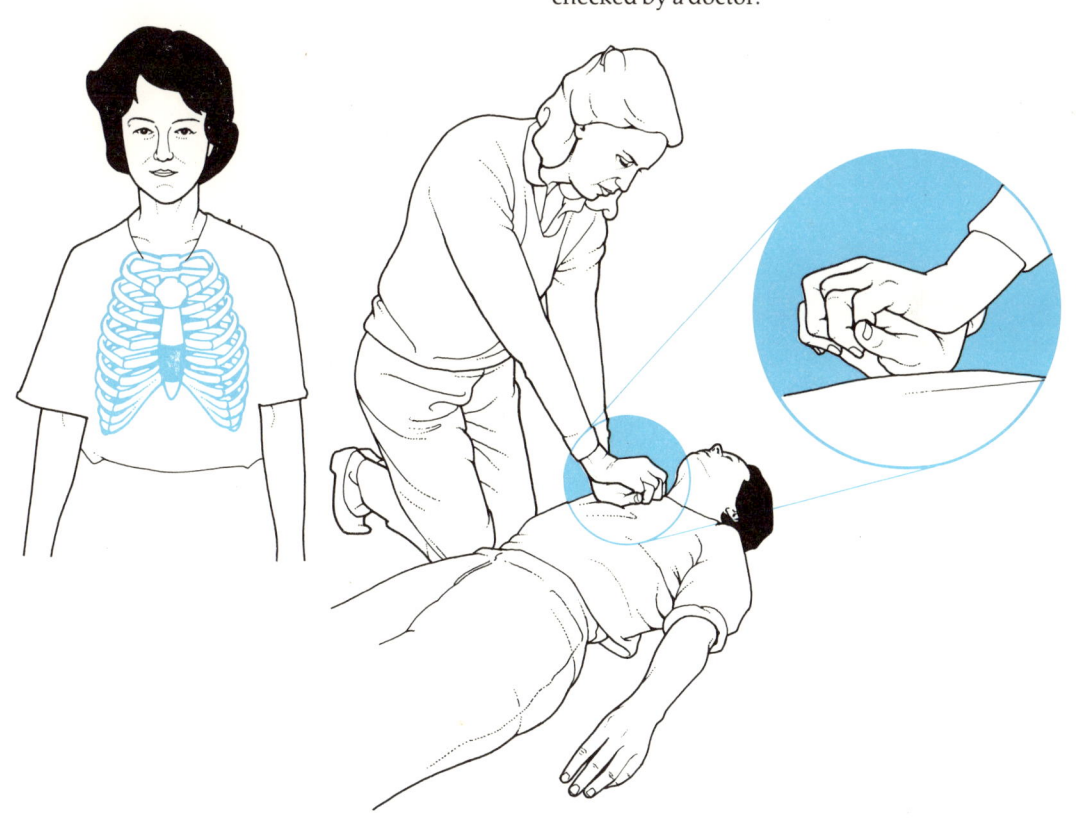

THE RECOVERY POSITION

This position prevents the person choking on his or her tongue, as it falls forward naturally, and also prevents him or her choking on blood or vomit, as this drains out of the side of the mouth.

1 Kneel down beside the person, turn her head toward you and tilt it back, keeping the jaw forward in the open airway position (A).

2 Place her arm nearest you straight down along her side and her hand under her buttock. Place the other arm across her chest.

3 Cross her furthest leg over the leg nearest you at the level of the ankle.

4 Support her head with one hand and, with the other hand, get a firm grip of her clothing or grasp hold of her far hip and pull her toward you, supporting her body against your knee (B).

5 Bend her uppermost arm and leg so that she does not roll onto her face. Gently pull out her lower arm from under her body and place it in a comfortable position (C).

6 Check that her head and neck are in the open airway position (see page 194).

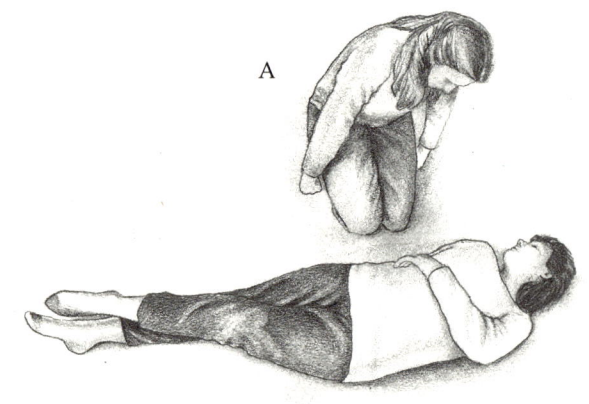

A

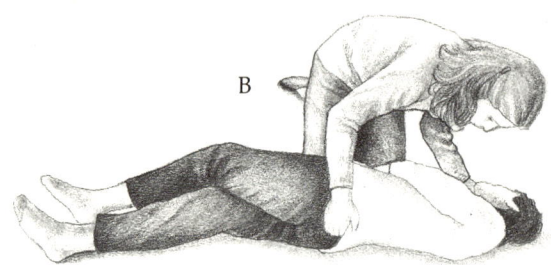

B

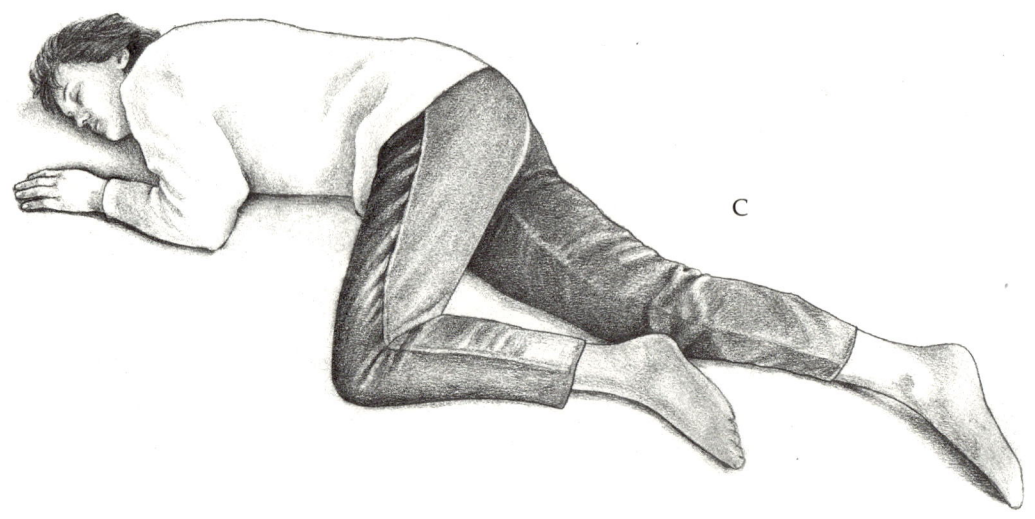

C

UNCONSCIOUSNESS

There are various stages or levels of responsiveness through which someone passes when they are losing consciousness. He or she:

○ Responds normally to questions and conversations
○ Then answers only direct questions
○ Then responds vaguely to questions
○ Then obeys commands only
○ Then responds to pain only
○ Finally, produces no response at all

During the first two or even three stages, efforts should be directed toward keeping the person awake. Once the last two stages have been reached, the person should be placed in the recovery position shown on the previous page.

1 An unconscious person should be placed in the recovery position, unless there are signs of a fracture to the spine (see page 209). If a fracture is suspected, do not move the person but hold his or her head in the open airway position (see page 194).

2 Check for anything which might indicate the cause of unconsciousness, such as drugs or alcohol, an identity bracelet indicating that the person suffers from diabetes or epilepsy, or signs of a fall.

3 Remain with the unconscious person, if possible, and send someone else to get help.

HEAD INJURIES

Head injuries can be very serious as they may lead to the brain becoming compressed. Compression occurs when there is bleeding within the brain and in the space between the brain and skull, causing increasing pressure on the brain.

Most head injuries are minor and have no ill-effects on the brain. However, you should take the injured person to see a doctor, if he or she shows any of the following signs or symptoms: loss of consciousness, even if only momentarily; altered level of consciousness; confusion; persistent vomiting; increasing headaches; clear fluid oozing from the nose or ears; weakness in movement and power of limbs; or deformity of the bones of the skull.

1 Prevent or minimize shock (see page 200).

2 If unconscious, place in the recovery position (see page 198) and send for medical help.

3 Dress any wounds (see page 214) to protect the skull and brain from infection.

4 If there is blood or clear fluid oozing from the nose or ear, this may be an indication that the skull is fractured. If the person is conscious, lie him or her down with head and shoulders raised and head inclined to the bleeding side to allow it to drain.

Watching for signs of brain compression

If you have to wait some time for medical assistance to arrive, check every 15 minutes the levels of responsiveness and note any changes.

Signs that the brain is becoming compressed include: noisy breathing; a rise in temperature; a flushed face and dry skin; a pulse which is full and bounding but slow; pupils of different sizes; and possible weakness or paralysis on one side of the body. As compression develops, the casualty's level of responsiveness falls. Treat as for unconsciousness and arrange for the injured person to be taken to hospital as soon as possible.

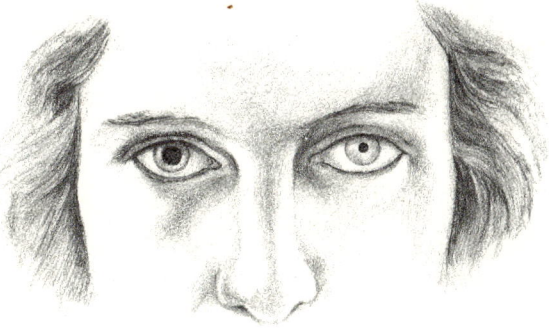

Concussion

Concussion results from a disturbance of the functioning of the brain following a knock on the head or jaw, and can occur without the person becoming obviously unconscious, or else unconsciousness may be only momentary. A concussed person may have a pale face, cold, clammy skin, shallow breathing and a weak but rapid pulse. He or she may feel sick or even vomit and may not remember anything about the accident which caused the concussion. Alternatively, the person may have a delayed reaction and seem quite all right immediately after the knock, but feel sick and giddy later on – normally within the next 24 hours. Treat as for a head injury.

SHOCK

'Primary', or emotional, shock develops as a nervous reaction to bad news or an emotional upset. The person feels dizzy and faint but will recover quickly if you sit him or her down with a hot drink and talk reassuringly. As no physical illness or injury is involved, it is quite safe to give something to drink.

Traumatic shock

A far more serious condition known as traumatic shock results from severe blood or fluid loss, extreme pain, sudden illness or prolonged exposure to cold. This is a very serious condition which can lead to death and requires urgent medical attention. Your aim should be to minimize shock or to prevent it from worsening but you are in no position to treat shock.

The following symptoms are all indications that the person may be suffering from shock: pallor; cold and clammy skin; an increase in the pulse rate which is weak and irregular; thirst, faintness, nausea and even vomiting; restlessness, confusion, slurred speech and possible loss of consciousness.

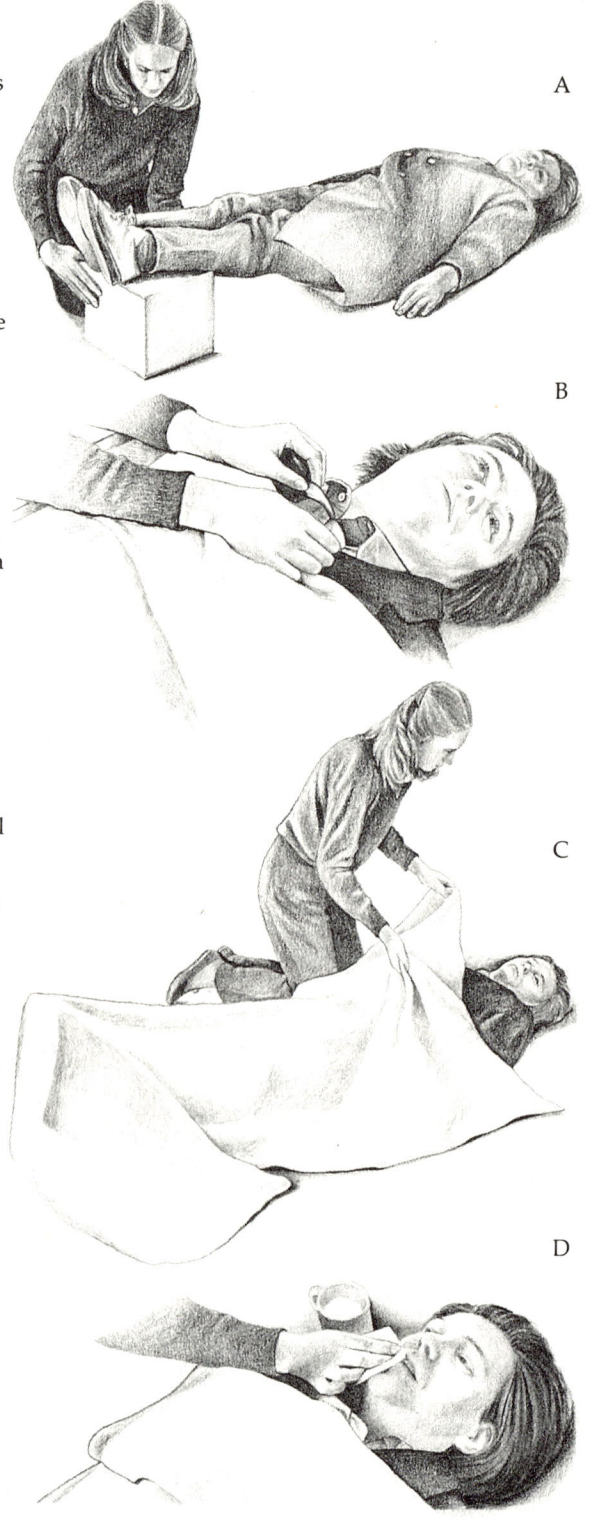

A

B

C

D

1 Stop any bleeding (see page 203). The more blood lost, the more in shock the person will be.

2 Lie the person down with her head low and turned to one side in case of vomiting or loss of consciousness, with her feet slightly raised: this will increase the blood supply to the heart and brain (A).

3 Loosen any tight clothing around the neck, chest or waist (B) but do not move the person or remove clothing unnecessarily.

4 Cover with a blanket to prevent her body losing heat (C) but do not apply direct heat or give alcohol or hot drinks as this will take the blood to the skin's surface or to the stomach and deprive the heart and brain of blood.

5 Do not give anything to drink, as an anaesthetic may be needed after arrival in hospital and any fluid taken may then be vomited. If she complains of thirst, moisten the lips with water (D).

6 Do not give anything to eat or smoke.

7 Check the pulse and breathing rate frequently and observe the level of consciousness.

CHOKING

Choking may be caused by any object blocking the person's airway, including a piece of food which has been inhaled.

1 Bend the person over so that her head is face downward and lower than her chest. Remove any obstructions from the mouth.

2 Slap the person sharply between the shoulder blades with the heel of your hand up to four times to dislodge the object.

3 If this does not work, try four abdominal thrusts (below): stand behind the person, place one arm around her abdomen and clench your fist between the person's navel and breastbone. Bring your other hand round to grasp your fist and pull both hands toward you with a quick upward and inward thrust. Repeat sequence if necessary.

4 Give artificial respiration after the object has been dislodged, if necessary (see page 194).

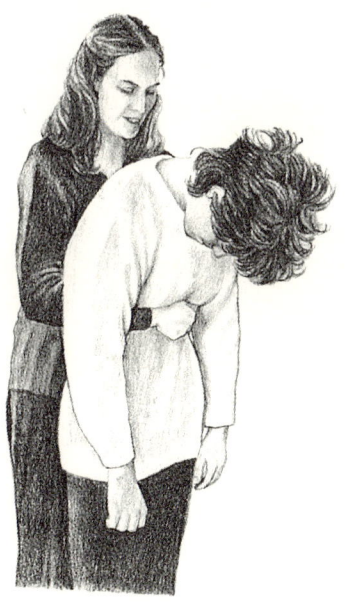

DROWNING

Get the person out of the water, remove any obstructions from the mouth and begin resuscitation (see pages 194-197): if possible, begin resuscitation in the water. Seek medical advice.

POISONING

If you suspect that someone has taken poison, get him or her to hospital as quickly as possible. Look for signs of poisoning: burns around the mouth, unusual sleepiness, rapid deep breathing, stomach pain, vomiting or retching, diarrrhoea, convulsions or a red face. There may be an empty bottle or container nearby. If the person is still conscious and able to talk, find out what was taken, how much of it and when. The person may lose consciousness at any time.

1 Keep a sample of vomit and look for evidence of what was taken. If you find anything, keep a sample or the container.

2 If breathing or heartbeat have stopped, start resuscitation (see pages 194-197), using the mouth-to-nose or Silvester methods if there is any risk of contamination.

3 If the person is unconscious, place in the recovery position (see page 198). Do not give fluids or attempt to induce vomiting. If possible, stay with the person and send someone else to get urgent medical help.

4 If the person is conscious and has swallowed a corrosive poison such as acid, alkali, petrol or fuel oil, do not try to make him or her vomit. Give plenty of fluids slowly, such as milk and water, in an attempt to dilute the poison and lessen the damage.

Poisoning from gas or exhaust fumes

1 Take a couple of deep breaths before going into the fume-filled area to bring the person out into the fresh air.

2 If it is not possible to remove the person immediately, turn off the gas tap or engine and open the windows and doors to let in fresh air. Do not do this in the case of a fire.

3 Resuscitate if necessary (see pages 194-197).

4 If he or she is breathing but unconscious, place in the recovery position (see page 198) and seek medical advice.

BURNS OR SCALDS

Burns may be caused by heat, chemicals or radiation. They can cause serious damage under the surface of the skin and in many cases will require medical attention.

1 If you can do so quickly, put out the fire with water or any other non-inflammable liquid.

2 If the person's clothes are on fire, get him or her onto the ground as quickly as possible, using a blanket, thick cloth or rug – do not use anything made of nylon or other inflammable material. Lay the person down with the burning area uppermost.

3 Smother the flames with the blanket: protect the person's face by bringing the blanket down over the face first. You can also use the blanket to shield yourself from the flames. If possible, do not roll the person around on the floor as this may spread the flames.

4 Place the burnt area in or under cold water for 10 minutes or until the pain has stopped. Do not try to remove any burnt clothing. If a young child has a burnt limb, put it in a plastic bag full of water so you can keep the child on your knee and give reassurance. If the skin is broken, cover with clean, non-fluffy material but do not immerse in water.

5 Prevent or minimize shock (see page 200) and, in the case of severe burns, send for medical help immediately.

6 In the case of minor burns, seek medical advice only if you are worried that the tissues underneath the skin have been damaged. Otherwise, cover the burn with a sterile dressing (see page 215) and leave untouched for 4 to 5 days. Never put oil or grease on a burn or attempt to prick any blisters which may form.

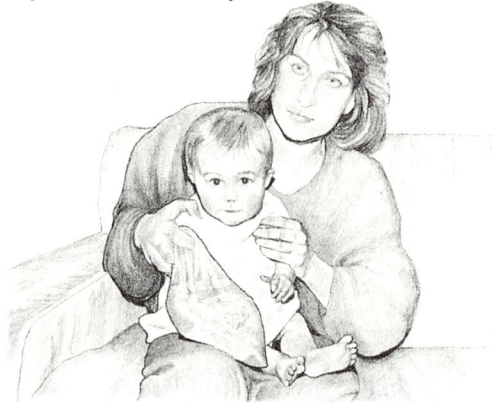

ELECTRIC SHOCK

Electric shocks can vary greatly in intensity and may cause serious injuries which can be fatal. Breathing and heartbeat may stop and severe burns may occur where the electricity enters and leaves the body. The higher the voltage, the more serious the burns. In the case of a high voltage electrical shock, you should not approach the person until you are sure it is safe to do so.

1 Do not touch the person until you have switched off or disconnected the appliance.

2 Use a wooden chair or piece of wood to move the source of electric current away from the person. Never use anything made of metal.

3 If breathing and heartbeat have stopped, start resuscitation (see pages 194-197). If the person starts to breathe again but is still unconscious, place in the recovery position (see page 198).

4 Observe and dress the burns (see left).

5 Seek medical advice as the burn may have damaged the tissues underneath the skin.

BRUISES

Bruising may result from a fall, bump or blow which causes blood to escape from the circulation and to collect under the skin. The bruised area will become purple or blue, turn green or yellow and then fade. Where bruising is minor, apply a cold compress (see page 100).

Severe bruising

Bruising may be severe if the person has fallen from a height. There may be no sign of a cut but if there is swelling, a great deal of blood may have escaped from the blood vessels.

1 Minimize or prevent shock (see page 200).

2 If unconscious, place in the recovery position (see page 198), unless a fracture is suspected.

3 Seek medical advice.

4 When medical help arrives, ensure that the injured person is moved on a stretcher.

BLEEDING

The adult body contains about 5 litres (10 pt) of blood and the rapid loss of even a litre (2 pt) is enough to threaten life. Blood which is bright red and spurts out in time with the heartbeat comes from an artery. Blood which is darker red and gushes out comes from a vein. Both these types of bleeding need urgent attention and must be stopped as quickly as possible.

Applying direct pressure
Venous bleeding can usually be stopped by applying direct pressure over the wound and by elevating the bleeding part above the level of the heart. You may not be able to stop arterial bleeding by direct pressure, in which case you will have to apply indirect pressure by compression of the injured artery.

1 Sit or lie the sick person in a comfortable position and, if possible, raise the injured part. In this position less blood is needed to supply the main organs of the body so blood pressure is lower and bleeding slower. Do not move the person if a fracture is suspected (see page 207).

2 Act quickly and restrict the flow of blood by pressing with your finger or hand directly over the bleeding area. If you have a clean cloth or dressing, place this over the bleeding site.

3 Press hard for 10 minutes. If the bleeding has not stopped, continue pressing until it does so. If the bleeding is coming from an arm or leg, lift the limb with one hand and press hard over the wound with the fingers of your other hand.

4 Once the bleeding is controlled, cover the wound with a sterile unmedicated dressing (see page 215) or a clean cloth and bandage. Do not bandage so tightly that you stop the circulation.

5 Avoid moving the injured part once a clot has formed as this may cause bleeding to start up.

6 If any blood comes through the dressing, put another dressing on top and continue to apply pressure. Do not change the dressing as you will disturb the clot that is forming.

7 Seek medical advice if you are unable to stop the bleeding or if you are worried that the wound may become infected.

Applying indirect pressure
If you cannot control the bleeding by direct pressure then apply indirect pressure by pressing on the artery supplying blood to the bleeding area for 10 minutes. If the arm is wounded, slide your fingers up the inner side of the upper arm, pushing the artery against the bone. If the leg is wounded, feel for the pulse of the artery in the groin and press it against the rim of the pelvis with your fist or the heel of your hand. Do not apply indirect pressure for more than 15 minutes at a time. This method should only be used as a last resort.

Tourniquets are dangerous if wrongly applied as they can deprive the whole limb of blood and cause gangrene. They should only be used by someone with specialist training.

Bleeding from the mouth
Bleeding from the mouth can be very heavy owing to the abundant blood supply to the area. Injuries are usually caused by the person's own teeth biting into the tongue, lips or inside lining of the mouth during, for example, a fall.

1 Ask the person to sit down. Place a towel across the chest and ask the person to bend his or her head forward over a bowl and to tilt it toward the injured side.

2 Give him or her a cloth to hold, with pressure, over the bleeding area. Giving ice to suck may help to stop the bleeding.

3 Ask him or her to spit any blood into the bowl and to avoid swallowing it as this may cause vomiting later on.

4 If the bleeding goes on for more than 20 minutes, or if the wound is large and gaping open, seek medical advice.

5 Once the bleeding has stopped, do not give any liquid for 2 hours as this may re-start bleeding. Do not give hot drinks for a period of 12 hours. If the person is thirsty, give water or cold, soft drinks.

Bleeding from a tooth socket
This type of bleeding may result from having a tooth extracted. Treat as for a bleeding mouth but ask the person to hold a thick pad of dressing or a clean handkerchief over, but not in, the socket for 10 to 20 minutes or until bleeding has stopped. Resting his or her jaw in cupped hands will make it easier for the person to hold the dressing or handkerchief in place.

Bleeding from the nose

If you suspect that the person's nose is bleeding as a result of a fractured skull, see page 199. A nose bleed should be treated in the following way.

1 Ask the person to sit down. Place a towel across her chest and ask the person to bend her head over a bowl. Loosen any tight clothing around the person's neck.

2 Tell the person to breathe through the mouth and to pinch the soft part of the nose, as shown below, firmly for 15 minutes. If bleeding has not stopped, continue pressing for a further 5 minutes.

3 If bleeding was caused by a blow to the nose, pinching it may only make the damage worse. Instead, place a piece of ice wrapped in a handkerchief over the nose.

4 Never be tempted to plug a bleeding nose with cotton-wool as the fibres may become detached and be inhaled into the lungs.

5 Ask the person to spit any blood into a bowl and to try not to swallow it as this may cause her to vomit later on.

6 Once bleeding has stopped, the person should avoid touching her nose for a period of 4 hours so that the clot is not disturbed.

7 A handkerchief or tissue held under the nose will absorb any spots of blood.

8 If bleeding has not stopped in 30 minutes or if it recurs again within 30 minutes, seek medical advice.

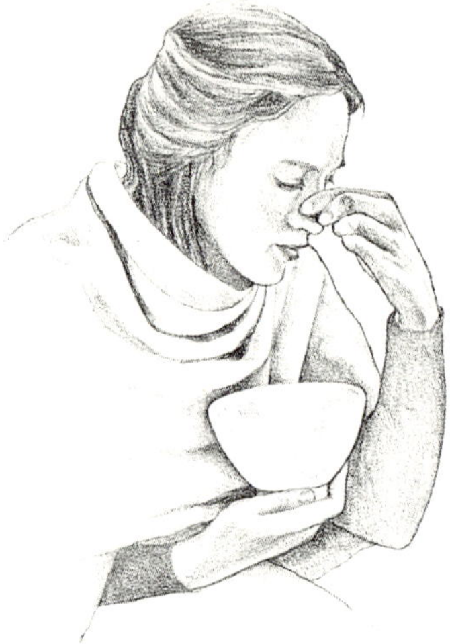

Bleeding from an ear

Bleeding from the ear can be the result of a fractured skull: if you suspect this to be the case, see page 199. Bleeding may also be caused by a ruptured eardrum which can result from an object being pushed into the ear, from a fall or dive into water, or from being too close to an explosion. The person may experience pain inside the ear as well as deafness. An injured eardrum, an acute infection of the ear or a scratch in the ear may also cause bleeding. You should seek medical advice.

1 Sit the person in a semi-upright position with his or her head to one side so that the blood can drain out of the injured ear.

2 Cover the ear with a sterile unmedicated dressing and keep it in place with a bandage. Do not plug the ear with cotton-wool as any attempt to stop the blood from draining out may cause pressure to build up in the ear.

3 Prevent or minimize shock (see page 200).

4 Seek medical advice.

Internal bleeding

Bleeding in the abdomen may be caused by disease or by crush or blow injuries. There may not be any outward sign of bleeding nor any pain but the person will be shocked and his or her abdomen will be firm and rigid.

1 Minimize or prevent shock (see page 200).

2 Ask the person to lie down with legs raised and head lowered and turned to one side in case of vomiting.

3 Cover with a blanket, placing a small table or chair over the abdomen to take the weight of the blanket off the stomach.

4 If unconscious, place in the recovery position (see page 198), unless a fracture is suspected.

5 Call for an ambulance or ask someone else to go and call for one: the injured person should only be moved by professionals.

OPEN WOUNDS

There are various types of open wound.
□ A graze is a superficial wound where several layers of skin have been scraped away.
□ A incised wound is caused by a knife or other sharp instrument and may bleed copiously.
□ A laceration is the result of skin being torn, for example by an animal, barbed wire or machinery. The jagged edges of this type of wound are more likely to become infected and may leave a scar.
□ A puncture wound is a deep wound which may be the result of an injury from a nail, needle, tooth or other sharp object. This type of wound carries a high risk of infection as germs may be carried deep into the wound. If somebody has a puncture wound which is deep and dirty, clean and dress it (see page 214) and find out from the doctor whether or not protection against tetanus is necessary.

1 Act quickly to stop any bleeding (see page 203).

2 Wash your hands thoroughly and, if the wound is dirty, clean with a sterile swab or gauze and apply a dressing.

3 If there is an object embedded in the wound, use a ring pad (see page 217).

Wounds to the eye

1 Do not put any drops in the eye without first consulting a doctor.

2 Place a large dressing over the eye and apply a bandage to keep it in place, until help arrives.

3 If one eye is badly injured or has an object embedded in it, bandage both eyes to prevent the wounded eye from automatically following the other eye when it moves. Make sure that no pressure is exerted on the embedded object and, if necessary, use a ring pad over the whole eye (see page 217).

4 Send for medical help.

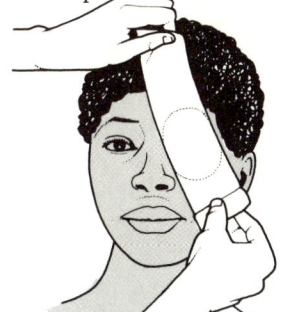

Wounds to the abdomen

Any deep wound in the abdomen (the area at the front between the chest and the hips) can be very serious because internal organs may be damaged and may even protrude from the abdomen.

1 Lay the person on her back with shoulders raised and head to one side in case of vomiting.

2 Place some cushions under the person's knees so that they are raised and bent; this will prevent the wound from gaping open. If the person is not placed in this position, the abdominal muscles will be stretched and the wound may be pulled open.

3 If the abdomen has been pierced by an object such as a knife which is still embedded, do not try to remove it as you may.cause more damage.

4 Dress the wound with a sterile dressing (see page 215).

5 If the contents of the stomach wall are protruding, *never* touch them or try to push them back in. Cover them with a damp sterile dressing or a damp clean cloth.

6 Prevent or minimize shock (see page 200) and send for medical help immediately.

7 If the person becomes unconscious, place something soft under the wound before placing her in the recovery position (see page 198), or just make sure that her head is in the open airway position (see page 194).

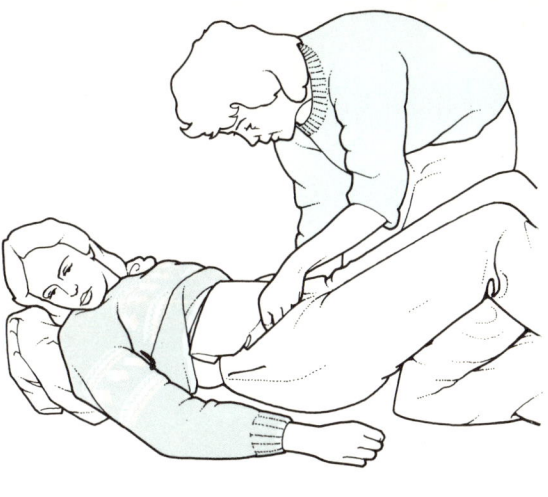

Wounds to the chest

As a result of a penetrating wound to the chest, one lung may be damaged and collapsed while the other may still be functioning and taking in oxygen. However, air may be sucked in through the open wound filling the chest cavity and preventing the sound lung from expanding as it should: this means that not enough oxygen is reaching the bloodstream.

1 Lay the person down with head and shoulders raised and body slightly inclined toward the injured side.

2 To prevent air from being sucked into the chest cavity, cover the wound with a firm, clean dressing (see page 214) and make an airtight seal with a plastic bag secured with adhesive tape.

3 If the person becomes unconscious, place in the recovery position (see page 198) with the injured part of the chest resting on a pad or cushion: this will make it easier for the sound lung to continue functioning.

4 Arrange for urgent removal to hospital.

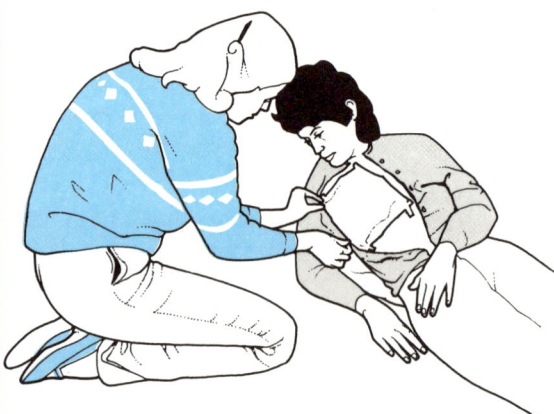

CRUSH INJURIES

This type of injury occurs when someone has been crushed under a heavy object. When released the crushed part may look quite normal but it may swell gradually and quite considerably over the next few hours owing to fluid being lost through the damaged walls of the blood vessels. This fluid loss can also lead to shock.

1 Prevent or minimize shock (see page 200) and arrange for the injured person to be taken to hospital as soon as possible.

2 Support the injured limb but leave uncovered, if possible. Do not allow the limb to get warm or the blood vessels will dilate causing more fluid to be lost. If you have to cover it, use a light dressing.

3 If the crush injury is minor and involves the hand or foot, place under cold running water or apply a cold compress (see page 100).

BLAST INJURIES

Blast injuries are caused by explosions. Various organs in the body may be damaged by the blast, including the lungs. Other possible injuries include broken bones, burns, wounds embedded with glass or other objects and damaged ear drums with possible bleeding from the ear. The person may also show signs of shock.

1 Lay the person down with head and shoulders raised and supported. If conscious, he or she may be more comfortable sitting half-upright. Loosen tight clothes and ask him or her to stay still.

2 Check to see what injuries have been sustained. Stop any bleeding (see page 203); dress any wounds (see page 214) or burns (see page 202) and immobilize broken bones (see page 207).

3 Check pulse and breathing rates every 10 minutes and assess the level of consciousness (see pages 86-87 and 199).

4 If the person becomes unconscious but is still breathing, place in the recovery position (see page 198). If breathing stops, start artificial respiration (see page 194). If heartbeat stops, start external chest compression (see page 196).

5 Get the person to hospital as soon as possible.

BROKEN BONES OR FRACTURES

Pain following a fracture may not be severe but will get worse on movement of the injured area. If the person is unable to move the limb or if it is swollen or deformed in any way when compared to the uninjured limb, the bone may well be broken. Feel very gently and carefully over the injured area; an irregular knobbliness will indicate where the fracture is and the surrounding area may be a red or bruised colour and tender to the touch. If in doubt, treat the injury as a fracture until a doctor tells you otherwise; it is difficult to tell if a bone is fractured without the aid of an X-ray.

1 Stop any bleeding. If a bone is protruding from the skin, control any bleeding by indirect pressure (see page 203).

2 Cover any open wound with a dressing (see page 214). Use a ring pad if the bone is protruding (see page 217).

3 If necessary, immobilize the broken bone as described here. Never move a fractured limb unless necessary.

4 In the case of all fractures, bear in mind that there may be internal bleeding.

5 Seek medical advice.

Tying a reef knot
Pass the right-hand end over the left end and then the left over the right so that a knot is formed which will remain firmly in position when pressure is applied.

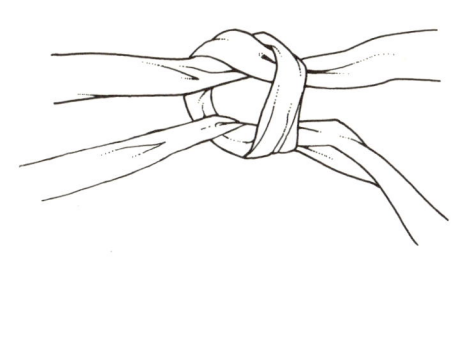

How to immobilize a broken bone

Immobilizing the joints above and below a broken bone will prevent movement of the fracture and at the same time help to reduce pain and lessen the risk of further complications. Complications can result if a jagged bone is moved as it may cause further tissue damage and even pierce through a nerve or blood vessel or through the outer skin.

Immobilize a broken bone only if you are waiting for an ambulance to arrive and it is likely to be delayed in getting to you, or if the injury does not warrant an ambulance – as in the case of a broken ankle, arm, hand, wrist or collar bone – and you are taking the injured person to hospital yourself.

1 Tie the injured part of the person's body to an uninjured part of his body, using bandages, handkerchiefs, scarves or any other suitable material.

2 A pad of any soft material between the limb and the part of the body acting as a splint helps to make the person more comfortable.

3 Use wide bandages or pieces of material and bandage around the limbs very carefully, taking care not to move them. The bandaging should be firm but not too tight and tied with a reef knot on the side which is not injured. Do not bandage directly over the site of a broken bone.

4 Check the colour of the fingers or toes: if they look blue, your bandaging is too tight.

5 An alternative to using the person's body as a splint is to use anything that is rigid and long and wide enough to prevent movement, such as the handle of a broom, a rolled-up newspaper or a piece of wood. Then secure as above.

6 Reassure and prevent or minimize shock (see page 200).

7 Seek medical advice.

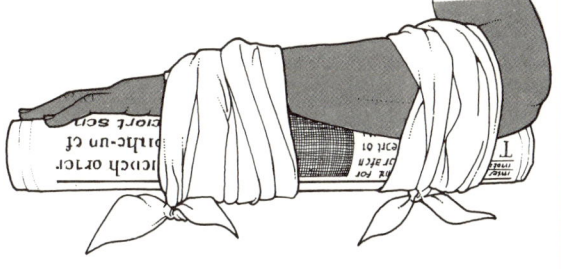

A broken lower jaw

1 Place a pad under the broken jaw and hold it in place with a bandage tied over the head.

2 Make sure that the person's airway is not blocked.

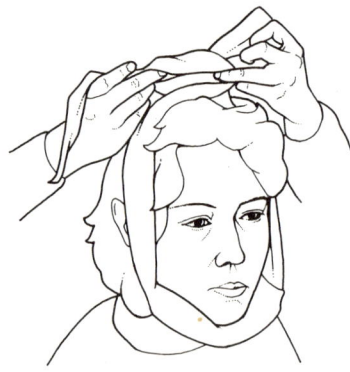

A broken upper jaw and cheek bone

There is no need to immobilize this type of fracture. Just hold a cold compress over the site (see page 100).

A fractured skull

See under head injuries, page 199.

A broken upper arm or forearm

1 Place a soft pad under the injured arm.

2 Move the forearm carefully across the chest until the hand reaches the opposite armpit or is as near as is comfortable. Do not move the arm if you suspect that the elbow is broken.

3 To support the arm pin the sleeve of the injured arm to the person's clothing or use a sling (see page 217). If the elbow is painful, you may have to immobilize the limb in the position in which you found it.

A broken collar bone, wrist or hand

1 Place soft pads under the injured person's armpit on the side of the fractured collarbone.

2 Lay the arm gently across the chest so that the person's fingertips are almost resting on the opposite shoulder.

3 Support the arm in this position with a sling (see page 217) or by pinning the person's sleeve to his or her clothing.

A broken pelvis

Apart from feeling pain and tenderness in the area of the hips, the injured person may also feel the need to pass water if the fracture is a serious one. Ask the injured person not to pass water if at all possible until he or she has been seen by a doctor. If he or she does have to pass urine, it may be bloodstained. If there is going to be a long wait for the ambulance or if the person has to be moved, you will need to immobilize the pelvis.

1 Place two wide bandages around the pelvis, one overlapping the other.

2 Put some padding between the person's legs and do a figure of eight bandage around the ankles and feet (see page 216), followed by a further bandage around the knees.

3 Raise the injured person's knees slightly, if this feels more comfortable.

A broken hip, thigh or leg

If the thigh bone is broken, the affected leg may appear shorter than the other. If the hip or neck of the thigh bone is broken the foot may be turned outward. If the shin bone is broken, the bone may come through the skin, in which case a ring pad (see page 217) and clean, preferably sterile, dressing should be applied and any bleeding stopped by indirect pressure (see page 203).

1 Bring the undamaged leg alongside the fractured leg and place padding in between the legs.

2 Secure the padding by bandaging the feet and ankles and then the knees together. One bandage should be placed just below the fractured site and the other one just above.

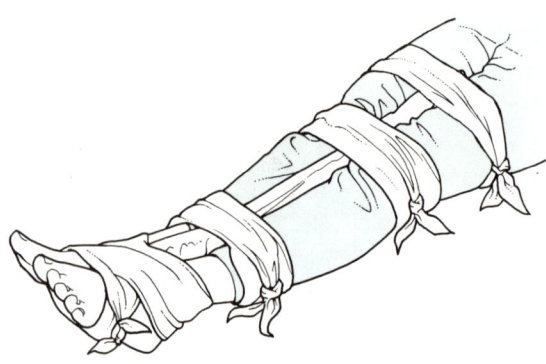

A broken foot

1 Protect the foot with a folded blanket or cloth, or a small splint, such as a hard-backed book, on the sole of the foot. Place padding between the foot and splint, if used.

2 Bandage the foot and ankle in a figure of eight (see page 216), starting and finishing at the base of the foot. Make sure that the bandage is tied on the opposite side from the fracture.

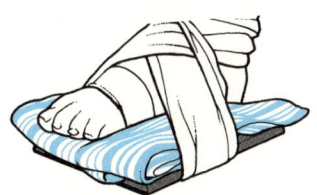

Broken ribs

There may be sharp pain over the site of the broken ribs which is made worse by breathing or coughing. The arm on the injured side should be supported in a sling (see page 217).

A broken back

Damage to the cord of nerves which runs through the spine can lead to total loss of power and sensation in all parts of the body below the injured area. There may even be paralysis. Never move someone with a suspected broken back as if you move them incorrectly, paralysis may result.

You should suspect a broken back if the person complains of severe pain in the back and feels 'cut in half', or if he or she is unable to move wrists, ankles, fingers or toes or cannot feel you touching his or her arms or legs.

Place some rolled-up clothing or blankets along both sides of the person's body to provide support and cover with a blanket.

A broken neck

You should suspect a fracture of the neck if the person has sustained a head injury; is complaining of pain in the neck followed by pain in the arms; has a sensation of tingling in the arms or legs or is unable to move them at all.

A collar is necessary to support the neck so that it cannot be moved in any direction. If you are on your own, do not attempt to put on a collar; just hold the injured person's head still until professional help arrives and ask him or her not to move. If there is someone who can help you, hold the injured person's head while your helper puts a collar on. Do not attempt to move the injured person.

1 Fold a newspaper to a width of about 10 cm (4 in).

2 Wrap it in a triangular bandage or the leg of an old pair of stockings or tights.

3 Hold the person's head and get your helper to wrap the collar carefully around the fractured neck, taking care to tie it at the front.

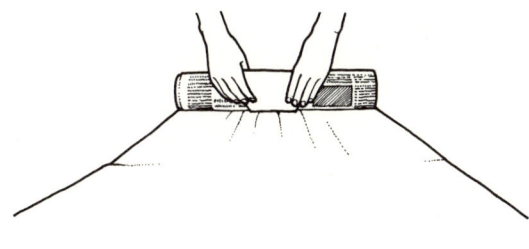

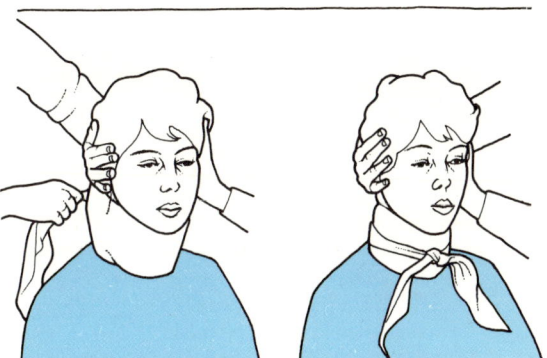

DISLOCATIONS

Dislocations occur when ligaments are torn and a bone is pulled out of its normal position. The pain is usually severe at or near the dislocation and the person may not be able to move the joint. The joint may appear deformed and there is usually swelling and later bruising over the surrounding area. A dislocation can look very like a fracture, so if in doubt treat as a fracture (see page 207). Do not make any attempt to put the joint back into position, and do not move it.

1 Support the joint with pillows or cushions or a sling (see page 217) and immobilize, if necessary (see page 207).

2 Prevent or minimize shock (see page 200) and seek medical advice.

SPRAINS

A sprain is caused by stretching and tearing of the ligaments around the joint as the result of a sudden wrench. There will be pain and tenderness around the joint followed by swelling and bruising. A sprain can look very like a fracture, so if in doubt treat as a fracture (see page 207).

1 Ask the injured person to sit or lie down and raise the injured limb.

2 Carefully remove any clothes and put on a cold compress (see page 100). Place a thick layer of padding around the joint and keep in place with a crepe bandage (see pages 216-217). If the foot is sprained, do not remove the person's shoes but give extra support by applying a figure of eight bandage over the footwear (see page 217).

3 Seek medical advice.

SUNBURN

If unprotected skin is over-exposed to the sun, this may produce redness, itching and tenderness. In severe cases of sunburn, the skin may become bright red, blistered and very painful.
☐ In cases of mild sunburn, cool the person's skin by sponging it down with cold water.
☐ In more severe cases, it is advisable to seek medical advice.

HEAT EXHAUSTION

This condition develops slowly and is caused by loss of water and salt from the body in the form of sweat as a result of intense physical activity in a hot environment. Someone who is suffering from water depletion will be thirsty and may become dehydrated. He or she should be given plenty of fluids in any available form, except alcohol. Someone who is suffering from salt depletion or a combination of salt and water depletion will experience the following symptoms: weakness, headaches, vomiting, cramps in the legs and abdomen and low blood pressure causing faintness on standing. Any sudden movement may lead to the person fainting.

1 Let the person lie down in a cool place and give salt in large amounts of water or any other fluid available, except alcohol.

2 If the person becomes unconscious, place in the recovery position (see page 198) and do not attempt to give fluids.

3 Seek medical advice.

HEAT STROKE

This condition may develop fairly rapidly when the body can no longer regulate its own temperature by sweating due to the extreme heat of the surrounding atmosphere. It can develop in anyone who is exposed to heat and high humidity for too long. Symptoms of heat stroke include feelings of dizziness, restlessness, irritability and confusion; a hot, dry, flushed skin; over-breathing; a full and bounding pulse and a raised temperature of up to 40°c (104°F). The person may become unconscious.

1 Seek medical advice as quickly as possible.

2 Move the person into a cool place and take off most or all of his or her clothes.

3 If conscious, sit in a semi-upright position; if unconscious but breathing, place in the recovery position (see page 198).

4 Give tepid sponging (see page 101) to reduce the temperature gradually, allowing the water to evaporate on the skin. Alternatively, place the person in a cool or tepid bath and fan him or her. Never use ice as this will lower the body temperature too fast.

5 Aim to reduce body temperature to about 38°c (101°F).

6 Take and record the temperature every few minutes.

FAINTING

Someone may feel faint owing to lack of food, tiredness or as a nervous or emotional reaction to bad news, a dreadful sight or pain. Long periods of sitting or standing in a hot, stuffy atmosphere can also lead to fainting. Someone who has fainted will have pale, cold, clammy skin, shallow breathing and a weak, slow pulse which will soon increase.

1 If someone feels faint, give him or her room to breathe and plenty of fresh air.

2 Sit the person down with his or her head between the knees to increase the flow of blood to the head. Loosen any tight clothing.

3 When the person's colour returns, let him or her sit upright again. Do not give anything by mouth until he or she is fully conscious: then give sips of water. Do not give alcohol.

4 Should the person actually faint, lay him or her down and raise his or her legs to drain the blood back to the heart.

5 The person will quickly recover but should only resume normal activity after a few minutes rest in a chair.

OBJECT IN THE EAR

1 Do not try to remove the object as you may push it in further.

2 Turn the person's head to the affected side to see if the object drops out.

3 If it does not drop out, seek medical advice.

OBJECT IN THE NOSE

1 Do not try to remove the object as you may only push it further up, and it may be inhaled into the lungs.

2 Try blocking the unobstructed nostril and breathing out through the obstructed nostril. If this does not work, ask the person to continue breathing through his or her mouth and seek medical advice.

OBJECT IN THE EYE

1 If the object is on the eye or is sharp, do not try to remove it; cover both eyes to prevent the damaged eye moving and seek medical advice.

2 If the object is loose under the lower lid, pull down the lid and, if you can see the object, try to remove it with the moistened corner of a soft handkerchief or a wisp of cotton-wool.

3 If the object is under the upper lid, ask the person to look down and then pull the upper lid down over the lower lid to remove the object.

4 If the pain continues, cover the eye with a dry dressing (see page 214) and seek medical advice.

5 If corrosives are splashed into the eye, wash the chemical out quickly with cold water, taking care not to wash it into the other eye. Tilt the person's head down on the affected side and wash out the affected eye so that the water runs away from the other eye. If running water is not available, ask the person to sit or lie down and squeeze a wet cloth over the injured eye so that water pours from the inner corner of the eye outward.

6 Cover the eye with a clean cloth and seek medical advice as to what to do next.

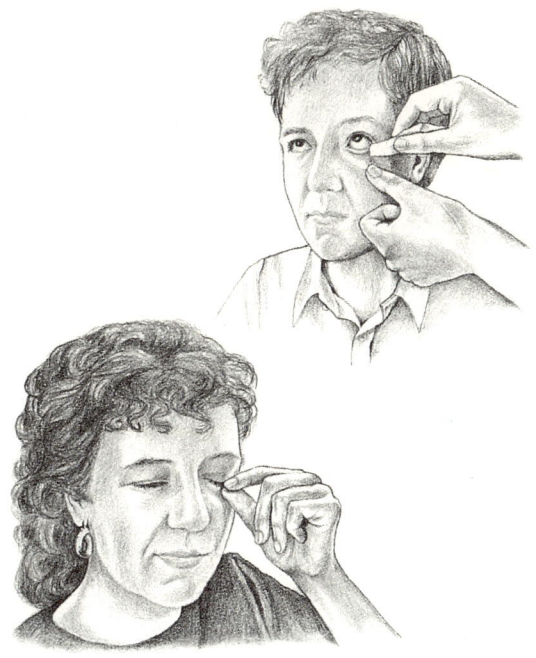

BITES OR STINGS

Animals harbour all sorts of germs in their mouths and bites from their sharp teeth may inject these germs deep into the tissues of the body. If someone is stung in the mouth, tongue or throat, seek medical advice immediately and be prepared to resuscitate the person if necessary (see pages 194–197). If the person is conscious and there is a lot of swelling in the mouth, give him or her ice to suck. If the person is unconscious, place in the recovery position (see page 198). Use a cold compress to reduce swelling and irritation around the eyes (see page 100).

Animal bites

1 Stop the bleeding (see page 203) and clean and dress the wound (see page 214).

2 Seek medical advice in case an anti-tetanus injection is needed.

Insect bites and stings

1 If the sting is still in the skin, remove it with clean fingers or tweezers. Do not attempt to squeeze or force it out.

2 Cold water or an ice pack (see page 100) will help to reduce any irritation.

3 If the sting becomes more painful over the next few days, seek medical advice.

Some people are highly sensitive to stings and may collapse or become very ill. If possible, remove the sting with tweezers or clean fingers but do not force or squeeze it. Minimize shock and seek medical advice immediately or take the person straight to hospital.

Snake bites

1 Attempt to identify the snake so that the correct antidote can be given if necessary. If possible, kill it and take it to the hospital for identification.

2 Lay the person down and ask him or her to keep still: this will help to prevent the spread of poison.

3 Immobilize the bitten part as you would a fractured bone (see page 207) to prevent the spread of poison, and cover with a clean, sterile dressing (see page 214).

4 Minimize or prevent shock (see page 200) and get the person to a hospital as quickly as possible.

EMERGENCY CHILDBIRTH

Women sometimes go into advanced labour unexpectedly fast. If you are faced with such a situation, there is no need to be frightened: giving birth is a natural process and is usually straightforward.

The first stage of labour, during which the cervix dilates, normally takes about 10 hours, or longer for a first baby, so you should have ample time to get the pregnant woman to hospital. If, however, the mother feels the urge to push down with each contraction, she is probably in second-stage labour, during which the baby is pushed out of the uterus, down the birth canal and out through the vagina. The second stage of labour normally lasts about an hour, but may be faster, especially in the case of a second or subsequent birth.

If you find yourself in a situation in which you have to deliver the baby without medical assistance, try to find someone else who can assist at the birth; if this is not possible, you can still manage alone.

Delivering a baby

1 Place some waterproof sheeting, or layers of newspaper covered with sheeting, over the bed, floor or any flat surface.

2 Get the pregnant woman to lie on the sheeting on her back or side, whichever is the most comfortable.

3 Give yourself 4 minutes in which to wash your hands and nails thoroughly. Do not dry them on a towel or touch anything other than the baby. If your hands become contaminated, wash them again.

4 Ask the mother to spread her legs apart as the contractions become stronger so that you can see the baby's head emerging.

5 When the head appears, ask the mother to stop pushing so that the baby does not come out too fast. To prevent the baby from shooting out, place your cupped hands over his head.

6 Once the head is out, do not interfere, just hold the baby's head. If you can see or feel that the cord is around the baby's neck, act quickly and ease it gently over the baby's head before it tightens with the next contraction. Ask the mother not to push while you do this.

7 Gently support the baby's head, until the next contraction pushes his shoulders out.

8 Hold the baby firmly but gently under the armpits and lift him onto the mother's abdomen, with his head down so that any mucus can drain out of his mouth and nose. Take great care not to let the baby slip or to pull on or stretch the cord. Cover the baby with a warm blanket, towel or shawl. There is no need to tie or cut the cord at this stage – just be careful not to pull on it.

The newborn baby
The baby will start by making gasping noises and crying as he or she begins to breathe. Once he or she is breathing, clear out his or her mouth and wipe away any fluid with a clean soft cloth. If the baby does not start crying or breathing, the airway may be blocked with mucus: clear the airway with your little finger covered with a dry cloth. If the baby is still not breathing, start artificial respiration immediately.

Artificial respiration and chest compression on a baby
Act quickly as you only have 4 minutes before the brain is damaged by lack of oxygen.

1 Lay the baby on his back or hold him in your arms so that his head is tilted back to open the airway (see page 194). Check that the mouth is clear.

2 Cover the baby's mouth and nose with your mouth and blow gently to inflate the chest at the rate of 20 breaths a minute.

3 Watch the baby's chest rise as you blow in and fall as you stop to take another breath. Give the first four inflations rapidly, then check for the heartbeat by feeling the pulse in the baby's neck or in the soft part on top of his head (fontanelle). The baby's colour will be pink if the heart is beating.

4 If the heart is beating, continue artificial respiration. If you cannot feel the pulse and the baby is grey and cold with pale lips, his heart has stopped beating: start external chest compresion immediately.

5 Lay the baby on a firm surface so that his head is tilted in the open airway position (see page 194).

6 Use two fingers of one hand to compress the chest very gently to a depth of 1.5 to 2.5 cm (0.5 to 1 in).

7 If you are on your own, give 15 compressions to two inflations at the rate of 100 compressions per minute. If there are two of you, alternate, with five compressions to one inflation at the rate of 100 compressions per minute.

8 Continue to check the pulse every 2 minutes. Once you can feel the pulse, stop the chest compression but continue the artificial respiration until the baby is breathing again.

9 Once the baby is breathing, place in the recovery position (see page 198).

10 Observe the baby closely and once you are satisfied that the baby is breathing regularly, wrap in a towel and give to the mother. Make sure both the mother and baby are covered and warm.

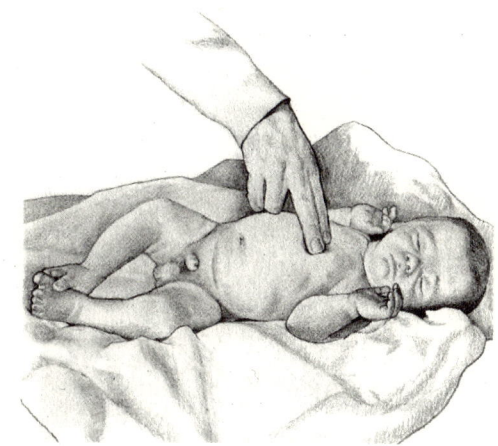

The third stage
This stage may last from 5 to 25 minutes as the afterbirth or placenta is expelled by the mother after a few further contractions. You can help the expulsion of the afterbirth by massaging the mother's lower abdomen above the pubic bone; this encourages the womb to contract. There is no need for the cord to be tied or cut at this stage.

1 Keep the placenta and place it in a plastic bag.

2 If there is a lot of bleeding after the delivery, raise the foot of the bed and massage as above. This will help to heal any bleeding areas.

In most cases it will do no harm to leave the baby attached to the cord until medical help has arrived. The mother may let the baby suckle at her breast while still attached to the cord.

DRESSINGS

Dressings are used to prevent a wound becoming infected, to control bleeding, to absorb any discharge and to protect against further injury. There are three principal kinds: adhesive dressings or plasters, gauze dressings and sterile unmedicated dressings.

Points to observe when cleaning and dressing a wound

☐ Use a dressing which is large enough to overlap the wound by 2.5 cm (1 in) all the way round.
☐ Never touch a wound with your fingers and avoid touching any part of the clean or sterile dressing which is to cover the wound.
☐ Never talk or cough over a wound or dressing.
☐ When swabbing a wound, use a piece of cotton-wool or sterile gauze once only and in one direction only.
☐ Use cotton-wool for swabbing a wound and as an absorbent, protective padding over gauze and non-adhesive dressings to absorb further bleeding or discharge, but never place directly over a wound as the wool fibres detach fairly easily and will become embedded in the wound, causing infection.
☐ Always place a dressing directly over a wound. Do not slide it into position, as any contact with the unclean area surrounding the wound may cause the wound to become infected.
☐ If the dressing slips off the wound before you are able to secure it with a bandage or adhesive tape, dispose of the contaminated dressing and start again with a clean dressing.
☐ If you are dressing the wound of someone who is in bed, make sure that at least an hour has passed since making the bed or cleaning the room so that any dust has had time to settle.

Cleaning a wound and changing a dressing

Collect together
● Six cotton-wool balls (or as many as you need to clean the wound and surrounding area)
● Small bowl of warm water
● Small bowl of soapy water or antiseptic in water as a cleaning solution
● Paper or plastic bag for disposal of used dressing materials
● Clean towel
● Dressing to be applied to the wound
● Strips of adhesive tape or bandage
● Pair of scissors
● Disposable gloves

1 Explain clearly to the sick person what you are going to do.

2 Clean the area on which you are going to place the equipment.

3 Wash and dry your hands.

4 Collect together all the necessary equipment. Make sure that the solution for cleaning the wound is made up correctly.

5 Prepare the sick person for the dressing by removing any clothes which are in the way; make sure he or she is warm and comfortable. Loosen the old strapping or remove the old bandage and, if there is already a dressing in position, loosen the edges.

6 Place a towel over the sick person's clothes, or bedclothes, to prevent them from becoming wet or soiled.

7 Wash and dry your hands, put on disposable gloves and remove the soiled dressing by holding an edge or corner with your fingertips. If the dressing is stuck, cover with a wet piece of cotton-wool and soak off gently.

8 Soak a cotton-wool ball in cleaning solution, squeeze it out, and, holding it between your fingers, swab the wound with one downward movement. Dispose of the cotton-wool ball into a paper or plastic bag.

9 Repeat this step with another cotton-wool ball soaked in cleaning solution, and then twice more with plain water, using a new cotton-wool ball each time. Finally, swab the wound with a dry cotton-wool ball.

10 Cover the wound with a dressing, an adhesive dressing and, if necessary, a bandage secured with strips of adhesive tape. Dressings must be secure but never too tight.

11 Replace any clothes or bedclothes and make sure the sick person is comfortable. Clear away, clean or dispose of any used equipment and wash and dry your hands.

Applying an adhesive dressing

Adhesive dressings are very useful for dressing small wounds with only slight bleeding. Available in a variety of shapes and sizes, they consist of a gauze or cellulose pad with an adhesive backing and are supplied in sterile packs. If the sick person is allergic to adhesive tape or has to have a dressing changed frequently, special strips of adhesive paper (Micropore) may be more suitable and can be bought from your local chemist.

Applying an adhesive dressing in the following way will prevent the wound becoming infected.

1 Wash and dry your hands.

2 Remove the outer wrapping and hold the dressing, gauze side downward, by the protective strips.

3 Peel back the protective strips without completely removing them, taking care not to touch the gauze pad.

4 Lay the dressing pad over the wound. Carefully remove the protective strips and press down the edges firmly.

To remove an adhesive dressing, pull off quickly from one corner, following the way the hair grows.

Applying a sterile unmedicated dressing

Sterile unmedicated dressings are made up of several layers of gauze covered with a pad of cotton-wool attached to a roller bandage. They are ideal for dressing arm and leg wounds. They can be bought from a local chemist and come in sealed packs which ensure that the dressing is completely sterile. If, on removal of the outer wrapping, the seal is broken, the dressing is no longer sterile and must not be used. Apply the dressing in the following way to prevent the wound becoming infected and to ensure that the dressing remains in position.

1 Remove the outer wrapping and, holding both ends of the bandage, place the dressing directly over the wound, with gauze side downward.

2 Hold the dressing in position with one hand, and with the other, wind the rolled-up bandage over the dressing and round the limb in order to secure the dressing. You will need to hold the end of the bandage in position along with the dressing to prevent it slipping.

3 Finally, tie the two ends together.

Applying a gauze dressing

This type of dressing can be adapted for use anywhere on the body and consists of an absorbent type of cotton-wool with a wide mesh which allows air through to promote healing. Packets of gauze can be obtained from any chemist and are generally clean but not sterile; they can also be obtained in sterile packets. Pads of gauze can be bought from your local chemist but should be used only when a light dressing is required, or when no sterile dressings are available. Apply a gauze dressing in the following way to ensure that it is effective.

1 Remove the outer wrapping and, holding the gauze square by the edges, place it directly over the wound (A).

2 Cover with more gauze, if necessary. If there is still bleeding or a discharge, cover with a further layer or two of cotton-wool and finally another gauze dressing (B).

3 Use a couple of strips of adhesive tape to secure the dressing. Do not use too much tape as it will have to be removed when the dressing needs changing (C).

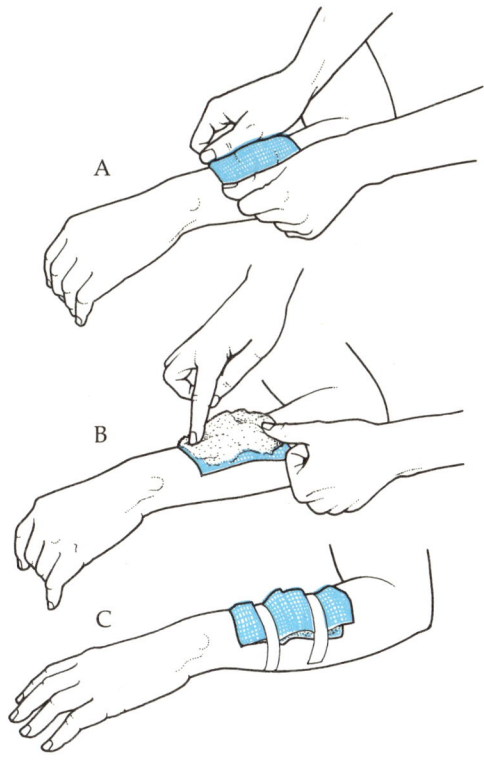

BANDAGES

Bandages are made of cotton, calico, elastic net or crepe and come in various widths. The size you need depends on the area to be bandaged. They are used to keep dressings in position, to support and prevent movement of an injured limb or joint and to prevent swelling.

Points to observe when applying bandages
☐ The sick person should be sitting or lying down.
☐ Make sure the limb is well supported in the position in which it is to be bandaged.
☐ The bandage should be tight enough to hold the dressing in position or to immobilize the limb, but not so tight as to restrict circulation.
☐ Fingers and toes should be left exposed as their colour will indicate whether or not the bandage is too tight. If the bandages are too tight, the sick person's fingers or toenails will start to go blue and he or she may complain of tingling or numbness or be unable to move his or her fingers or toes.
☐ Tie the bandage on the opposite side of the body from a break, fracture or wound.
☐ If the bandage is being used to control bleeding, tie the knot over the dressing covering the bleeding point to apply direct pressure.

Types of bandages
The two principal types of bandage most commonly in use are the roller and triangular bandages.

Roller bandages are made of cotton, gauze or linen and are usually sold in 5 m (5 yd) rolls. Stretchy crepe roller bandages are extremely useful as they stretch to fit the injured limb exactly and thereby ensure that the dressing is held firmly in place.

When applying a roller bandage, work from the inner side outward, holding the head, or roll, uppermost. Make a fixing turn to hold the bandage in place and then work from below the injury upward. Bandage in such a way that each new layer covers two thirds of the previous layer.

Triangular bandages are usually made of linen or calico and can be improvized by using a piece of linen or calico not less than 1 m (1 yd) square and cutting it in half diagonally, or simply folding it in half diagonally.

To make a broad bandage, fold the tip of the triangle over to the base and fold again. To make a narrow bandage, fold as for a broad bandage and then fold again.

Bandaging a joint
The figure of eight style of bandaging described below can be used to bandage and to apply pressure over an extended joint or to bandage a leg, foot, hand or arm where movement is required.

1 Using a roller bandage, start off with a single fixing turn below the joint.

2 Take the bandage up around the front of the limb, down round behind the limb at the same level, then across the front of the limb and back over the first turn as in a figure of eight.

3 Repeat this figure of eight several times until the whole joint is covered.

4 Finish by making one straight turn above the wound and fasten with a safety pin.

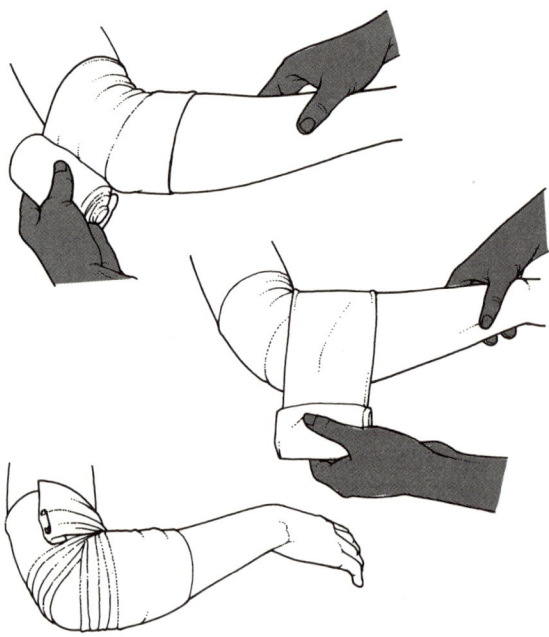

A simpler style of bandaging can be used to hold a dressing in position over a joint while applying very little pressure. Make two straight turns around the joint, then pass one turn above and one below the joint – covering half of each previous turn as you bandage.

Bandaging fingers
To bandage fingers correctly takes time and practice. You may find it easier to use Tubegauz, which you can buy from your local chemist as a 'finger' pack with instructions enclosed.

Bandaging a hand

1 Using a triangular bandage, place the person's hand palm upward so that the wrist is level with the base of the triangle.

2 Fold the tip of the triangle over the person's hand so that it touches the base of the triangle.

3 Take hold of both of the outer ends of the bandage and fold them round the hand until it is securely bandaged.

4 Tie off over the back of the wrist with the point of the triangle protruding.

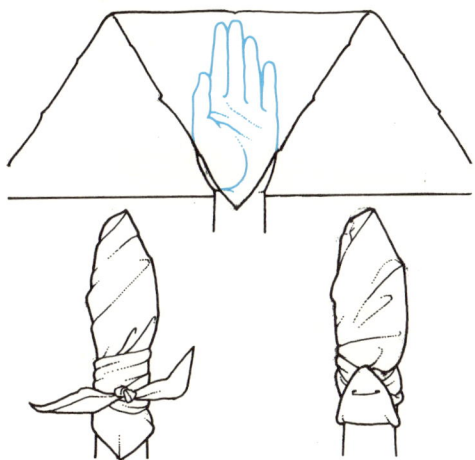

Use of a ring pad

A ring pad is used to help reduce pain and to prevent the wound becoming infected when an object has become embedded in part of the body. A piece of gauze is placed over the embedded object, followed by a ring pad and then a bandage; this ensures that the wound is protected without any pressure being exerted on the embedded object. Simply bandaging over the object will only push it in further and cause more damage; attempts to remove it may also do more harm than good.

A ring pad can be improvised by using either a narrow roller bandage, or a triangular bandage which has been folded to make a narrow bandage.

Make a circle large enough to surround the wound and wind the rest of the bandage round the circle until it is well padded. Tuck in the end.

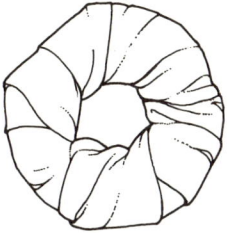

Slings

Slings are normally made from triangular bandages. If the injured person is in need of an arm sling, the arm should be placed across the chest so that the wrist and hand are slightly higher than the elbow.

1 With the point toward the elbow of the injured side, pass one end of the bandage between the person's chest and injured forearm taking the end up toward the shoulder.

2 Bring the lower end of the bandage up over the injured arm and tie off in the hollow above the collar bone.

3 Bring the tip of the triangle over the elbow and pin it securely to the front of the sling.

If the injured person needs the hand and forearm raised, so that the hand is practically at the height of the shoulder, the loose ends of the sling are tied in a knot just above the collar bone of the uninjured arm.

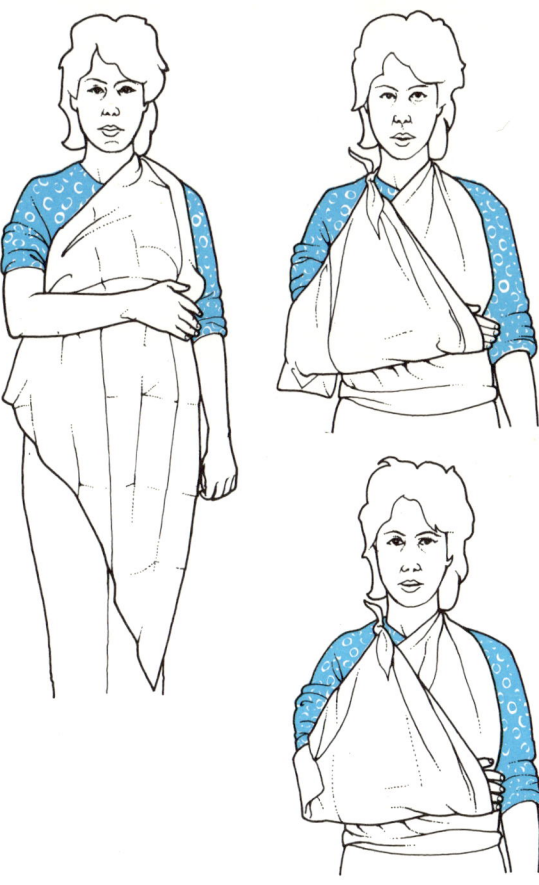

Where to Find Help

In the UK, medical and social services are provided by the Department of Health and Social Security (DHSS) in an attempt to ensure that the sick, the elderly and the handicapped are adequately cared for in their own homes, and also to facilitate the task of those who care for them. The health services are there to deal with physical and emotional problems arising from illness, handicap or disability as well as providing information on general health care, while the social services are responsible for the care and welfare of people, particularly where there are difficult home circumstances.

COMMUNITY HEALTH SERVICES

Your general practitioner (GP) will be able to tell you which services are available in your area and whether you are entitled to any. If you need help from any of the following people, he can arrange for you to receive it.

□ A district nurse will call regularly at the sick person's home to perform basic nursing procedures.

□ A health visitor (a qualified nurse specializing in the care of babies and pre-school children) will visit mothers with young babies at regular intervals after the birth, as well as the elderly in need at home. With children, she concentrates on preventive care, ensuring that the mother is well-informed in the handling and care of young children. She is also there to answer any queries and to respond to any complaints or demands the sick person may want to make to her.

□ A community midwife will visit mothers with young babies to give nursing care and any information the mother may require on the handling and care of young babies.

□ A physiotherapist will rehabilitate a patient by aiding healing and recovery of an injured or diseased part of the body with the aim of restoring it to its previous function.

□ An occupational therapist will help with the invalid's rehabilitation by suggesting alterations to the home or useful equipment which may help to make life easier for him or her. An occupational therapist has an important role to play in the life of the elderly and the handicapped.

□ A community psychiatric nurse will give advice and support to those suffering from psychiatric problems.

□ A speech therapist will help children with speech problems, and adults who have developed speech difficulties as a result of a stroke or other illness.

□ A chiropodist will call at the home of an elderly or disabled person to ensure that his or her feet are properly cared for.

□ A dentist and optician will pay regular visits if the person is unable to leave his or her home.

□ Some areas also provide geriatric visitors: these are trained nurses specializing in the care of the elderly.

SOCIAL SERVICES

A social worker will visit families and individuals with personal or social problems to give support and advice and to help them make good use of existing services. Outlined below are some of the principal services available.

Services for children

There are various services available to assist parents in the care and upbringing of their children. Parents are however unlikely to make use of the full extent of medical and educational services available unless their child is suffering from a serious handicap or a prolonged physical or mental illness.

□ An educational welfare officer from the Department of Education and Science (DES) may visit your home if your child is likely to be away from school over a long period. He or she is primarily responsible for monitoring the child's attendance at school.

□ A social worker may visit your home if your child has a particular problem which requires specialist help, if relations between you and your child are difficult or if you as parents require financial assistance in any way. He or she may also put you in touch with the Education Department, should your child require specialist educational provision.

Services for the elderly

An elderly person who is incapacitated in any way by age, infirmity or illness will have his or her situation assessed by the doctor, who will then recommend that appropriate services be made available to him or her. Your local Citizens Advice Bureau or Social Services Department can advise you as to what financial help is available and whether you are likely to receive extra assistance in the form of help with heating, travel, outings or holidays. If the elderly person is not satisfied with the service obtained from government sources, he or she should contact the local Citizens Advice Bureau and ask for the address or telephone number of any local voluntary schemes. In most areas the Old People's Welfare Committee – co-ordinating the work of a number of voluntary bodies – will give information on recreational and other services for the elderly. The following services may also be available.

☐ A home help who will assist the elderly person with housework and essential shopping. A charge is made for this service based on what the elderly person can afford.

☐ Meals-on-wheels, a service that brings hot meals to the elderly in their homes. A small charge is made for this service.

☐ 'Good neighbour' schemes which arrange for people from the community to visit the elderly on a regular basis to help with shopping, light household chores, gardening, etc.

☐ Home care programmes which provide a home help, meals and home nursing when an elderly person is first discharged from hospital following an illness or operation.

☐ Peripatetic services – available in some areas – provide round-the-clock nursing assistance in emergency situations. This service is only made available in cases of extreme need where the person is not receiving the care he or she requires. The emergency nursing care is provided for a maximum period of 3 weeks.

☐ Day or night sitters – available in only a few areas – to ensure that the caregiver has a chance to get out or just to get some rest.

☐ Visits from a social worker to discuss any particular problem the elderly person may have and to ensure that he or she is receiving the full benefit of any services to which he or she is entitled.

☐ Laundry service for those caring for someone who is incontinent, or free supply of incontinence pads – available in some areas only.

☐ Geriatric day centres where the elderly can spend the day. A meal is provided and various activities, such as handicrafts, are encouraged.

☐ Organized visits to clubs for the elderly and to handicraft centres.

Services for the disabled

The following services or special facilities are available for people suffering from blindness, deafness with or without speech, all types of physical handicap, cerebral palsy or epilepsy. The doctor will assess the extent of the person's handicap and decide which services he or she is entitled to. Dial UK (Disablement Information Advice Line) offers a free advisory service on what facilities exist within the health service and what your entitlements are (see page 220). The following services may also be available.

☐ Practical assistance in the home in the form of home helps and meals-on-wheels.

☐ Help with the installation and payment of the rental of a telephone and any special equipment necessary.

☐ Assistance in obtaining a television, radio, books or other recreational facilities.

☐ Organized visits or transport to parks, sports centres and club activities.

☐ Assistance in using educational facilities.

☐ Travelling facilities for individuals and groups.

☐ Financial and other assistance with holidays.

☐ Visits from social workers to discuss any particular problems.

Help with running a household

If someone is unable to look after the home because of age, illness or confinement, he or she may be entitled to assistance from a home help, whose duties include cleaning, preparing and cooking meals, shopping, lighting fires and looking after children. He or she may also be entitled to help through the good neighbour scheme or to help from day or night sitters in the few areas where this service exists.

Help with acquiring equipment

Medical loan services are run by the Red Cross and the local District Health Authority, supplying equipment for the bedridden and handicapped, including backrests, commodes, bedpans, urinals etc. Equipment is not usually loaned over long periods but only to cover an emergency or to provide temporary help when a disabled person comes to stay. If you require further information, your local doctor, district nurse or occupational therapist may be able to help you further.

If you are interested in buying equipment, there are many firms which manufacture equipment especially designed for use by the handicapped in their homes. The Disabled Living Foundation (see page 220) will be able to recommend reliable firms to buy from. Always check that any equipment you buy is safe and in working order and if it is not exactly what you want, send it straight back.

Resources

The support groups listed below deal with specific illnesses, handicaps or disabilities and can provide valuable advice and assistance for the sufferer and those involved in caring for him or her. They will be able to tell you where you can go for specialist help or more information on your particular problem and may also put you in touch with a local contact.

Allergy
Action Against Allergy
43 The Downs
London SW20 8HG
01.947.5082

Arthritis
The Arthritis and
Rheumatism Council
41 Eagle Street
London WC1R 4AR
01.405.8572

Asthma
Asthma Society and
Friends of the Asthma
Research Council
St Thomas' Hospital
Lambeth Palace Road
London SE1 7EH
01.928.3099

Autistic children
National Society for
Autistic Children
276 Willesden Lane
London NW2
01.451.3844

Back pain
Back Pain Association
31-33 Park Road
Teddington
Middlesex TW11 0AB
01.977.5474

Bereavement
CRUSE (The National
Organization for the
Widowed and their
Children)
126 Sheen Road
Richmond
Surrey TW9 1UR
01.940.4818.

The Society for
Compassionate Friends
(help for bereaved parents)
Mrs Jill Hodder
5 Lower Clifton Hill
Bristol 8
0272.292778

Blindness
The Royal National
Institute for the Blind
224 Great Portland Place
London W1N 6AA
01.388.1266

Cancer
Cancerlink Ltd
46 Pentonville Road
London N1
01.833.2451

Cancer Help Centre
Grove House
Cornwallis Grove
Bristol BS8 4PG
0272.743216

Care of the dying
British Hospice
Information Centre (BHIC)
St Christopher's Hospice
51-53 Lawrie Park Road
London SE26 6DZ
01.788.1240

Colostomy
Colostomy Welfare Group
38-39 Eccleston Square
London SW1
01.828.5175

Deafness
British Deaf Association
38 Victoria Place
Carlisle CA1 1HU
0228.48844

Diabetes
British Diabetic
Association
10 Queen Anne Street
London W1M 0BD
01.323.1531

Disabled — physical and mental handicap
Dial UK (Disablement
Information Advice Line)
117 High Street
Clay Cross
Chesterfield
Derbyshire S45 9DZ
0246.864498

Disabled Living
Foundation
380-384 Harrow Road
London W9 2HU
01.289.6111
(provides Incontinence
Advisory Service)

MENCAP (Royal Society
for Mentally Handicapped
Children and Adults)
123 Golden Lane
London EC1Y 0RT
01.253.9433.

Eczema
National Eczema Society
Tavistock House North
Tavistock Square
London WC1H 9SR
01.388.4097

Elderly people
Age Concern England
Bernard Sunley House
60 Pitcairn Road
Mitcham
Surrey CR4 3LL
01.630.5431

The National Council for
Carers and their Elderly
Dependents Ltd
29 Chilworth Mews
London W2
01.262.1451

Epilepsy
British Epilepsy
Association
New Wokingham Road
Wokingham
Berkshire RG11 3AY
0344.773122

Haemophilia
Haemophilia Society
PO Box 9
15 Trinity Street
London SE1 1DE
01.407.1010

Heart disease, high blood pressure and strokes
British Heart Foundation
102 Gloucester Place
London W1H 4DH
01.935.0185

Chest, Heart and Stroke
Association
Tavistock House North
Tavistock Square
London WC1 9JE
01.387.3012

Hysterectomy
Hysterectomy Association
Rivendell
Warren Way
Lower Heswall
Wirral LH10 9HV
051.342.3167

Kidney disease
British Kidney Patient
Association
Bordon
Hants
04203.2022

Mastectomy
The Mastectomy
Association
26 Harrison Street
London WC1
01.837.0908

Migraine
British Migraine
Association
178A High Road
Byfleet
Weybridge
Surrey KT14 7ED

Mental Health
Mental After Care
Association
Eagle House
110 Jermyn Street
London SW1Y 6HB
01.839.5953

MIND (National
Association for Mental
Health)
22 Harley Street
London W1N 2ED
01.637.0741

The National
Schizophrenia Fellowship
78 Victoria Road
Surbiton KT6 4NS
01.390.3651

Multiple sclerosis
Multiple Sclerosis Society
286 Munster Road
London SW6 6BE
01.381.4022

Parkinson's disease
Parkinson's Disease
Society of United Kingdom
36 Portland Place
London W1
01.323.1174

Psoriasis
Psoriasis Association
7 Milton Street
Northampton NN2 7JG
0604.711129

In most countries the
names and addresses of
any existing support
groups can be obtained
from the appropriate
Department of Health.

Australia
Department of Health
McKell Buildings
Rawson Place
Sydney 2000
New South Wales
217 6666

Department of Health
State Health Building
147-163 Charlotte Street
Brisbane 4000
Queensland
224 0515

Public Health Promotion
Services
Savings Bank Buildings
158 Rundle Mail
Adelaide 5000
South Australia
218 3211

Health Department of
Western Australia
Curtis House
60 Beaufort Street
East Perth 6000
Western Australia
328 0241

Health Commission of
Victoria
555 Collins Street
Melbourne 3000
Victoria
616 7777

New Zealand
The Director General
Department of Health
PO Box 5013
Wellington
New Zealand

South Africa
The Director General
The Department of Health
and Welfare
Private bag X63
Pretoria 0001
Transvaal
South Africa

FURTHER READING

Ansell, B. and Lawton, S.,
Your Home and Your Rheumatism,
Available direct from The Arthritis and
Rheumatism Council.

Brackenridge, R. G.,
Essential Medicine,
MTP Press, 1980.

Bradshaw, J.,
*Incontinence, a burden for families with
handicapped children,*
Available direct from the Disabled Living
Foundation, 1978.

Carr, J.,
Helping your handicapped child,
Penguin, 1985.

Chilman, A. M. and Thomas, M.,
Understanding Nursing Care,
Churchill Livingstone, 1981.

Copperman, H.,
Dying at Home,
John Wiley, 1983.

Downie, P. A. and Kennedy, P.,
Lifting, Handling and Helping Patients,
Faber and Faber, 1981.

First Aid Manual,
The Authorised Manual of St John Ambulance,
St Andrew's Ambulance Association,
The British Red Cross Society,
Dorling Kindersley, 1982.

Hollis, M.,
Safer Lifting for Patient Care,
Blackwell Scientific, 1985.

Incontinence: a very common complaint,
Health Education Council, 1978.
Available direct from your Local Health Education Unit.

Introducing Arthritis,
Available direct from The Arthritis and
Rheumatism Council.

Kubler Ross, E.,
On Death and Dying,
Tavistock, 1973.

Lewer, H. and Robertson, L.,
Care of the Child: The Essentials of Nursing,
Macmillan, 1983.

Sanctuary, G.,
*After I'm Gone: What will happen to my
handicapped child?,*
Souvenir Press, 1984.

Informative books and publications on different aspects
of health can be obtained from:

The Health Education Council
79 New Oxford Street, London WC1A 1AH
01.631.0930

Index

Editor	Clare Mitchison
Art editor	Anne Fisher
Text editors	Gian Douglas-Home
	Sarah Mitchell
	Jo Christian
	Anne Forsyth
Designer	Bob Gordon
Editorial assistant	Amanda Malpass
Art director	Debbie MacKinnon

The publishers would like to thank the following for their help:

Medical Consultant: Michael Modell FRCGP MRCP DCH.

Photography: Nancy Durell McKenna.

Illustrations: Elaine Anderson; Andrew Farmer; Andrew Popkiewicz.

Additional artwork: Alicia Durdos; Andrew McDonald; Ann Winterbotham; Sandra Pond.

Editorial assistance: Elizabeth Fenwick; Joanna Jellinek; Joanna Chisolm; and to Pippa Rubinstein for original work on the book.

Typing: Chris Bowles; Gillian Bussell; George and Elizabeth Galfalvi.

Photographic prints: John Mallow.

Retouching: Nick Oxtoby.

Typesetting: SX Composing.

Reproduction: Newsele.

The publishers would also like to thank the following for allowing themselves to be photographed for this book:
   Martha Alexander; John and Shirley Benson; Cathy and Margaret Berry; Joyce and Rachel Dick; Pamela Fisher; Joseph Herman and William McKenna; Anya and Andrew Innes; Yolande Mebius; Alexander Monro and Bill McKenna; Christopher Ogilvie-Thompson; Zero Page and Joyce Cross; Christopher and Hannah Pugsley; Fermin and Florence Robertson; Jean and Camilla Rowland; Michael, Joanna and Caroline Sale; Martin and Simon Stirrup; Donna Taylor; Stephen and Alison Zollner. Special thanks to Kathy Ogilvie-Thompson for advice and help. Also, thanks to Dorset County Hospital and Lewisham Hospital for loan of space and equipment and to The American Red Cross, F J Payne Ltd., DMA Ltd., and Stannah Ltd., for reproduction of illustrations.